D1414192

THE TYPE C CONNECTION

THE
TYPE C
CONNECTION

THE BEHAVIORAL LINKS
TO CANCER AND
YOUR HEALTH

**Lydia Temoshok, Ph.D.,
and Henry Dreher**

 RANDOM HOUSE NEW YORK

Library of Congress Cataloging-in-Publication Data
Temoshok, Lydia.
The type C connection: the behavioral links to cancer and your
health/Lydia Temoshok and Henry Dreher
    p.   cm.
    Includes bibliographical references and index.
    ISBN 0-394-57523-7
    1. Cancer—Psychological aspects. 2. Cancer—Risk factors.
I. Dreher, Henry. II. Title.
RC262.T38 1991
616.99′4′0019—dc20   91-48186

Manufactured in the United States of America
98765432
First Edition
The text of this book is set in Times Roman

To Herbert Lehmann, M.D.,
who helped me to merge compassion with science
—L.T.

For Deborah Chiel
—H.D.

AUTHORS' NOTE

Although *The Type C Connection* is a collaborative effort by Dr. Lydia Temoshok and Henry Dreher, for the sake of clarity and simplicity we decided to use the pronoun "I," for Dr. Temoshok, throughout, particularly because the scientific and clinical findings herein are a product of her research. The names and identifying details of the patients discussed in this book have been changed to protect anonymity. (The only exceptions are those instances where both first and last name are given.)

The sections in this book on changing the Type C pattern, and other therapeutic or preventive suggestions, are offered as health recommendations to enhance well-being, not as medical cancer treatment or as substitutes for such treatment. We recommend that anyone with cancer be treated by a physician or cancer specialist, and the suggestions in this book should be considered strictly supplemental.

ACKNOWLEDGMENTS

Bruce W. Heller was there with me at the very beginning of my research endeavor into cancer and the mind. His ideas contributed to the elaboration of the Type C behavior pattern; his friendship and support were invaluable. Richard W. Sagebiel and the late Marsden S. Blois provided the original stimulus for my work on malignant melanoma. From Paul Ekman, I learned a great deal about human emotion, its measurement, and its vicissitudes. Over the years, I have discussed and debated, sometimes furiously but always engrossingly, theoretical ideas about mind and cancer connections with Bernard H. Fox, George F. Solomon, Hans J. Eysenck, and the late Norman Cousins. Jane M. Zich, David M. Sweet, and Andrew W. Kneier are among the research collaborators to whom I owe a large debt of gratitude.

—Lydia Temoshok, Ph.D.

Deborah Chiel helped me in countless ways. She read portions of the manuscript and invariably pointed me in the right direction. More important, she gave me the support I needed, time and time and time again. Certain friends and family members were there during the good times and the hard times associated with this project: my sister and brother-in-law, Stephanie and Ira Krotick; Barbara Miller, John Bean, and Diane Dreher. Barbara Gess listened, cheered me on, and offered helpful advice during countless dinners, many of which were brightened by the presence of Drago.

—Henry Dreher

We both wish to thank our editors: Susan Kamil, for her enthusiasm, her instincts, and for challenging us to do better; and Olga Tarnowski, for her care, patience, and perspicacity. We owe a special thanks to Karen Rinaldi of Turtle Bay Books for her support above and beyond the call of duty.

Our agent and friend, Chris Tomasino, has been a trusted and ardent advocate from day one. Her tireless efforts on our behalf made this project not only possible but considerably more pleasurable.

A number of professional associates helped us enormously by contributing time and ideas. We particularly thank Ronald B. Herberman, John Hiserodt, Sandra M. Levy, Charles Weinstock, Jane G. Goldberg, Eve Boden, and Warren Berland. We owe a special debt of gratitude to Steven Greer, friend and colleague, who gave unstintingly of his time and energy. His theoretical and empirical contributions to the development of the Type C concept also helped to make this book a reality.

Linda Weill is a fine transcriber and also very patient. Our copy editor, Karen Richardson, was superb.

Vanessa Lynn, Phyllis Aron, and Barbara Genest told us their stories and added life to our book.

Finally, we wish to express our deepest appreciation to all the individuals with cancer who were participants in the research described in this book, whose stories inspired us, and whose generosity of time and spirit helped us to better understand some of the myriad connections among mind, body, and illness.

CONTENTS

PART I

THE TYPE C
BEHAVIOR PATTERN

CHAPTER 1

When old words die out on the tongue, new melodies
break forth from the heart; and where the old tracks are
lost, new country is revealed with its wonders.

—*Rabindranath Tagore*

Introduction

In early 1979, I began a series of research projects concerning the role of the mind in cancer. Without fully realizing it, I had stepped right into the middle of a fiery medical controversy, one which burns to this day. Can emotions and behavior affect our risk of cancer, or our recovery should we contract the disease? After a decade of study, I am convinced that a specific behavior pattern, which I named "Type C," does indeed alter both cancer risk and recovery. My own results converged with findings from scores of other published studies to paint a striking picture of how the mind may influence cancer development. As in a jury trial in which there is no eyewitness to a crime but there is a trail of persuasive clues, I believe that the mind can be implicated in cancer when we examine *all* of the evidence.

I first entered the fray in December 1978. That's when I received an intriguing phone call from Richard Sagebiel, M.D., codirector of the Melanoma Clinic at the University of California, San Francisco. Dr. Sagebiel knew that I was conducting research at UCSF on stress and health, and he wanted to meet with me. He told me he was beginning to suspect "a strange pattern of stress and coping" among his patients. He thought he might have chanced upon a significant connection between behavior and cancer, and wanted to discuss how he could follow this lead in a scientific fashion. I was fascinated by his story and ready to offer my assistance.

I met with Dr. Sagebiel and Marsden S. Blois, M.D., the other director of the melanoma clinic. We discussed their patients, all of whom had melanoma, a form of skin cancer that is extremely aggressive and often lethal if not detected in its early stages. The "strange pattern" was most apparent among their melanoma patients who were faring poorly—the ones with the thickest tumors and the worst prognosis. Sagebiel and Blois saw that these patients handled the stress in their lives, and the stress from their illness, in an oddly similar fashion. The two doctors sensed something emotionally "flat" about their patients' reactions, but beyond that they could not pinpoint the precise nature of this pattern. They wondered aloud if I could set up a scientific study of their patients to see if there was a mind-body connection. Although I wasn't yet sure if a systematic study was possible, I was ready and willing to undertake a preliminary investigation.

I decided to spend as much time as possible at the melanoma clinic getting to know the patients. After talking with scores of patients for many hours over several months, I detected a striking and very specific behavior pattern among them. I arrived at the rather unnerving realization that almost all the patients were extremely nice. The characteristics they shared were so pronounced, and the implications so potentially rich, that I decided to devote all my research at that time to the psychology of cancer patients.

The melanoma patients had come to the clinic to have their lesions assessed by the physicians or to hear the results of their biopsies. They would receive more precise diagnoses and recommendations for treatment. Most of them faced the prospect of surgery, and a minority would undergo chemotherapy, radiation, or experimental treatments. Needless to say, they were living with a degree of stress ranging from unpleasant to agonizing. And there I was, in no official capacity, asking to speak with them, taking up their time. All they knew and all I could tell them was that I was a psychologist interested in how people cope with cancer. Nonetheless, these patients were perfectly willing to spend prolonged periods of time answering my questions.

They didn't seem to have any burning need to talk. Above all, I sensed that they simply didn't want to disappoint me. They would routinely miss lunch to finish a conversation. On several occasions, patients canceled what sounded to me like important appointments in order to continue talking. One patient offered to stay late at the clinic even though he would miss his ride and would have to take a taxi to the opposite end of San Francisco.

But their willingness to talk was only one telltale sign of their overriding behavior. Patient after patient appeared to be more concerned about their loved ones than they were about themselves. Ted, one of the first melanoma patients I talked to, had just been diagnosed with life-threatening cancer when he told me, "I'm fine. But I'm really worried about my wife. She takes things so hard."

I recognized in Ted's response a form of denial. He had shelved the reality that caused him overwhelming anxiety and focused instead on his wife's feelings. Many people use denial to cope with the initial shock and anguish of a cancer diagnosis. Much like the effects of a narcotic drug, the anesthesia of denial is transient and slowly wears off as the person accepts his illness and his own emotional responses.

Soon I was to discover that an extraordinary percentage of the melanoma patients I met used denial as a coping strategy. This alone seemed unusual, but it also became clear that even the *form* of denial from patient to patient was strikingly similar. Ted, it turned out, was only the first to say "I'm fine. But I'm really worried about my wife." As more patients told me they were fine, that they were more concerned about their spouses or parents than they were about themselves, I began to suspect that more than simple denial was involved. Why did all these patients ignore their own discomforts and divert their anxiety by dwelling on the reactions of their immediate loved ones?

Here was a clue to the emerging Type C pattern. When I delved more deeply, I found that these patients had always been completely devoted to pleasing their spouses, parents, siblings, friends, or coworkers. Their very identity seemed to depend wholly upon the reflected acceptance of those people significant in their lives. In *The Lonely Crowd,* David Riesman coined the phrase "other-directed" to describe this ongoing psychological reflex. Psychotherapists recognize that their other-directed patients have an underdeveloped sense of self. Out of touch with their primary needs and emotions, they look to others for signals on how to think, feel, and act.

Here, it seemed, was a group of other-directed people who had just been diagnosed with cancer. Already distanced from their own feelings, they handled fear and sadness by intensifying their focus on loved ones. They seemed to project their distress onto family and friends, and then nurtured *them* instead of themselves. I saw how mixed were the results of such coping methods. The patients' over-concern for others drained off some of their anxiety but still left their own needs sorely unattended.

Throughout this early phase of my research, I never thought I had stumbled upon a tragic psychological blueprint whereby a person's character led him inexorably toward malignant disease. The cancer patients did not share similar personalities or life histories. What they shared was a manner of handling life stress. The melanoma patients coped by keeping their feelings under wraps. They never expressed anger, and rarely did they acknowledge fear and sadness. They maintained a facade of pleasantness even under the most painful or aggravating circumstances. They strived excessively to please the people they cared about, to please authority figures, even to please strangers. These are the essentials of the behavior pattern I would soon name "Type C."

Type C behavior is an extreme version of coping methods many of us employ—we appease others, deny our true feelings, and conform to social standards. But my study of the melanoma patients led me to convincing evidence that our physical health is compromised when we chronically repress our needs and feelings to accommodate others. I was able to find evidence that this coping style weakens our immune defenses and leaves us more vulnerable to cancer progression. This does not mean repression causes cancer; it means that a specific behavior pattern is one of many factors in cancer risk and recovery.

I devised a plan for a series of scientific studies of the relationship between Type C and cancer development. My formal research began the same way my informal investigations did—by talking to patients. But this time I carefully interviewed them, using an extensive list of prepared questions. I videotaped the interviews so that my colleagues and I could later study them intensively and objectively. This was a crucial yet sensitive phase of research, because I had to keep a scientific distance from the patients while remaining open to understanding their emotions and behavior. I could not interact with them the way a therapist would—that would be tampering with the objective reality I was studying. I did, however, create an interview that delved deeply into their experiences so that my data would be ample and rich. This allowed me to develop a theory explaining the Type C phenomenon from a psychological, social, and biological perspective.

These interviews (and the medical information provided by the patients' doctors) yielded the data I needed to establish a scientific link between Type C behavior and cancer. I also became privy to an invaluable treasure trove of information about these patients, their stories, and their particular ways of meeting life's challenges. My understanding of the patients, the environments that fostered their behavior, the stuggles they endured—mostly silently—and the way their behavior affected their daily lives grew not from standard psychological tests but rather from these encounters. I used psychological tests later to confirm what I had discovered by simply asking patients probing questions about fundamental issues in their lives.

In Part II, "The Type C Connection," I will describe my series of studies that forged scientific connections between Type C behavior and cancer. Yet another critical issue must be addressed, and I will do so throughout this book and especially in Chapter 9, "Type C and Mind-Body Science": How, exactly, do mind and body interact in the development of disease? What are the biological pathways between mind and body? The answers are beginning to be understood, in the wake of a veritable scientific revolution in the study of psyche and soma.

In Appendix II, I will provide references for every study mentioned in this book—my own and others'—and extensive notes on my research methods. Anyone interested in the scientific background of the research described in this book should consult this section.

Our entire view of health and illness is undergoing a seismic change. The strongest wave of change is the recognition that mind-body relationships can have a profound effect on our state of health or disease. A new science—psychoneuroimmunology—is charting a labyrinth of mind-body connections involving brain structures, chemical messengers, and immune cells. Researchers in this young field are discovering that how we think and feel alters the strength of our immune system, the body's network of defense against disease.

The question is, How far, and how deep, does the mind-body connection go? Does its influence extend to the mechanisms of a disease such as cancer? Could the tendrils of the mind reach down to the level of cells and molecules whose behavior determines whether a tumor develops? Recently, mind-body researchers have turned up evidence that supports a qualified yes to all these questions. But uncertainties linger, and the incendiary nature of the mind-cancer controversy has led to polarization in the medical community and the public.

Cancer patients, their families, physicians, scientists, journalists, and the health-conscious have taken sides in a passionate argument about cancer and the mind. The believers are often uncritical in their thinking, causing harmful misunderstandings about how attitudes or emotions influence cancer. But many of the critics are close-minded, and beneath their opposition they appear to be shocked—even appalled—by the idea of a relationship between cancer and the mind. Both sides have bypassed the truth. In so doing, I believe they have missed the opportunity to apply groundbreaking knowledge of the mind-body connection in a rational and compassionate way.

The discovery that emotions can influence cancer risk and recovery means that we all have potentially powerful allies against cancer: our own hearts and minds. Yet many people reflexively interpret the mind/cancer link pessimistically: "You mean I'm doomed to cancer because of my state of mind?" I answer them with an emphatic "No!" The existence of psychological risk factors does not mean we're fated to get cancer—they are but one piece of a dizzyingly complex puzzle. Cancer is really a collection of more than one hundred diseases, and for each type, countless factors interact to cause the disease and determine its course. The mind does not play a part in all cancers, but my research showed that it is a significant contributor to *certain* cancers in *certain* individuals.

I also learned that *people did not bring cancer on themselves.* Their Type C behavior began unwittingly and persisted without conscious volition. No one can be blamed for mind-body factors in cancer, because no one intentionally develops the cancer-prone behavior pattern. Furthermore, without knowledge of the Type C-cancer link, how could someone realize that his behavior might impact his cancer defense system on a *molecular* level? In Chapter 10, "Blaming the Victim and Other Traps," I will explain why a compassionate self-awareness of Type C behavior, and transformation to a healthier pattern, can help free people from self-blame over their illness or their behavior. I will also attack the myths that have caused some to interpret the mind-body connection as blame-inducing.

Type C behavior is not a shameful distortion of one's personality. I realized early in my research that Type C behavior had been each person's best attempt to cope with the pains, stresses, humiliations, and unmet needs of early childhood. Later in life, this coping method had liabilities—both mental and physical—that the person could become aware of and change in order to lead a healthier and more meaningful existence. In Chapter 9 and elsewhere, I will explain why Type C behavior is associated not only with cancer but with many other diseases caused by immune dysfunction. (It may even influence the progression of HIV and AIDS.)

The discovery of disease-prone behavior offers renewed prospects in the fight against cancer and other illnesses. We've always known that we could stop smoking, change our diets, and avoid certain environmental carcinogens. These actions will reduce our risk of cancer. But many of us also know someone with a spanking-clean health record—who never smoked, drank, or ate junk foods, yet who still contracted cancer. This causes us to throw up our arms in surrender—"There's nothing I can do!" We ponder the imponderables, the things we can't change: our genetic heritage, pollutants we can't avoid, past exposure to agents we never knew were carcinogens. The mind-body cancer connection means that we have one more important lever of control over our fate.

As I will show, the Type C behavior pattern is one potential cancer risk factor that people can do something about. I have seen people reshape their pattern, and I have helped others, through a program of behavior transformation, to bring about this change in themselves. The result, I am convinced, is a reduced risk of the onset and growth of cancer. Part IV, "Type C Transformation— For Recovery," is devoted to helping cancer patients change their behavior, both as a boon to their well-being and a potential boost to their recovery. Part V, "Type C Transformation—For Prevention," describes my approach to helping healthy people change their Type C pattern in order to achieve psychological wholeness and the prevention of diseases such as cancer.

From the beginning, I did not expect to uncover such a discrete behavior pattern among cancer patients. Nor did I expect to find an open door to new vistas for controlling the threat of malignant

disease. These realizations came to me over time, as a slowly dawning surprise. Before telling you about my formal scientific studies,
I want to convey to you my clinical impressions from the initial
interviews I conducted with more than 150 melanoma patients.
These impressions, and the insights gleaned from hearing the patients' striking and often poignant life stories, led me to the slowly
dawning surprise that was the Type C behavior pattern.

CHAPTER 2

If I closely examine what is my ultimate aim, it turns out
that I am not really striving to be good and to fulfill the
demands of a Supreme Judgment, but rather very much
the contrary. I strive to know the whole human and
animal community, to recognize their basic predilictions,
desires, moral ideals, to reduce these to simple rules and
as quickly as possible trim my behavior to these rules in
order that I may find favor in the whole world's eyes.

—Franz Kafka

From the reconstructions available through analyses, I
have gained the impression that there are children who
have not been free to experience the very earliest feelings,
such as discontent, anger, rage, pain, even hunger and, of
course, enjoyment of their own bodies.

—Alice Miller

I saw a vision of us move in the dark, all that
    we did or dreamed of
Regarded each other, the man pursued the woman,
    the woman clung to the man, warriors and kings
Strained at each other in the darkness, all loved
    or fought inward, each one of the lost people
Sought the eyes of another that another should
    praise him; sought never his own but another's.

—Robinson Jeffers on the myth of Orestes

Portrait of the Type C Individual

Martin, a thirty-three-year-old man with his own graphic-design business, had suffered a relapse of cancer. His doctors considered his prognosis to be guarded, yet he was conspicuously calm in responding to the sudden return of this life-threatening illness. I asked Martin how he felt when he was first told that his cancer had spread. He said he was "somewhat surprised." His answer seemed strange to me, because his expression indicated a type of surprise one might associate with hearing a news flash about a world event that is unexpected, perhaps disturbing, but that has no direct impact on one's own personal life.

I asked Martin why he was surprised. "Well, because statistically—if you can quantify such things—it shouldn't have happened," he said. "But I wasn't terribly upset."

Martin was among the first patients I formally interviewed in my research on the role of the mind in cancer. When he told me he wasn't upset, I understood that Martin used denial as a way of coping with the awful terror of his serious relapse. But after a long and detailed interview, I saw that his detachment was not a symptom of the normal temporary denial that cancer patients often use as a coping strategy. Martin's behavior had deep roots. This was his *fixed* style of coping, an ingrained pattern of behavior that long predated his experience with cancer.

A year and a half earlier, Martin had noticed changes in a mole that was hidden by his beard, just below his jawline. It had darkened, become scaly, and a few black spots dotted its surface. He immediately consulted a dermatologist, who biopsied the mole and determined that it was a malignant melanoma. The doctor described it as a "thin" lesion and told him there was only a 10 percent chance of recurrence. Martin believed he'd never have to think about melanoma again.

Now, despite the odds, Martin was back at the clinic with swollen lymph nodes in his neck. The melanoma had spread and his doctors were debating the medical course of action. Eventually, Martin would undergo a subtotal neck dissection, in which most of the lymph nodes on one side of his neck would be removed. When I interviewed Martin, he had just been told that his prognosis was uncertain.

What exactly was he doing to cope with this news? He talked about gathering facts and information, consulting with his doctors, considering the crucial decisions on his horizon. These were valid and healthy ways of coping—many cancer patients are far more passive than Martin regarding their medical care. Yet Martin appeared to have no feeling reaction at all to his melanoma or its recurrence. The sudden and virulent return of this cancer would, for many patients, have been an emotional blow of huge proportions.

I wondered if Martin had reacted this way eighteen months earlier, when he was first told he had melanoma. "How did I feel?" he said. "Somewhat curious. It was sort of an intellectual exercise, in a way, that this was in fact cancer. It was a curious exercise at the time. I was not alarmed. I didn't see my life flash before my eyes or anything like that."

Martin's idea of cancer as an intellectual exercise struck me as powerful testimony to his need to view the world, and his own life circumstances, through extremely narrow blinders. Having cancer is anything but an intellectual exercise—it is a psychological and spiritual maelstrom. During the course of the illness, a patient must draw on his intellectual resources to sort out information and make decisions, but the essential experience is usually an overwhelming mixture of conscious and unconscious feelings. Martin saw cancer as a puzzle to be solved, and this was his way of distancing himself from inner experience.

I was soon to understand the wide variety of psychological

defenses that cancer patients use to keep from being overwhelmed. Patients need these defenses, but as I proceeded with my research, I discovered that defenses which helped patients cope in the early stages of illness might not work well in later stages. I also found that certain defenses—like Martin's detachment—had an upside and a distinct downside, both mentally and physically.

In my study of patients like Martin, I was the dispassionate observer, not the critic. My job was never to judge or criticize but rather to understand and describe their behavior as truthfully and precisely as I could.

Martin was pleasant and friendly at all times. I asked him if his cancer or its recurrence made him angry. Or depressed. Or frightened. He said he felt none of these. When I asked him an anxiety-provoking question—like, What is your worst fear about your illness?—he would smile ironically. At the same time, I would notice the blood draining from his face. This gave me the impression that anxiety registered below the level of his own consciousness. He laughed nervously every time he mentioned the prospect of death—a reaction I noted in many other patients.

In my interview with Martin, I asked him about his cancer, the various day-to-day stresses in his life, and other aspects of his behavior and personality. (We told him nothing about the nature of our Type C hypothesis—just that we were interested in how people cope with cancer.) Here are some telling excerpts:

LT: Now, at this point, have the doctors told you anything about your chances?
Martin: I discussed it with Dr. Sarnow today, and the chances seem good, but there's no way to quantify that. In the initial stages, after the biopsy and excision [of the original melanoma] there's a lot of literature quantifying people at different levels and their chances. At this point, though, I don't fit into any of those patterns, and so my chances appear to be OK. But already I've come to know that doesn't mean a great deal, because my chances were very good—even excellent—before the recurrence.
LT: What do you think now?
Martin: It means the disease can do any damn thing it wants to. It can go away or it can show up again. And no matter what the outcome of the surgery is, I'm not sure who's in the driver's

seat anymore. Because I thought I was, or the doctors were, after the original excision. So who knows.

LT: Can you tell me briefly some of the major stresses in your life?

Martin: Probably the single biggest stress is my work, in that I'm starting a new business. It's my own graphic-design studio. I have limited myself to doing annual reports and corporate logos for companies, which is a particular area that's very competitive. I've had this studio for two years now, and the stress is getting it off the ground. There's a lot of cash flow problems, and keeping clients coming in has been a serious stress. Prior to that I was a newspaper reporter, and there are obvious stresses in that job. You're always writing under deadlines, and that gets to you after a while. Although there's probably more adaptability to that.

LT: OK, I'd like to . . .

Martin: [Interrupting.] I would say I'm not a Type A personality by any means. I've worked with those people, so I really can contrast myself to them. In fact, most people think I'm quite mellow, they always say I'm too laid-back. That was a criticism when I worked in the newspaper, that I didn't seem to get all excited, jumping up and down when a big breaking story came in. And I felt there is a certain dispassionate third person standoffishness required when a big story is breaking, to report it accurately. So most people would say I'm fairly mellow, but I think I tend to internalize some problems. I would internalize stress and not, you know, show it so much.

LT: Tell me more about that.

Martin: Yes, doctor. [Laughs ironically—then turns serious.] I probably feel the same kind of stresses as everybody else, but I keep a more outward cool facade than do the other people who are leaping over desks and yelling and screaming. I am not a compulsive worker. I'm not a workaholic by any means, so there are some contrasts there too. But I'm sure I feel the stress of trying to get this business going.

LT: At this point, what is the most worrisome or troubling thing about having melanoma and getting treated?

Martin: Beyond the immediate anxiety about surgery . . . why, obviously dying, let's face it. [Laughs.] I mean, nobody wants to contemplate their death, and so I don't. That is not a fear at this time, it's more of an intellectual exercise. But I think that it has crossed my wife's mind, and she thinks about that. And my mother—it bothers her and consequently that's what bothers me. I'm thinking of them and how it affects them more than it does me.

LT: You're more concerned with how they're dealing with it?

Martin: Right. I'm not—I'm not afraid of dying, at this point. I don't think we've got to this point where I've been written off, or anything like that. I'm too intellectual at this point, hypothetical.

LT: What about when you have a moment when you feel down or anxious about it? How do you cope with that sort of thing?

Martin: [Long pause.] Uh, I don't know. I feel anxious about it from time to time but . . . how do I cope with it? I don't know. I don't know what that—I don't know.

LT: Have your friends helped at all?

Martin: Most people don't know too much about [my cancer]. They're not that up on melanoma—let's face it. [He laughs.] I would say most of my closest friends don't know a great deal about what's happening. Like I said, I'm a relatively private person. I'm not going to air all this until it needs to be aired.

LT: This question may seem unusual, but give it a bit of imagination. If that part of your body [where the cancer is] could speak, what might it say?

Martin: [Laughs bemusedly.] I should have a snappy comeback, right? Well, I don't know. I'm sorry that I don't have an imaginative response for that. I don't think it would say "help me," because we—it's already doing that, that's underway. It wouldn't say "look at me" or "help me" or anything like that. It might say "ow." I don't know.

LT: Can you remember a time when you were really angry?

Martin: [He puts his hand on temple, as if thinking hard. A long pause.] I should be able to think of some, but I can't right offhand, think of a time that strikes me as being real . . . demonstrative.

LT: It doesn't have to be demonstrative. It could be sort of a seething underneath.

Martin: Yeah, uh [Seems confused.] . . . I can't think of anything that's so out of the ordinary that would . . .

LT: It doesn't have to be out of the ordinary. What sorts of things in everyday life really make you angry, really get your goat, piss you off?

Martin: Um. [Pauses again.] Bank of America. [Laughs ironically.]

LT: Is there any specific example you can recall of being really mad at somebody, openly or on the inside?

Martin: [Long pause.] Boy, I've just drawn a blank.

THE SHIELD OF DETACHMENT

Martin was matter-of-fact about his prognosis, and he spoke in a detached manner about the fact that the doctors could not "quantify" his chances easily. While his words told me a great deal about his state of mind, I was able to glean even more from his body language. It was for just this reason that I had decided to videotape each patient interview. An interview transcript by itself lacks crucial information—that stemming from the subject's nonverbal behavior. Videotape enabled me to analyze later each patient's voice, movements, and facial expressions, revealing behaviors that either confirmed or contradicted the spoken word. For example, Martin made statements that on paper might seem angry, such as "the disease can do any damn thing it wants to," and "I'm not sure who's in the driver's seat anymore." However, his voice and body language betrayed not a trace of anger. Beneath his intellectual facade, Martin actually seemed resigned, powerless. The disease had fooled him once, and he knew he could be fooled again. He wasn't going to invest any hope or show any emotion about his prospects; it was better to remain cool and removed.

Yet this was the way Martin had always handled stress. Martin was forthright and articulate about his behavior, and his self-description matched my sense of him—he was a reliable, good guy who was "mellow," "laid-back," and tended to "internalize stress" and "not show it so much."

Martin had unknowingly provided a detailed verbal description of the Type C behavior pattern I was in the process of uncovering. I later interviewed patients who perfectly embodied the Type C pattern, but none of them provided me with such a clinical portrait of themselves. In his detached, objective way, Martin had a firm grasp of his own behavior. He didn't have an understanding of the forces that shaped his behavior nor an awareness of the emotions he so firmly denied. But he had been a journalist, and with a journalist's eye and ear, he gave me a meticulous picture of the external facets of his own character.

Martin had told only his wife and mother about his real condition, yet he wanted to protect them from further distress. So to whom could he turn if he were to become upset? Martin hid whatever pain and fear he had from the significant others in his life. This seemed to cause him little discomfort, because he hid these feelings from himself, too. When I asked him what the part of his body with melanoma might say if it could speak, he told me what it *wouldn't* say: "look at me," or "help me." I wondered whether, under his shield of detachment, there was a deeply buried voice wanting to cry out. If so, it was a voice Martin had totally disowned.

ANGER—THE PHANTOM EMOTION

When I asked Martin to recall a time when he felt really angry, his voice dropped and he fell silent for a long time. Even though I gave him every opportunity to remember an angry feeling or episode, he was confused—even bewildered—in his effort to produce such a memory. By this time I'd interviewed Martin for over an hour, and he had answered all my questions in great detail. For the first time he was utterly stumped, as if I'd asked him to solve a mathematical problem of the utmost complexity.

The fact that Martin drew a complete blank when it came to anger was striking. But after I had interviewed many more patients, I came to expect such reactions. I'd ask the person to recall a time when she was the most enraged. If she could not summon up her angriest moment, I asked her instead to remember any incident—whether a year ago or a week ago—when she felt anger. Many patients said, "You mean, where I got openly mad? I can't think of anything." I'd take another tack: It didn't matter whether the anger had been expressed. I asked them to think of a time when they simply *felt* angry or even just aggravated—whether or not it showed. Most patients *still* responded with long pauses, perplexity,

or blank looks. Often, their expression shifted from one of composure to blatant confusion, until they wound up uttering, "Angry. I
don't know. . . . I just can't come up with anything."

I found similar observations in the literature of medical psychology. In the mid-1970s, psychoanalyst Stephen A. Appelbaum
conducted a modest but painstaking psychological study of a group
of cancer patients. He wrote, "I am satisfied with regard to the
following: The intolerance of these patients for anger in themselves,
their fear of fantasied repercussions of the expression of such anger,
and the consequent submissiveness in the service of controlling such
anger are excessive, clear, dominating, and determining much of
their behavior."

Dorian was another melanoma patient I interviewed whose
behavior was stripped of any vestiges of anger. In her late sixties,
she was a handsome, upright woman, dignified in bearing and
attitude. Dorian ran charity drives, had a small group of close
women friends, and worked with them in local political campaigns.
She believed that her finest quality was her moral rectitude. She was
thoughtful, considerate, and buttoned-up in terms of emotional
expression. Her illness was her personal business, she thought, and
she never even mentioned it to anyone in her social circle.

As I spoke with Dorian, I realized that nothing ruffled her—
until I asked her to remember a time of anger. She chuckled nervously, her eyes widened, and her forehead began to twitch visibly.
"Oh, dear!" she proclaimed. "No, I can't!" It was as if I had asked
her to remove her clothes in public.

Although the melanoma patients' most common answer to the
anger question was "I can't think of anything," there were a variety
of other related responses. Here is a sampling:

"I'm slow to anger."
"I'm not the type who gets angry. I let things simmer."
"If I get upset, I don't say anything."
"Anger has not been a part of my life."
"I don't believe a person should go around being angry all the
time."

Barbara, a thirty-five-year-old patient, felt great empathy for her
fellowman and volunteered countless hours each week helping the
homeless. But Barbara had no resentment toward any person or

institution responsible for their condition. "I don't hold anyone responsible; I just want to help," she said. She was as devoted to her husband and family as she was to her community.

Barbara had a tranquil aura but I detected some turmoil beneath the surface. She said that being diagnosed with cancer did not cause her much anxiety. But the longer we talked, the more uncomfortable she seemed, shifting in her chair and squinting each time I asked a question about her illness. She nevertheless insisted that she wasn't frightened or upset. I asked her about the time she was most angry. "I can't really answer your question," she said. "I usually find a flower in each day and swing through the hours on it. I just don't let anger take up my world." Perhaps that worked well for Barbara, but my instincts as a clinician told me that she suffered by not recognizing and dealing with the feelings she harbored within.

Some patients could recall only one single incident in their entire lives when they had experienced anger. Georgia, a fifty-year-old woman who had never been married and was socially isolated, said that the one time she lost her temper was when her wallet was stolen from her purse. Other patients tied anger to extremely trivial incidents. Roger was a man approaching forty who had seen his share of hard times. Long before being diagnosed with melanoma, he had contracted colon cancer. A few years earlier, a motorcycle accident had caused neck damage because he wasn't wearing a helmet. Roger confided in me that he never felt close to his parents. He admitted being depressed about the future prospects for his health and happiness. After hearing all this, I asked him when was he the most angry. One day, a year earlier, he had hit his head on a hanging plant, he told me. I pressed him, but it was absolutely the only memory of anger he could produce.

Roger's hanging plant was emblematic to me. Through all his trials and tribulations, why hadn't Roger felt the least bit angry? Hadn't he been mad at the cards dealt him by fate? Hadn't he been furious at having to endure a second bout of a different cancer? What about the parents who he felt had never shown him affection? Wasn't he even angry with himself for injuring his neck because he had neglected to wear a helmet? No. But he was pretty upset with that hanging plant. Clearly, Roger could never acknowledge anger at those individuals or life situations that had seriously wounded him. Instead, he was perpetually depressed and unhappy with himself. That hanging plant probably tripped a hot wire inside him, and for once in his life he could lash out because the target was not a person who could turn around and hurt, abandon, or castigate him.

I was discovering that, for a majority of these patients, anger was the phantom emotion. They had no memories of anger and were perplexed, amused, or unnerved when asked to recall one. Psychologists generally recognize that anger is a natural component of everyone's emotional repertoire that is an appropriate and biologically rooted response to situations of physical danger or emotional insult. In the patients I interviewed, the capacity to respond with anger was seriously hampered. Sensations and memories associated with anger seemed to have been excised from their consciousness.

Everyone controls their anger to an extent—we learn to manage our aggression during the process of socialization. However, few of us receive a balanced education on how to properly regulate anger. The result for many of us is the overcontrol of anger and the repression, or gradual blocking from consciousness, of angry emotions. Never is this tendency our *fault,* it is simply a legacy we carry from our early years, when we learned to accommodate our parents, siblings, peers, and teachers.

ARE EXPRESSIONS OF ANGER *NATURAL*?

When I discuss "repressing anger" as a mind-body problem, people often ask about the naturalness of anger. This summons up age-old arguments about the nature of human aggression. Many psychobiologists view aggression as a genetically ingrained instinct. We have come to understand aggression in most animal species as stemming from the "fight or flight" response. In the face of danger, an animal must fight or flee to survive. We also know that, despite epochal changes through the course of evolution, human beings still possess the fight or flight response.

Anger is a "higher level" human emotion that draws its biological force from our aggressive instinct. Unlike "raw" aggression, however, it involves the cerebral actions of judgment and choice. Humans can bring their cognitive powers to bear when faced with danger. We know how to control and channel our anger to ensure gratification of our physical and social needs. For example, if an employer promises us a raise and never delivers, we'd defeat our purpose by following our instinct to walk into his office and dump the contents of his wastebasket on his head. On the other hand, if we tactfully but forcefully confront him, we stand a chance of getting the promised raise.

The anger response becomes dangerous primarily when social conditions are chronically frustrating. In these circumstances, our self-protective impulses transform into destructive violence. We can lose the ability to manage anger properly, whether by implosion or explosion.

I wouldn't presume to resolve these complex issues here, but I share the view of many biologists and psychologists that the human emotion of anger is based on survival instincts. Rollo May and other social philosophers have tried to clear up our society's confusion between the constructive aspects of anger and the destructive aspects we rightly fear. May argues that our understandable fear of the violence of unbridled rage causes us to forget that plain anger is a biologically based emotion designed to preserve our integrity, not to make us kill. He makes the point that when anger is allowed appropriate expression, it rarely turns into brute force or cruelty. Indeed, our cultural tendency to prohibit natural expressions of anger may feed the dammed-up hatred that breeds violence.

Chronically repressed anger also breeds simmering resentment. "No one can arrive at real love or morality or freedom until he has frankly confronted and worked through his resentment," wrote May. ". . . one will not transform those destructive emotions into constructive ones until he does this. And the first step is to know *whom* and *what* one hates."

I agree with Dr. Anthony Storr, a renowned psychologist and author, who describes how inhibited anger creates the preconditions for violence. "One reason why aggressiveness is a problem to modern man," writes Storr, "is that the natural exploratory urge to grasp and master the environment has perforce to be limited in a way which is bound to cause frustration. There are far too many things which children must not do or must not touch; so that within all of us who have been brought up in Western civilization, especially in urban civilization, there must be reserves of repressed, and therefore dangerous, aggression which originate in early childhood."

A person who erases anger from his emotional palette will, over the years, experience psychological repercussions. He will miss the biological cues that an insult or threat is present in the environment. He's lost a spur to action, a vital mechanism of self-defense. But, is it possible that the loss of anger could affect more than behavior—that it could somehow bring on a physical disease such as cancer?

WOODY ALLEN'S ANGER PROBLEM—AND OURS

I remember a line in Woody Allen's movie *Manhattan* that touched lightly on the link between repressed anger and cancer. His girlfriend, played by Diane Keaton, not only breaks off their relationship, but in the same moment announces that she is returning to her former lover—his best friend. Allen responds passively, while Keaton waits for a big fight to resolve the tension building between them. "Why don't you get angry so we can have it out, so that we can get it out in the open?"

"I don't get angry, okay?" replies Allen. "I mean, I have a tendency to internalize. That's one of the problems I have. I—I grow a tumor instead."

The audience laughed at that line with a kind of knowing recognition. Somehow people accept the notion that bottling up one's feelings can throw the biological switch that turns cells malignant. It's a concept that strikes a chord, and a certain mythology has grown around the link between stifling anger and cancer. Does Woody Allen's line capture a belief that has any basis in scientific fact, or is it just a lot of psychosomatic hokum?

My experience with the patients at the melanoma clinic was lending eerie credibility to the anger hypothesis. After a search through the medical literature, I discovered that another researcher had turned up findings strikingly similar to my own. In the late 1970s, British psychiatrist Steven Greer, M.D., rigorously tested a population of women with breast lumps before it was known whether they had a malignancy. After the biopsy results were in, Greer compared those who turned out to have breast cancer with those who had benign tumors. Most of the women with cancer had "never or not more than once in their lives" lost their temper in anger. Greer identified "extreme suppression of anger" as a possible risk factor for the development of cancer.

Other researchers forged a broader connection: patients who

repressed emotions in general were more likely to develop cancer. I found in the work of psychologists Claus and Marjorie Bahnson a complex theory of how emotions are processed by different individuals. Put simply, the Bahnsons saw two markedly distinct modes of expression: people either "act out" or "act in" their emotions. The "act out" type is more prone to mental illnesses, while the "act in" type is vulnerable to certain physical disorders. The more severely conflicted a person is about expression, the deeper the physical effects of the repressed emotions. The Bahnsons believed that people who contracted cancer had, in a sense, "discharged" their frustrated drives on their own bodies, resulting in chaos on the lowest levels of cellular organization.

Looking strictly at anger, the Bahnsons saw most people conforming either to an anger-out or anger-in profile. When they studied the relationship of this profile to physical disorders, they found that subjects who tended to project anger outward were more prone to heart disease, while those who turned their rage on themselves were more susceptible to cancer.

Currently, I can find scant hard evidence—and no scientific theory—to explain how repressed emotions could *directly* fuel the machinery of cancer growth. We don't just "grow" tumors instead of getting angry, but complex scientific truths often underlie such simple metaphors. Mind-body researchers have found that a lifelong tendency to repress anger and other negative emotions may be one factor that gradually weakens our biological defense against cancer. I'll elaborate on this discovery, one which I confirmed in my own research, in coming chapters.

"THE NICEST PEOPLE I HAD EVER MET"

I clearly recall my impression, soon after arriving at the melanoma clinic, that the patients were among the nicest people I had ever met. After systematic interviews with more than one hundred, my impression was solidly confirmed. Along with nonexpression of negative emotions, their excessive niceness was a key element of the emerging Type C pattern.

What do I mean by "excessive" niceness? To many, this phrase alone is an odd comingling of terms. Describing a person as *too* nice seems absurd, like saying someone is too good, too compassionate, too worthwhile. Good-guy behavior is so praised in our society that there seems to be no upper limit on how nice we can or should be. Yet I believe we can draw a line between nice and too nice.

Obviously, nice behavior is not—in and of itself—pathological. A pleasant demeanor in work and personal relationships can be a sign of adaptability to one's environment. The capacity to serve, to please, to compromise, and to smooth over differences has great value in establishing and preserving strong social ties. On the other hand, a person who exhibits *compulsive, unyielding* niceness in any situation—no matter how stressful, insulting, or dangerous—has a sizable gap in his emotional repertoire. You can usually recognize this style of niceness in yourself or others—it has a forced, unnatural quality. The nice guy who can't protest when he's been abused is vulnerable to lasting abuse. The nice guy who's afraid to push for a raise or vacation time will neither advance his career nor enjoy the pleasures he deserves. The nice guy who sees the world through rose-colored glasses will be blind to the malicious intent of the con men who, in one guise or another, he'll meet at various times in his life. The nice guy who's trying to please everyone will rarely please himself.

In *Doctor Zhivago,* Boris Pasternak wrote a passage that captures the price paid by people who are locked into the Type C pattern:

> The great majority of us are required to live a life of constant, systematic duplicity. Your health is bound to be affected if, day after day, you say the opposite of what you feel, if you grovel before what you dislike and rejoice at what brings you nothing but misfortune. Our nervous system isn't just a fiction, it's part of our physical body, and our soul exists in space and is inside us, like the teeth in our mouth. It can't be forever violated with impunity.

I interviewed one cancer patient after another whose nice-guy behavior went deep, having originated long before he or she was diagnosed. These were people who, as Pasternak wrote, had lived against the grain of their feelings "day after day," until their physical defenses seemed to collapse under the strain.

There was Leonard, the rabbi who had recently lost his father, to whom he was deeply attached. This was a painful time for him, made more stressful because he felt he had to remain strong and supportive for his entire family. He was also on the brink of losing financial backing for the new temple he was hoping to build—a lifelong dream about to go up in smoke. On the cusp of all this stress, he developed cancer. Leonard could not think of a time in his entire life when he had lost his temper in anger.

I asked Leonard if he was having any problems in his relationships. He said he was quite troubled by the well-meaning friends and congregants who were coming to him with all sorts of medical advice. Some of them prompted him to explore way-out alternative cancer therapies. Leonard didn't want the advice but felt compelled to be the good rabbi and listen to their prolonged exhortations. He didn't know how to sidestep these people without offending them. "I just don't want to hurt anyone," he said. Leonard's sentiments were admirable. But he was trapped between his need for respite—after all, he had just lost his father, his dream, and his good health—and his need to protect everyone else's feelings.

Leonard kept counseling the members of his temple, listening to their advice, tending to his duties, and taking care of his bereaved family. For several months before he was diagnosed, Leonard felt he was at the end of his tether. He had exhausted himself in his role as the beneficent rabbi ready to serve at the drop of a hat, regardless of his own physical or emotional state.

Coincidentally, another patient I interviewed was a Catholic priest with a story similar to Leonard's. Raymond was soft-spoken, sensitive, compassionate toward all his parishioners, open to all points of view. To Raymond, being a priest entailed a "fierce sense of obligation" to his congregation. His biggest stress in life, he said, was the terrible infighting among his staff members. Raymond was the one who "bore the brunt of the stress" by mediating the conflicts, listening to each staff member's complaints, and absorbing the tension. He recalled being upset when passed over for a position in another parish, but he kept his feelings to himself. "In my business, you repress these feelings. You learn not to show emotions, especially anger. It's unpriestly."

Although certain occupations and social roles demand repression more than others, no one develops a pattern of holding in feelings without an earlier predisposition. Raymond stifled his anger long before he entered the priesthood. (At one point in our conversation, I asked Raymond how his body felt when he was upset. He explained to me why he couldn't answer: "When you repress all your feelings *your whole life,* you're not in the habit of identifying them.") Perhaps he gravitated toward the priesthood not only because of his deep faith and innate compassion but also because he was in some sense comfortable with its restrictions on emotional expression.

One patient made a powerful statement that stayed with me— she articulated the existential bind of the nice guy. Naomi was a middle-aged woman who told me she'd spent her whole life trying to please her mother. After contracting cancer, she felt the first stirrings of a desire to free herself from her "good girl" persona. Naomi's mother visited her often after her surgery, and it only added to her suffering. She felt harangued by her mother, who made unreasonable demands and expressed subtle disapproval of Naomi's life-style. Despite these realizations, Naomi said that changing her old behavior was one of the hardest things she'd ever attempted. "I would rather have died than tell my mother to leave me alone," she said.

I have found precise descriptions of Type C–like behaviors in the psychiatric literature. Perhaps the writer who most accurately portrayed this pattern in a purely psychological (not mind-body) context was the renowned psychoanalyst Karen Horney. In several of her books she described in detail an appeasing, passive, nonexpressive character type. Here, in *Our Inner Conflicts,* Horney captures the nuances of the nice-guy syndrome:

> He tends to subordinate himself, takes second place, leaving the limelight to others; he will be appeasing, conciliatory, and—at least consciously—bears no grudge. Any wish for vengeance or triumph is so profoundly repressed that he himself often wonders at his being so easily reconciled and at his never harboring resentment for long. Important in this context is his tendency automatically to shoulder blame. Again quite regardless of his real feelings—that is, whether he really feels guilty or not—he will accuse himself rather than others and tend to scrutinize himself or be apologetic in the face of obviously unwarranted criticism or anticipated attack.

As Horney explained, extreme nice-guy behavior is directly associated with repression of one's darker impulses. While these individuals may harbor genuine empathy and goodwill, they are also hiding negative emotions from themselves and the world. The human animal was not biologically designed for saintliness, and it's safe to wonder what kind of psychological and physical price is paid by those who conform to an impossible ideal.

Consider the case of Jessica. After her doctor diagnosed her with melanoma and told her it was life-threatening, she was overcome with depression. She was a cashier in an all-night convenience store at the time, and phoned another cashier—a woman she thought of as a friend—to cover her shift for the night. Jessica explained her ordeal, but the cashier would not take her place. She offered a flimsy excuse, but Jessica didn't press her. A few hours later, with no replacement to be found, Jessica reluctantly reported to work. She told me about the gut-wrenching strain of that night. She'd been wounded by the double affront of her doctor's diagnosis and her friend's callousness. Several days afterward, she crossed paths with the woman and they exchanged pleasantries. Jessica was shaking inside but said nothing. Instead, the friend's insult ate away at her for several weeks.

It may seem like a minor instance of covering over bad feelings, but for Jessica, this was a common occurrence. She had always maintained a nice front for others—even those who had caused her pain. The most glaring instance occurred two years before she developed cancer. Jessica worked as a bank teller, with a boss—and a salary—that she liked very much. But her boss's wife was difficult, paranoid, and made her presence known at the bank. One day, she falsely accused Jessica of trying to seduce her husband. This led to a period of great stress, during which the wife put pressure on her husband to fire Jessica. He finally caved in and told Jessica she was being "terminated." Jessica wasn't furious; rather, she was gravely hurt by her boss's betrayal and by his wife's viciousness. Still, she never confronted them. Tears welled in her eyes when she told me that she had lodged no protest—this despite the fact that she desperately wanted to keep her job and was innocent of the allegation.

"How did you cope?" I asked her.

"You just go ahead," she said. "You go out and find another job."

Throughout my interview with Jessica, I sensed an ongoing internal battle between her strong emotions and the conscious mental forces she used to keep them at bay. I asked her how she was coping with cancer. "Everything is fine," she murmured. Moments later, she literally fought back tears. I asked her if friends were helping her through this crisis. She said they were, but inexplicably, she began to cry softly. Once again she fought the sadness, dabbing her eyes constantly with a tissue to prevent tears from streaming down her cheeks.

I asked if she needed more from her friends. "I'm a private person," she replied.

Jessica's niceness, which helped her function in some areas, also caused her to accept subtle and not-so-subtle abuse from others. She had bottled up her sadness and anger to the point of bursting but still kept a tight cap on her feelings. Now, with the advent of her cancer, the lid was coming unglued. Jessica was depressed and confused. I read her behavior and picked up the message she unwittingly transmitted: "My way of coping has failed me, and I don't know what to do now."

Jessica's story brought home to me that the nice-guy accommodation to the world could, at a certain point in a person's life, cease to function effectively. Jessica thought her behavior was functional, and so did the people in her environment. But the current crisis had shaken her to the roots, and her niceness prevented her from securing the social support she desperately needed.

SELF-SACRIFICE: A FORM OF SELF-NEGLECT?

The melanoma patients reminded me of certain people from my youth. I thought of the neighbors I liked so much because they were relentlessly helpful and friendly. I recalled the sweet, grandmotherly women from my hometown who organized the local charity drives.

Likeability has its place—it greases the wheels of social interactions, making them more pleasant and trouble-free. A person can minimize the possibility of being rejected or socially humiliated by always appeasing others. And many of us have had parents and schoolteachers who taught a rigid gospel about being kind, considerate, and helpful. The confusion may start there, because who can argue with being kind, considerate, and thoughtful? It was the *inflexibility* that confined us, the fact that we had to be considerate no matter what was done to us, what we needed, what we felt. "Self-sacrificing" is a most appropriate description—for if we continue to embrace such behavior rigidly throughout our lives, we may end up losing our selves.

Elizabeth was a case in point. She was a caregiver for elderly people with Alzheimer's disease, and a deeply religious person devoted to helping others. In many respects, she was coping well with her illness. Although she denied any anger, sadness, or fear, she was optimistic about her chances and determined to recover. Like many other cancer patients, Elizabeth seemed to believe that the only way to stay strong and positive was to erase negative feelings from her mind and heart. And I believe this was true *for her*—she was so unaccustomed to such feelings that, had she abruptly allowed herself to experience them, she might have become overwhelmed and unable to cope.

With the support of her family and her religious faith, Elizabeth was untouched by fear. "I face the fear with faith," she told me. She repeated these words like a mantra throughout our interview. I asked her what else, besides faith, helped her to cope. Elizabeth's guiding light was her concern for other cancer patients and her desire to educate them and their families about the disease so they would never become "paralyzed by fear." Whatever minor anxieties she felt—and she assured me they were minor—could be alleviated by serving others. Like every other person with cancer, Elizabeth brought her lifelong coping strategies to bear in dealing with her illness. She'd lived her life to give care, and saw her illness as another opportunity to reach out to people in need. "Maybe this is a way for me to be even more compassionate in my work with Alzheimer's patients," she said.

Elizabeth was more concerned with what her family was going through than what she had to endure. The one problem area she acknowledged was the solicitude of some friends and coworkers. She did not want any special attention or doting concern from others; it made her feel that they were unintentionally robbing her of dignity.

After our lengthy interview, it was clear to me that Elizabeth's bout with cancer had triggered in her less a transformation than an intensification of the way she'd always lived. Her compassion and commitment were real and moving, but I wondered: where do her needs fit into this equation? Is it possible for someone to escape the cancer experience unscathed by the discomfiting sensations associated with sadness, anger, and fear? Is religious faith such an effective balm that it cuts these feelings off at the pass, preventing them from reaching the conscious mind or sensate body?

We all use denial (or repression) under extreme stress. This psychic defense sometimes acts as a bridge over troubled waters. It gets us through turbulent times until we reach the other side, where relative peace can reign again. Once we've traversed that bridge, we can reflect on our stressful experience and recover our fully feeling selves. That's why we so often experience a delayed reaction after shock, trauma, or loss. Days or weeks later, we'll cry over the death of a friend, rage over the loss of a job, or weep with joy over a personal victory. (Positive changes can be stressful, too.) For some of us—like Elizabeth—the bridge goes on indefinitely. We never get to the other side, where we can safely integrate the intense emotions triggered by stressful life events.

Elizabeth's self-sacrifice served to keep her attention and energies firmly focused on others and off herself. She was loathe to ask for help and was much more comfortable giving. In Elizabeth's worldview, her own pains and fears didn't matter. What mattered was alleviating the pains and fears of others in the same boat. It was a strange paradox, because her empathy grew from her capacity to understand what others had to endure—as if she identified with the very suffering she had denied in herself. I believe that Elizabeth saw her suffering self mirrored in others and doled out loving support as a symbolic way of nurturing herself. Over the years her efforts had indeed brought an indirect form of love and support—namely, gratitude.

You may ask, what is wrong with this way of coping? Again, my observations were not judgments. Elizabeth's style had served her well and I saw nothing "wrong" with her self-sacrifice. There was certainly a lot right about it, both for Elizabeth and for the objects of her care. She had given her disabled patients genuine love and support. But her behavior was part of a pattern that included denial of her own needs and feelings in favor of others'. Elizabeth admitted that for several years before she developed cancer, she experienced great stress and had pushed herself far too much in care-giving activities.

Also, Elizabeth's brush with cancer had been relatively minor—fortunately, her prognosis was good and surgery was expected to cure. But what if her melanoma had been much more serious? What if she'd been incapacitated for weeks or months? Her outlet of care-giving would have been cut off. And she'd have required a great deal of rest, care, and emotional support. Elizabeth would have had to change her style drastically to get these needs met.

Elizabeth's history brought home to me the need for proper balance between attention to self and attention to others. Those who work ceaselessly for their fellow human beings while neglecting themselves suffer silently in both mind and body.

I encountered many self-sacrificing patients who tended to live vicariously through others. Pauline, a sixty-one-year-old nurse, had spent her life as a caretaker. She revealed to me that her raison d'être was helping her daughter, who was soon to give birth to her second grandchild. Pauline said that her "every waking minute" was involved with her daughter, her six-year-old granddaughter, and their needs. Although Pauline had been wrapped up in her daughter's life for years, since her diagnosis her involvement had intensified. It was her way of dealing with the illness.

At first, Pauline's story didn't seem unusual—many people in the face of great stress find one activity to occupy their time. Many people are intimately involved in the lives of their children and grandchildren. But for Pauline, immersion in her daughter's life was coincident with her neglect of her own needs. Pauline hadn't told anyone—except her husband and daughter—about her recently diagnosed cancer. She chose not to share this information with friends or other family members, and she hadn't even revealed the seriousness of her condition to her husband. "I don't want him to worry," she said.

How did she cope? "I just push it aside," she said. "Like Scarlett in *Gone with the Wind*, I say to myself, 'I'll worry about that tomorrow.' "

It must have been a heavy burden for her to keep her anxieties so completely wrapped up. It was a burden she handled by funneling all her energies into her daughter. Another clue to the price exacted by such self-sacrifice was Pauline's lack of pleasure in other areas of life. She admitted a certain unhappiness because, she said, "I can't seem to get excited about anything." I, too, sensed her lack of affect. Pauline's life was missing emotion, color, and meaning. Perhaps she had expended so much energy care-giving, and shared so few of her own needs and fears, that not much was left for her to enjoy for herself.

Patients like Pauline led me to consider a fundamental aspect of mind-body health: the ability to stay in contact with one's own needs and take control of meeting them. Ralph Linton, a famous anthropologist, once wrote, "The role of physical and psychological needs in human behavior is strictly that of first causes. Without the spur which they provide, the individual would remain quiescent." I was confronting patient after patient who embodied that phrase: out of touch with their needs, they remained quiescent.

Many of us stay in the background, afraid of appearing the least bit demanding or narcissistic. We only feel safe stepping out into the world to lend a hand, never to ask for one. The quiescent Type C patients personified these traits, with no room for deviation. For them, admission of need was undignified, a form of selfish indulgence, a sign of flagging strength. Paradoxically, their inability to express need was perhaps their greatest weakness.

SADNESS, FEAR, AND ANXIETY

For the melanoma patients, anger was not the only phantom emotion: many patients also had trouble experiencing and expressing sadness, fear, and anxiety.

I had asked Martin, the Type C patient described earlier who kept up a facade of detachment, whether he could recall an experience of extreme fear. He went on to describe, in verbal Technicolor, an extraordinary near-death incident that occurred when he was river rafting in Idaho. Martin and his friends hit extremely turbulent rapids, then suddenly found themselves cascading over a steep waterfall. They all managed to swim to safety, but for several minutes the outcome was uncertain. Martin told me proudly that he'd actually enjoyed the experience. Never for a moment, he said, had he been seized by fear.

Martin's response was quite typical. I asked him when he was most afraid, and he told a tale of fearlessness. Often, patients had difficulty differentiating one emotion from another. I would ask about anger, and they'd tell a story of sadness; I'd ask about sadness, and they'd describe a time of anxiety. Another patient, Betsy, answered the fear question by telling me about a walk she took with her husband in a dangerous neighborhood. "My husband said it was a bad neighborhood, so for a moment I was worried. But it lasted a second because I don't let myself get scared. It turned out to be the most enjoyable walk. The air was fresh and it was great."

Betsy's story is a reminder that fear serves a vital purpose. If Betsy had entertained even a modicum of fear, she'd have made her husband join her in a walk elsewhere. Fear is the spark for our self-protective impulses, and it's a spark we need to keep alive. As with all primary emotions, the rule of thumb is balance: if one is overly sensitive to signals of fear or trapped by past experiences of fear, one can readily become paralyzed. But a fine-tuned sense of fear—an ability to sense and recognize situations of danger and act accordingly—is a survival mechanism.

Many patients told me they weren't the least bit anxious about having cancer. They used the defense of denial to completely block awareness of fear. These were individuals who could not tolerate fear, and my impression was that they'd been that way since childhood. Morton, a forty-year-old maintenance man, lived alone with his mother and sister. He told me that finding out he had cancer "didn't bother me, didn't faze me." He added, "I don't really think I have cancer anymore." The only thing about cancer that made him anxious, he said, was the big-city traffic he would hit on his way into San Francisco for doctor's appointments.

Anxiety, too, is a signal that tells us something in our world needs to be rectified. For people just diagnosed with a life-threatening illness, some anxiety is both understandable and useful: it goads the patient to take proper action to reduce that anxiety. This can mean getting the best medical care, adhering to the doctor's prescriptions, researching alternative therapies, or just asking for support. Taking control reduces anxiety in real, practical ways. Complete denial reduces anxiety by suspending it in a web of illusion. When patients resort to complete denial, the anxiety never really vanishes.

I encountered patients who could not either experience or express sadness. Though not an uncommon psychological defense, this tendency was marked among the melanoma patients. I asked Sean, a middle-aged security guard, to tell me the time when he felt most sadness.

"I don't experience it very often," he said. I pushed for an answer. "Well, my father passed away fourteen years ago."

"Did you cry at the time?" I asked.

"Not really. A little, I think."

"How did you handle the sadness, what did you do?"

"I kept busy. I rationalized it. I tried not to think about it."

"How did you rationalize it?"

"I thought, well, we were never really that close. Why should I get too upset over it, when we weren't that close?"

"Did you have any bodily sensations during that time?"

"Yeah. All I can remember is a kind of sick feeling."

"Tell me more."

"I guess I must have felt worse than I thought. I do recall a sick feeling in my stomach for quite a while. When I look back, I think I must have been more upset than I knew. There were a lot of things I wanted to tell him that I never got a chance to. Maybe I was sad over what could have been, instead of what was. But I didn't want to dwell on it."

Sean was describing, in clear terms, what psychologists call "repressive coping." He handled the stress of his father's death, and the emotions it triggered, by keeping a firm cover on his feelings. During the course of bereavement, this period of denial and/or repression is normal and necessary. If it never lifts, however, a person never experiences the sadness of loss, and he circumvents the natural process of grieving. He is left with unconscious, unresolved feelings that affect mind, body, and spirit in subtle ways for years to come. The result may be low-grade depression, loss of affect, chronic stress-related physical symptoms, or a suppressed immune system.

I was also struck by the fact that many patients expressed sadness in situations that one would normally expect to arouse anger. I call this the "sad instead of mad" syndrome—the person uses sadness as a kind of defense against her own anger. Tara, a young woman who had just been left by her boyfriend of three years, described his injustices against her. The list was lengthy. She said she was never more angry than when he unilaterally broke off their relationship. What did she say or do? "I just stayed in my room and cried," she said. "I felt so terrible. I talked to him and let him know how depressed I was. I begged him to change his mind." Tara never once directly expressed anger to her boyfriend; her rage was turned against herself. At the time of the breakup, she felt guilty, worthless, and needy. The impulse to confront him, to get her feelings off her chest, transformed into tears and pleading.

I was beginning to see that, in general, these patients had

difficulties expressing all "negative" emotions, including sadness, fear, anxiety, and anger. (I use *negative* in quotes because it carries the implication that such feelings are somehow bad or destructive. This is a creeping form of critical judgment aimed at our own natural emotions. The clinical term for such emotions is *dysphoric*, which simply implies that they are experienced as unpleasant. However, in deference to the conventions of language, I'll use negative— though under protest.) From the earliest days of infancy, negative feelings have survival value—they are psychobiological alarm bells. A clear and present danger is near or nurturance is lacking or food is not forthcoming or abandonment has occurred. The word *emotion* comes from the Latin root meaning "to move." Threatening or disturbing circumstances cause us to be moved to fear, anger, or sadness, and these emotions involve complex chain reactions by our nervous and endocrine systems. If the feelings cannot be experienced, discharged, or properly managed, a biological imperative is blocked. The long-term consequence is mind-body imbalance.

From studying melanoma patients, I also learned about the short-term consequences. The repressive coper has narrow options for handling a crisis. He may not be able to defend himself with anger when attacked. He may not be able to fully grieve over a loss. He may not be able to express a strong need for support if such an admission belies his facade of contentment. What I call the Type C behavior pattern has ramifications in terms of physical health, psychological well-being, and spiritual development.

TYPE C: A WORLD APART FROM TYPE A

My insight into this behavior pattern was enhanced by an experience I had months earlier. I had taken a course on the Type A behavior pattern with cardiologist Ray H. Rosenman, M.D., who along with Meyer Friedman, M.D., had written the landmark book, *Type A Behavior and Your Heart.* Type A individuals are hostile, competitive, hard-driving, and suffer from "hurry sickness"—a kind of pathological impatience. Friedman and Rosenman demonstrated that Type A's had a far greater than normal risk for developing heart disease.

The two cardiologists devised creative methods for measuring Type A behavior, which included analysis of vocal patterns recorded on audiotape. Type A's spoke rapidly and explosively, sometimes sputtering words and sentences in machine-gun fashion. During my course with Dr. Rosenman, he had expanded the repertoire of Type A research by using videotape to study the body language of these tense and often combative people. I was learning to identify Type A's by their words, actions, voices, movements, and facial expressions.

Now, after interviewing scores of melanoma patients, I was impressed by the marked contrast between them and the aggressive Type A people. (It was no surprise that Martin, the cancer patient who was so accurate in his self-description, took great pains to contrast himself to the "Type A personality.") I realized that the cancer patients were not just different from the Type A's—*they were the polar opposite.* The primary polarities I found were:

- The melanoma patients were cooperative and appeasing, unassertive, patient, and utterly compliant with external authorities. The Type A patients were highly charged competitors, struggling fiercely to achieve or maintain a top-dog position in their careers or relationships.
- The cancer patients did not express negative emotions, especially anger. Rosenman's Type A subjects were often overflowing with anxiety, hostility, and anger.
- The melanoma patients were more involved in meeting other people's needs than their own. The Type A people were self-centered, focusing incessantly on their own needs and how they could meet them.

When Rosenman and Friedman discovered the Type A behavior pattern, they expressed the view that there existed a contrasting, healthy, Type B pattern. Type B's were genuinely relaxed, noncompetitive, and never had out-of-control temper tantrums or hostile episodes. They were at peace with themselves and their environments. According to Friedman and Rosenman, everyone was either a coronary-prone Type A or a healthy Type B with no increased risk of heart disease.

On the surface, the melanoma patients had Type B–like qualities. They were not driven overachievers. They never had rageful outbursts. They *seemed* perfectly relaxed. But as I studied them scientifically, it was clear that their lack of anger did not stem from a sense of inner peace. Their inability to assert themselves was extreme and I did not see it as a healthy departure from the rat-race mentality. Underneath their facade, there was a great deal of *unexpressed* anger, carefully guarded feelings of anxiety, and in many cases, I was to discover, a deep-seated feeling of despair. Put simply, these people were no Type B's.

This is why I named the behavior pattern exhibited by our cancer patients *Type C*. The group of behaviors I observed was utterly distinct, diametrically opposed to Type A, and strongly associated with cancer. Type B's, I believed, represented the healthy middle ground between the extreme, unhealthy Type A and Type C patterns, which anchored opposite ends of a continuum of how people cope with stress.

Here is the sum of my initial findings, based on interviews with more than 150 melanoma patients. Approximately three fourths of the patients demonstrated the Type C behavior pattern, which means that they displayed most or all of the following behaviors:

1) They were nonexpressors of anger. Often, they were unaware of any feelings of anger, past or present.
2) They tended not to experience or express other negative emotions, namely anxiety, fear, and sadness.
3) They were patient, unassertive, cooperative, and appeasing in work, social, and family relationships. They were compliant with external authorities.
4) They were overly concerned with meeting the needs of others, and insufficiently engaged in meeting their own needs. Often, they were self-sacrificing to an extreme.

TYPE C BEHAVIOR: THE PRIMARY COLORS

The Type C patients I met and studied were all confronted with similar levels of stress from having cancer. What really distinguished them was how they coped with these circumstances: they kept their feelings in check, maintained a pleasant demeanor, never complained, and focused selflessly on the needs of those close to them. As I conceived it, the Type C pattern was a way of thinking, feeling, and behaving in response to life's tribulations.

I was learning the lesson that mind-body researchers today

have fully embraced. Stress per se is not a critical factor in illness—it's the strength or weakness of one's coping mechanism. We all have stress, and scientific attempts to link stressful life events with illnesses such as cancer have had ambiguous results at best. It's our psychological resources that determine how healthfully we will endure the death of a loved one, the loss of a job, or a physical illness.

For some patients, the Type C style "worked" to a degree—it helped reduce stress through various stages of the life cycle. But for many of them, I observed that the Type C style had profound psychological and physical deficits. Type C coping was like a weak foundation for a building: it held up for a certain number of years until one day it cracked, revealing its essential fragility. A person who doesn't assert his needs or express emotions appropriately may remain functional for decades. But eventually, the psychological and/or physical strain will manifest itself, and the person's health and day-to-day functioning will suffer.

During the initial phase of my research, I excavated every available study of psychological factors in cancer. With varying degrees of scientific rigor, previous investigators had uncovered psychological states and traits shared by cancer patients. Many of these states and traits bore an uncanny resemblance to aspects of the Type C pattern emerging from my studies of melanoma patients. David Kissen, M.D., a physician from the University of Glasgow, forged the first bona fide scientific link between nonexpression of emotions and cancer. Kissen was a specialist for the Scottish mining industry during the 1950s. He conducted careful interviews and tests on almost one thousand miners who came to one of three chest units for diagnosis and treatment. Kissen compared those with lung cancer with those who were healthy or had other lung ailments. The lung cancer patients had "poorer outlets for emotional discharge." This held true even after he controlled for the effects of cigarette smoking. The smokers had a higher risk of cancer, but those with normal outlets for emotional expression had a better risk profile than those with "poor" outlets.

Kissen was not the only researcher who studied repression and other psychological factors in cancer patients. A number of investigators had confirmed parts of the Type C hypothesis. (I will describe the key studies of other researchers throughout this book.) Their findings overlapped with each other and with my own observations. I began to sketch a picture of how the mind influences cancer. The picture was highly complex, with a great deal of lush background detail. But the foreground—the "primary colors" of the mind-body-cancer relationship—was bright, strong, and clear. The Type C pattern was composed of these primary colors.

CHAPTER 3

So many of my patients have experienced a neglect of
their most basic, deepest human needs—for touching and
for companionship, for sharing inner feelings, for
expressing creative energy, for sexual fulfillment, for
personal validation, and for the giving and receiving of
love. Instead, their lives were characterized by duty and
obligation to the very people who gave them little or
nothing in return.

—*Dennis Jaffe*

Some people never learn that their organism has the right
to take up space without shrinking, to assert itself
without feeling guilt. . . . Anger for most people is an
alternative to fading away.

—*Ernest Becker*

The defensive pattern does not define the person. The
core does. A person in treatment . . . is a human being
whose functioning has gone awry, and whose soul has an
inborn brilliance and beauty . . . that the therapy is
designed to release.

—*John Pierrakos*

Shared Patterns, Unique Personalities

The more patients I studied, the more certain I became that Type C was not a personality. It was a behavior pattern, a coping style. Type C was not who people were; it was what they did to cope with outer stress and inner distress. Type C was an early conditioned response that had become their accommodation to the world. The negative feelings they banished from consciousness had not disappeared, they were hidden away. The "real person" was locked up, and I could often sense the unhappiness, confusion, melancholia, or pent-up rage they carried with them in a remote inner place, a place neither they nor I could easily contact.

Definitions of *personality* differ from one expert to another, but to most people, personality is an aspect of selfhood that is rather all-encompassing and unalterable. I don't use Type C *personality* because Type C is *not* all-encompassing and it *is* alterable. Type C is not the whole person. Rather, it's a major part of the individual's psychic defense against emotional threats from within and without. The use of *personality* could lead some to believe that a person's core identity—who they are—plays a role in his getting cancer or even dying from it. I don't believe that is possible—it carries implications that are false and even cruel. But I do believe that how a person characteristically handles stress *can* affect his biological defense against cancer. This is verifiable, and it can be a source of hope and empowerment for cancer patients or anyone wishing to stay healthy.

This is because the way we handle stress—our coping style—can be transformed. We can't abruptly restructure our personality (certainly not without long-term psychotherapy, and perhaps not even then). But we can change our behavior patterns.

Through the course of my research, I learned that some people cannot change their Type C behavior, for reasons that were hard to discern. Whatever the reasons, which were undoubtedly hidden in the folds of each person's life history, their difficulty was beyond judgment of any kind.

Although it's important to recognize that some Type C individuals can't change, most can transform their behavior and their lives. I have seen them do it with and without psychotherapy. They become more expressive, assertive, and self-nurturing. They bring about a fundamental shift in their relationship to self and to the world—by deepening their awareness of inner needs and feelings and by expanding to make more genuine contact with others. And I have witnessed the results: a healing of the split between mind and body, and a remarkable improvement in emotional and physical health. I'll describe the process of Type C transformation in the last two sections of this book. But I found clues to the healing potential of change in my early investigation of Type C melanoma patients.

THE FLEXIBILITY FACTOR

Although I could identify the "primary colors" of the Type C pattern in most patients, the pattern occurred in as many different configurations as there were individual cancer patients. My search for a pattern was not a search for rigid uniformity, and I did not find rigid uniformity. The melanoma patients were a diverse population in many respects. They had differing interests, habits, family relationships, life-styles, values, and dreams. The only thing they had in common was their Type C pattern. Even there, the intensity of Type C behavior and the degree to which they exhibited one strand of Type C more than another (say, repression of anger more than self-sacrifice) varied greatly from patient to patient.

These variations were more than just individual idiosyncracies. I saw that subtle differences among the patients held important information about the health and state of mind of each one. Analyzing these differences was a form of prognosis, much the way biomedical doctors analyse blood fractions for variations that indicate a patient's potential for disease—i.e., a cholesterol count over 200 is considered a mild risk for later heart disease; a count over 240 is considered a far more serious risk.

I realized that the sheer *intensity* of Type C coping was a clue to the role of this behavior pattern in a person's cancer or his recovery. For example, Martin was an extreme Type C coper who kept an airtight lid on his feelings. He never acknowledged any fear, anger, or sadness, and didn't share his experience with others. Two months after I interviewed Martin, he died. I was stunned—the doctors had not expected him to succumb so quickly. From a strictly medical standpoint, they thought he had a reasonable chance to survive five years.

Scientists are quick to criticize anecdotal evidence. We know that one case like Martin's does not prove a theory. But I felt a shock of recognition at Martin's death because he had so conspicuously personified the Type C pattern. I knew that Type C behavior could, theoretically, play a role in both the onset of an individual's cancer and in his chances for survival. In Martin's case, it may have influenced both disease onset *and* progression. And the intensity of his Type C coping could have contributed, in some measure, to his rapid decline.

As depressing as Martin's outcome was, I knew that seeds of hope could be found in understanding this connection. For other Type C's were not as extreme as Martin, and perhaps their prospects for health and longevity were better. The less intense Type C's had the quality I refer to as *flexibility*. Flexible Type C's tended to be passive and held in their anger. But sometimes they could rise to an occasion and stand up for themselves. In an interview, a flexible Type C person might reveal a lifelong pattern of nonexpression, then let down her guard and express unpleasant feelings.

This led me to investigate the diversity of Type C behavior among the melanoma patients. The flexibility factor, I surmised, made a crucial difference in how well people thrived and survived with cancer.

An attractive woman in her late forties, Yolanda had experienced severe stresses in the five years prior to her developing melanoma. It all began with a wrenching divorce and continued when her teenage daughter became addicted to drugs, which precipitated her mental breakdown. More recently, her son had been hospitalized with kidney disease. How had she coped with all this? "I developed a really thick shell," she said. I was impressed by her directness. Yolanda was very controlled throughout our interview. She wasn't telling her family or friends about her illness, for fear of disturbing them. "I always keep things very close to the vest," she remarked.

Yolanda's honesty was the first clue I had to her flexibility. The second came when I asked her a question that I asked every cancer patient I interviewed—a question designed to bypass the conscious mind and poke through into the unconscious: "If the part of your body with melanoma could speak, what would it say?" Yolanda thought hard for a second, then said, "It would be outRAGED!" The "RAGED" burst out of her mouth with such unexpected force that I was utterly surprised.

"A lot has come together in my life just now, and I just can't believe there's a possibility that I won't be able to enjoy it." She was visibly quaking. Yolanda had seen her children through their crises and she had survived her own. Now it was her time to find pleasure in life.

Until that moment, Yolanda *had* kept everything close to her vest, but my question broke through her rationality. She was furious at the thought of losing her life, and when her imagination took flight for a moment, she spoke a truth she would not have otherwise divulged. No other Type C patient answered my question with such passion. Perhaps Yolanda's passion made a difference, for she has survived her cancer without a recurrence.

Yolanda's nonverbal responses, and her description of herself, told me that she had always been a Type C coper. But her forthrightness and sudden departure from the Type C norm told me that she also had flexibility. She had what I call a *wider repertoire* of emotional expression, when compared with an extreme Type C coper like Martin.

Renata was a person who, for most of her life, handled hard times by sweeping her feelings under a rug. Although she had no idea that I was investigating a possible behavior pattern in cancer, at one point in our interview she blurted, "I haven't figured it out yet, but I think my pattern is to bury things and keep them buried."

Renata worked as housing coordinator for an international

students' summer arts program in San Francisco. A few years earlier she found out about a student who was being psychologically and physically abused by the father of her host family. On several occasions, the father had belittled and struck the fifteen-year-old girl. Renata made efforts to get the father to stop his abuse, but it went on unabated.

"I don't get angry very often—like every ten years I'll get furious at something," Renata said. "I'm not one to blow off steam. But that pushed my buttons."

"What did you do?" I asked.

"I really would have loved to obliterate him," she said vehemently. "But instead I put my foot down and extricated that girl from the situation."

"How did your body feel when you were most angry at the man?"

"I surprised myself. Lots of adrenaline was pumping. I really wanted to liquidate him the quickest way possible," she said, laughing. "But that wouldn't have solved the problem."

Renata had acknowledged to herself the intensity of her rage, then channeled it into appropriate action. Though this deviated from her usual pattern, she had risen to the occasion in a remarkably healthy way. It was as if there were cracks of light streaming through her psychological armor, small fissures that allowed her to feel anger and use it wisely in a crucial situation. I believe it was Renata's flexibility that enabled her to cope so well with her recently diagnosed cancer. The experience of cancer actually expanded Renata's capacity to express her needs, emotions, and creativity.

Renata's flexibility served her so well, in fact, that she was able to admit to the depths of fear about her cancer while retaining a steadfast determination to fight the disease and win. This is a rare quality in anyone, and especially a person who generally wears a mask of contentment.

I asked her how she felt when she first found out she had melanoma.

"Fear, right up front. Fear right from the top of my head down to my feet. Then I went through what I suspect is fairly common. Your mind ponders the worst. When you first drive away from the doctor's office, it's ridiculous, it's this Technicolor movie going on in your head. It's very scary and sad. You think about all the things you might have done to prevent this. You think about all the things you desperately want to do with your life. All the things you've bypassed."

Like many other patients, Renata saw cancer as an opportunity to grow. Scores of popular books counsel sick people to do just that—view their illness as a positive turning point instead of a hopeless ordeal. But I believe it was Renata's emotional flexibility that allowed her to adopt that life-affirming position. Otherwise, no amount of "positive thinking" would have gotten her there.

"This has made me think about the time I've wasted," she told me. "There are specific things I want to do with my life. Things I kept putting off because I place other people ahead of me. I've started to turn that around." Renata wanted to get more involved in the women's movement, and told me about her personal pledge to live out her commitment to social change. That, for Renata, was a sign of transformation.

The unwavering support of her husband and two daughters, and her own ability to accept their help enabled Renata to expand her horizons and remain hopeful. Another sign of her flexibility was the fact that Renata did *not* consider herself responsible for her family's feelings about her illness. This was in direct contrast to most other Type C copers.

"I haven't been able to be very helpful to them. I can't quite understand that. They knew I was really scared at the beginning, because I couldn't hide it. I wasn't as brave and wonderful as I thought I was or would be. I was really shook up by the experience. Perhaps if they hadn't witnessed me so scared I would have been more helpful to them. But they saw it and that's that and . . . so what."

Renata bore no guilt about her expressions of fear or the effect they had on her family. She only reflected on the possibility that it had been difficult for them. And she embraced the reality that what transpired was inevitable—she *had* been scared, her feelings *did* show, and "so what." Renata didn't feel like a failure; she felt like an imperfect human being and accepted herself as such.

Renata was a Type C coper undergoing a process of metamorphosis. I was sure that her flexibility—past and present—enabled her to blossom and mature in the face of her illness. What was it about her behavior that indicated flexibility? Renata had an awareness of her pattern. She had insight into how her coping style affected her life, and the function it served. She had the ability to let her emotions seep through her psychological defenses.

These were the criteria I looked for to gauge an individual's flexibility—a degree of self-awareness, insight, and emotional openness. Even if I saw only glimpses of these qualities, they told me that the person's coping abilities might not be overwhelmed by cancer. She might be able to seek support, express her feelings, and take care of her own needs. Flexibility became my litmus test for Type C individuals—the more flexible they were, the healthier their mind-body profile.

Flexibility was a sign of hope that Type C's could change without having to undergo a personality transplant. *They could change gradually, just by becoming more flexible.* The change might not be easy, but I observed it happening in a naturally occurring circumstance—i.e., in patients who had read no books and seen no therapists. These patients had only one prior advantage—a slight opening of the passageway to their own emotions. When cancer struck, the door opened farther to enable them—at least partially—to get their needs met and avoid the pit of hopelessness. As examples of flexibility, Yolanda and Renata not only showed evidence of psychological health but physical health as well. Both are alive and free of disease five years since my interviews with them.

I also observed extreme Type C patients—albeit not many—who loosened the rigid control they had always exercised over their feelings. These changes occurred without any psychological intervention. I wondered how much more open, expressive, and self-nurturing these patients could become with counseling or therapy. The possibilities seemed great, since I had seen that even small moves in the direction of change yielded substantial psychological and physical benefits.

REPRESSION OR SUPPRESSION?

I've mentioned that one of the factors I look for in emotional flexibility is awareness. Is the Type C individual aware of his anger, but hides it to remain in good social graces? Thus far, my research indicated that extreme Type C's were completely unaware of angry emotions. Does the Type C person know when he's sad, anxious, fearful? Again, he appeared to be unaware of such feelings, or simply did not experience them in situations where they would be appropriate.

What, then, happens to the anger, the fear, the sadness? What happens to the capacity to experience and act upon these basic emotions? For the answer, I must turn momentarily to the literature of psychotherapy and psychoanalysis, where the terms *repression* and *suppression* originated. *Repression* refers to the psychological defense mechanism whereby unpleasant emotions are completely blocked from awareness. Thus far, I have used *repression* because most Type C patients fully censored from consciousness their anger, their need for support, and their intense anxiety. By definition, the censored needs and feelings remain in the person's unconscious, where they affect mind and body in subterranean ways.

Suppression refers to the conscious holding back of an emotion. A person who has been slighted, knows he is angry, and intentionally stops himself from showing signs of rage is suppressing his anger. A minority of the Type C patients I studied were generally conscious of negative emotions but said they deliberately suppressed them.

In most psychotherapy patients, it's not hard to detect both suppression and repression. These psychological defenses are not monolithic; they shift in and out of power, change shape, and become more or less intense, depending on the person's past and present circumstances. (Later in this book, I will rely on the term *nonexpression* to cover both suppression and repression because, in both cases, the person does not express emotion.)

What I found striking about the Type C melanoma patients was the degree to which repression reigned. There were, however, suppressors among them—patients who remained conscious of negative emotions but chose to hide them from the world. Theirs was a more functional psychological defense. Why? Precisely because it involved more choice, less self-deception, and less alienation from self. These were the patients with flexibility. They displayed less extreme Type C behavior and were potentially more capable of change. Some of them had strong memories of earlier times when they felt rage or deep sadness. Gabrielle, a woman in her early thirties, was one:

I can't pinpoint a specific time in my past when I got really angry. Looking back on my childhood, I see it as a pleasant time. But when I stop and think hard about it, I do remember feeling a lot of anger and hostility. My mother used to say I woke up in the morning with a chip on my shoulder. [Note: her melanoma was on her shoulder.] And I felt a lot of anger at the time, I could identify it at the time, but I couldn't get it out. Nor could I explain it away or justify it. It was just there. I had a lot of jealousy toward my sister—much of it irrational, some of it based in fact. My father was an alcoholic and that created tremendous stress in our family. My mother was overbearing—always having to have her way. These must have been reasons for my anger, but I never blew up. Now, looking back, I wonder if all that hidden hostility had something to do with my arthritis when I was fifteen. I didn't drink, smoke, curse, "play around," or anything, so I think it was just held in. Perhaps the anger could only come out that way, in a physical illness.

When Gabrielle "thought hard," she remembered the anger that lay beneath the surface of her childhood. She also admitted that keeping her emotions under wraps had been her style ever since those early years. "I haven't ever seen myself as the kind of person that liked to open up a lot as far as my personal feelings go," she told me. "I talk objectively about things but not when it starts hitting the real nitty-gritty."

The Type C process begins at an early age when, like Gabrielle, the person still feels strong stirrings of anger or sadness. But, to use a metaphor coined by the poet Robert Bly, she is compelled by others to put her feelings and needs "in the bag." In the bag they remain for the course of a lifetime unless or until they reemerge. "We spend our life until we're twenty deciding what parts of ourselves to put in the bag," wrote Bly, "and we spend the rest of our lives trying to get them out again."

The child's decision, "I won't bother Mommy now by telling her I'm hungry," is a prototypic example of how needs are stifled to please others. The child who is roundly scolded for an angry outburst will think twice before having another tantrum. The child exposed to unremitting punishment, scorn, or indifference for expressing taboo feelings will begin to wear a poker face.

Sooner or later, though, the suppressor no longer recognizes in himself the biological signals of pain and distress. It would be hard for a child to maintain psychological balance, when she perpetually experiences emotions that can't be discharged, needs that can't be voiced. Eventually, the Type C person becomes numb to inner signals of pain and fatigue. Her stiff upper lip becomes frozen; her compliance becomes chronic; her anger and aggressiveness are squelched. That's when early suppression, or conscious control, gives way to repression—the erasure of feelings from consciousness.

For reasons we can never fully know, some people repress feelings more completely than others. A suppressor, like Gabrielle, held on to awareness of her feelings, even though they were painful. A repressor, like Martin, lost touch completely with the "negative" parts of himself. He had the more rigid, unyielding Type C defense. Martin maintained the increasingly precarious position of being numb to fear, sadness, and anger—emotions that are crucial feedback from our inner and outer environments.

I asked Vicki, one of the Type C melanoma patients, "What would the part of your body with melanoma say if it could speak?" Her answer revealed much about the Type C defense. Without hesitation, she said, "Go ahead and kick me around, because I can't feel it."

I view the extreme Type C person as being in the same kind of anesthetized state as a wounded racehorse that's been injected with painkillers so that it can compete in a big-money derby. The horse won't feel any pain and will finish the race, but after the drugs wear off its injuries could be dangerously aggravated. Likewise, the person who doesn't feel the emotional wear and tear of daily stresses will continue to endure a painful job, marriage, or life-style until he physically breaks down.

This analogy may even represent a biological truth. Mind-body research is revealing that the "numbness" of the repressor may be due to an increase in certain neuropeptides, called beta-endorphins, which are the biological equivalents of morphine. Yale University researcher Gary E. Schwartz, Ph.D., (now at the University of Arizona, Tucson) has concluded that repressors have unusually high levels of these painkilling chemicals in their bodies, which not only narcotize negative feelings but which may also suppress the immune system—our defense against cancer. We're beginning to understand the biological mechanisms by which repression leads to a kind of psychological anesthesia *and* to greater susceptibility to disease.

THE COPING CONTINUUM

Once I recognized the diversity among the Type C patients, I was prevented from lumping them into a uniform, simplistic category. *Type C* as a term is inordinately valuable because it represents the unmistakable strand of behaviors shared by these patients and offers the prospect of a unifying principle. At the same time, my observations of individual differences arose from, and reflected, the true complexity of the relationship between cancer and the mind. I realized from the outset that my research would not yield any simple equations, such as "Type C causes cancer." The shadings of behavior, the nuances of expression, and the underlying, unarticulated needs and disappointments had to be studied carefully, revealed, and respected. Indeed, I came to the realization that subtle behavioral variations held important clues to the mysteries of cancer and the mind, and pointed the way toward health and transformation.

The world is not made up of Type A's, B's, and C's. *A, B,* and *C* are descriptions of behavior and principles of mind-body health and dysfunction. Many people exemplify A-, B-, or C-type behavior but few embody every behavioral detail, as if they were living case studies. In terms of coping styles, most people can be described as falling somewhere along a continuum. Based on my own observations, studies, and the work of other mind-body researchers, I developed a specific *continuum of coping styles.* The Type A person, who is highly competitive, anxious, and overly aggressive, is at one pathological extreme. The quintessential Type C coper, passive and never angry, anchors the other end of the spectrum. The Type B person, who can express emotions appropriately and is relaxed and self-assured, holds down a healthy middle ground. Here is a diagram of the continuum:

THE COPING CONTINUUM

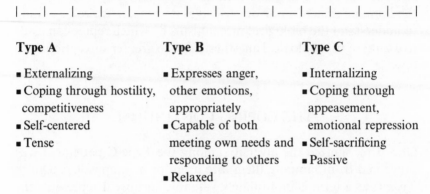

Type A	Type B	Type C
• Externalizing	• Expresses anger,	• Internalizing
• Coping through hostility, competitiveness	other emotions, appropriately	• Coping through appeasement, emotional repression
• Self-centered	• Capable of both	• Self-sacrificing
• Tense	meeting own needs and responding to others	• Passive
	• Relaxed	

As you can see, there is open space along the continuum for the many unique coping styles that fall between Types A and B and Types B and C. The continuum is a yardstick by which we can measure the intensity of a given individual's coping style and assess the possible impact on mind-body health. According to Type A researchers, extreme Type A behavior puts people at greater risk for a heart attack. How so? By mechanisms only beginning to be understood, the percolating hostility of the Type A person affects his *cardiovascular system.* According to my research (and others'), extreme Type C behavior puts people at greater risk of cancer development. How so? The nonexpression of the Type C person appears to weaken his *immune system,* which he counts on to protect him from cancer and infectious diseases. In coming chapters, I will discuss my research confirming the role of Type C behavior in impaired immunity and increased risk of cancer progression.

By contrast, the balanced Type B is someone who can express emotions *appropriately.* He is not brimming over with the rage that theoretically could damage his cardiovascular system. He has not stifled his feelings for years, and thus has not suffered the immune-damaging effects of long-term repressive coping. Type B's may therefore be at reduced risk for both heart disease *and* cancer.

A person who exhibits Type C behavior but has emotional flexibility—like Renata—would place somewhere between *B* and *C* on the continuum. The more aware the individual is, the more expressive and the closer she is to the Type B middle ground of health. Likewise, a high-strung Type A personality who is capable of relaxation, of occasionally letting go of his fierce competitiveness, would fall somewhere between *A* and *B*.

My continuum emphasizes the night-and-day differences between the way a Type C person copes and the way a Type A person copes. By placing Type B in the middle, I am emphasizing that mind-body health is a state of balance. The capacity for anger, striving to meet ambitious ends, and self-involvement are not by definition pathological. In moderation, and in their appropriate context, these are healthy ways of coping in the real world. When these same qualities are distorted or excessive—as in Type A's—they *are* pathological. Likewise, a pleasant demeanor, conscious control of anger, and temporary fearlessness in the face of trauma can be effective ways of coping. In a rigid or excessive pattern—as in the Type C person—these same behaviors can be disabling to both mind and body.

I was particularly concerned about the health ramifications for people at the far end of the Type C pole. These were individuals who exerted total control over emotions, who were largely unaware of their feelings, and thus could not get their underlying needs met. As a result, they suffered in silence. This sort of quiet desperation—a form of hopelessness—has been shown to damage the immune system.

At the same time, I observed that, in rare instances, even these rigid Type C's could relax the grip of repression on their hearts and minds. The more flexible patients were certainly more capable of change. But with psychological intervention, I saw reason to believe that almost any Type C person could move along the continuum toward the Type B center—the middle ground of health.

The *fluidity* of the coping continuum is perhaps its most useful advantage over other similar models. You can find your place on the continuum and define the steps you need to take to achieve a healthier balance in the way you express emotions and handle stress. In this way, you can progress along the continuum toward the Type B ideal. Even the most extreme Type C person can move toward healthy coping by becoming more emotionally flexible. *What matters is not where you end up, but how far you've traveled— how many small steps you've taken.* My program for Type C transformation (described in the last two sections) is essentially a guide to flexibility—an individualized approach to help you contact your feelings, soften your defenses, and change your relationships.

ORIGINS OF TYPE C BEHAVIOR: SOCIETY

How did the Type C pattern originate? How did this way of coping become so entrenched? At first glance, a sociological analysis enabled me to understand how an individual could develop the Type C pattern. For the incipient Type C coper, keeping negative feelings at bay made human interactions "easier." Type C behavior, with its niceties, conformity, and appeasement, helped the person make his way in the world with minimal opposition—the path of least resistance. It helped him maintain a sense of equilibrium in the face of internal or external threats. The Type C worldview is based on the belief that little harm can come when one plays the game of social interaction strictly by the rules of those in power. The worst that can happen is that you lose the game, but at least no one can accuse you of being a bad guy. You will be the object of no one's wrath, and you'll never get thrown out of the game, abandoned, or left to fend alone.

So Type C behavior was a trade-off, a way to gain assurance of minimal security. For Type C's, "Like me, don't leave me, and I won't rock the boat" is the fundamental social transaction. Notably, the Type C person doesn't ask for much—the other person can often exploit or abuse him as long as he doesn't abandon him.

The Type C person, with his covert pledge of compliance, makes an art of socially acceptable behavior. She usually possesses an extraordinary sensitivity to others' sore spots and makes it her business to avoid any behavior that inflames them. The Type C person is particularly attuned to other people's potential discomfort with her needs, her anxieties, and most especially her anger. Whether in social groups, at work, or in the family, she will conceal even the faintest sign of her discontent, for fear that she will be cast adrift, even momentarily, for allowing such unpleasantness to darken the relationship.

The Type C person keeps his angers and anxieties in so deep a hole that even he has no access. The loss of anger hinders healthy development, as psychiatrist Alice Miller explains so deftly in her book *For Your Own Good:* "Everyone must find his own form of aggressiveness in order to avoid letting himself be made into an obedient puppet manipulated by others. Only if we do not allow ourselves to be reduced to the instrument of another person's will can we fulfill our personal needs and defend our legitimate rights. But this appropriate form of aggression is unattainable for many people who have grown up with the absurd belief that a person can have nothing but kind, good, and meek thoughts and at the same time be honest and authentic. The effort to fulfill this impossible demand can drive sensitive children to the brink of madness."

And if such children do not go over the brink into madness—and most do not—what happens to them? Where do the pent-up drives and feelings go? In recent years, the emerging science of psychoneuroimmunology has begun to uncover the biology of repression. (See Chapter 9, "Type C and Mind-Body Science," for a discussion of recent breakthroughs.) Researchers have shown how our bodies, and immune systems, suffer when our pains and protests cannot be expressed, shared, and thus resolved.

ORIGINS OF TYPE C: THE FAMILY

The drama is this. We came as infants "trailing clouds of glory," arriving from the farthest reaches of the universe, bringing with us appetites well preserved from our mammal inheritance, spontaneities wonderfully preserved from our 150,000 years of tree life, angers well preserved from our 5,000 years of tribal life—in short, with our 360-degree radiance—and we offered this gift to our parents. They didn't want it. They wanted a nice girl or nice boy. That's the first act of the drama.

—Robert Bly

A number of the Type C individuals I interviewed grew up in families in which expressing anger was strictly forbidden. They had parents, siblings, or caretakers who had taught them to defer their needs in favor of meeting the needs of the other family members. As children, when they cried or complained, their parents reacted with punishment, frowns, or apathy. Their Type C behaviors had clearly been shaped by their parents through positive or negative reinforcement. But there was only a handful of patients who described their

upbringings. Most were not forthcoming about their family backgrounds. I therefore could not determine whether the majority of
Type C copers had similar early experiences. But I couldn't ignore
the anecdotal evidence that the Type C pattern was laid down at an
early age and reinforced by the family.

A handful of investigators have found that cancer patients
suffered emotional traumas in early life or had disturbed family
relationships. In these studies, the subjects were asked to assess
family patterns or early events with hindsight. The data they provide are interesting but not foolproof—it's impossible to objectively
verify the truthfulness of the patients' retrospective views of themselves. There exists, however, one compelling piece of scientific
evidence that cancer patients had troubled early lives.

In 1946, researcher Caroline B. Thomas at Johns Hopkins
evaluated thirteen hundred medical students, then tracked them for
fully three decades. She was searching primarily for psychological
traits that predispose people to heart disease, and never thought she
would find a cancer connection. After thirty-two years, she
analyzed her data and came up with "striking and unexpected
findings" regarding those students who developed cancer. *They had
reported a lack of closeness to their parents in their childhoods, and
described themselves as emotionally detached or "low-gear."*

In my population of cancer patients, I found unusual patterns
of early-childhood loss, dysfunctional family dynamics, and deaths
or illnesses in the family. There were a remarkable number of recent
tragedies. Commonly, someone in the person's family had been in
a terrible accident, developed a serious illness, or suffered a personally devastating loss. The Type C person was then saddled with an
even greater caretaking burden. As with Leonard, the rabbi who
nurtured his entire family after his father died, the person shoul-
dered all the tensions besetting the family.

I noticed a variety of patterns of family interaction around the
issue of anger expression. Some patients grew up in families in
which anger was disallowed because it was considered "bad" behavior. Daniel, a young man with a melanoma on his back, said
that his parents "were very quiet people, and my sister and I went
out into the world and were shocked at how raucous other families
seemed. We never even thought about shouting at each other. It just
wasn't done."

Lawrence came from a family in which his father, an alcoholic, was given to fits of violent temper. In this fearsome atmosphere, there was no room for anyone else's frustration or anger. Lawrence was still bedeviled by memories of his father's tantrums. Later in life, he suppressed his anger "because it always reminded me of my father's destructive violence." He sensed in himself the same potential, and it frightened him. Lawrence was right to be concerned about his own violence, because it's clear that victims of physical abuse—or even child witnesses of brutality against others—are themselves susceptible to becoming rage "addicts." Later in life, they inflict the same harm on others or their own children. But Lawrence had gone to the other extreme, denying even his rational anger and crippling his capacity for self-protection.

Lawrence told me that recently he'd begun to alter his pattern. "I have learned to realize that I can be angry and it's OK. I have a job that gets me angry at least once a week. I have to get mad when the people under me just aren't doing their job, and I must let them know that it's not all right for them to slough off. It's my responsibility to take care of that, and my anger is a tool, not a weapon."

He was another patient with flexibility. Lawrence had come from a family in which the slightest hint of anger had been squelched by a tyrannical father, yet he managed to develop an assertive stance in the world.

In other families, the members shared a rationalization for the prohibition of anger. Jane, thirty-five, said that her family had to suppress their anger because of her brother's mental illness:

> I grew up with my brother's mental illness, and things went on in my family that a normal kid wouldn't have to see or deal with. There was a lot of stress around that. I felt bad because his behavior hurt my folks, and I was too young to be very helpful. I could only stand around and watch. I felt angry and frustrated about not being able to do anything. And we were always expected . . . not expected, we *had* to be very quiet. Noise was a big factor. You see, my brother would have fits of rage. You had to understand that and to suppress what you may be feeling. A lot of times, I wanted to tell him to shut up. But of course, you can't because he'd get very, very angry. He might use your little outburst as an excuse to have a fit of his own. My whole family had to keep a lid on their emotions.

Jane's family faced a difficult situation. Yet it seemed that her brother had taken the role in the family of the angry one, while everyone else had taken the role of victim. He was allowed and expected to vent his rage; they sat on theirs. Jane described a harrowing incident in which her brother senselessly attacked and beat her mother while she and her father, who was in a wheelchair, watched helplessly. She was only twelve at the time, and she was able to get away to call the police. But neither Jane nor her parents were able to react emotionally to the brother's attack—they remained paralyzed by fear. Indeed, Jane had never in her life been able to express anger toward her brother.

While telling me this story, Jane was overcome with emotion and began to cry. Her rage had finally risen to the surface. So did a sense of heartbreak over the image of her defenseless father. Her tears surprised her—and me—because it was the first time she had ever shared her feelings about the incident.

For Jane, this discrete memory had been associated with a cluster of emotions. They included her feelings at the time—fear and helplessness—and the underlying emotions that were suppressed—rage and sadness. The entire cluster had smoldered underground in her psyche until this moment. I witnessed her heartbreak and frustration burst forth as if they'd been lying in wait ever since the day ten years earlier when her brother unleashed his violence.

Throughout her childhood, Jane's family members were tyrannized and afraid to express themselves. They shared the collective fallacy that the brother's mental illness compelled them to inhibit their own feelings. I sensed Jane's confusion and knew that her family was well meaning, but they suffered from lack of proper guidance. Certainly, the answer was not for them to indiscriminately vent anger at her brother (that would be the other extreme—blaming the victim). But their cloak of silence, their inability to properly defend themselves from his rage, needed to be rectified. Family therapy, for example, might have facilitated the brother's recovery and dispelled the emotional shroud around Jane and her family. Undoubtedly, the parents' belief in the need to inhibit emotions had earlier origins, in their own upbringings.

TRAUMAS, AND TUMORS IN STRANGE PLACES

My impression was that Type C copers were conditioned to suppress negative emotions through countless, mostly forgotten early experiences. For most, unremarkable events—minor but charged interactions, incessant teachings, hidden messages—helped to form the Type C pattern. For others, the causative events were quite traumatic. These were patients who had been victimized by psychological or physical abuse that carried the message "Get angry (scared, sad) and you're in big trouble." And I was intrigued by a small number of cases in which the very location of a patient's melanoma appeared to be related to a specific past trauma.

A majority of melanomas are found on exposed portions of skin, where the sun is thought to promote these cancers. Some develop at sites where sun exposure is less likely to play a causative role (the back, legs, etc.). But I came across several patients with tumors in very strange places where melanomas rarely occur.

Marilyn, a quiet, anxious young woman, was one of them. She had come to the clinic with a melanoma on the big toe of her left foot. She told me that the most stressful time in her life had occurred several years earlier, when she had had to take care of her mother, who was gravely ill with complications from diabetes. During her protracted illness, Marilyn had played the role of caretaker as best she could. She would do anything to help and please her. But the responsibilities had taken their toll, and she became emotionally and physically depleted as her mother's illness worsened.

At one point, because of her mother's circulatory problems, gangrene had developed in the big toe of her left foot. Her doctor removed the toe, but the surgery was too late. The gangrene had already spread up through her leg, so that the entire limb eventually had to be amputated. This was especially painful for Marilyn.

Now here was Marilyn, many years later, with a malignant tumor on the same toe. "I was terrified when I found out, because I had lived with my mother and saw what she went through," she said. "I was scared I would lose my leg, too. I don't know how I could have gotten cancer in the same spot."

Like many Type C patients, Marilyn sacrificed herself ceaselessly to care for her mother. She also demonstrated a form of "sympathetic suffering"—she seemed to overidentify with her pains and symptoms. Perhaps this psychological dynamic contributed to the location of her melanoma, although there is no known biological mechanism to explain this phenomenon.

There were a handful of other such cases. Wendy, a shy, attractive young woman, had come to the clinic with a melanoma within the fold of her vagina—an extremely rare occurrence. She told me about her strict upbringing in a Catholic family. Her parents were very moralistic, and sex was a hush-hush topic. Wendy and I talked for a very long time, and I sensed her defenses lowering as she became more comfortable with me. I asked her about stressful times in her past, and with much difficulty, she revealed her most painful memory. As a young girl, Wendy had been raped by her great uncle. She hadn't told anyone, and had kept her feelings of shame and anger locked inside. Because of her background, she was afraid of being accused of encouraging her uncle and being rejected by her family.

If there was a mind-body connection between Wendy's melanoma and her childhood trauma, it would be impossible to verify scientifically. However, for most of the melanoma patients, the Type C pattern was shaped by early events that carried a painful message: *your emotions must not be expressed.* Wendy's case showed a possible linkage between Type C coping and a singular trauma: she had repressed the searing pain associated with the rape, and years later developed a tumor at the very site of her violation. If Type C behavior increases the risk of cancer by depleting one's cancer defense system, is it possible that this weakness could be localized in one area of the body—an area where psychic tension has gathered from an unresolved trauma? The answer isn't clear, but the question is a valid springboard for further investigation. The cases of tumors in strange places provided hints of the power and concreteness of the mind-body connection.

Based on my study of developments in mind-body science, it appears that a lifelong pattern of repression can cause *a generalized deficiency in the cancer defense system.* For most patients, there is no locational, mystical, or metaphorical link between their tumor and a past event. However, there may be a connection between their illness and the systematic denial of parts of their humanity. Their denial has more than psychological consequences—it has material, physical consequences. In following chapters, I will demonstrate just how material these consequences can be.

PART II

THE TYPE C
CONNECTION

CHAPTER 4

While there are many ways you can participate in your fight for recovery, you don't have the power to ensure recovery. If you believe that recovery is guaranteed if you do it right, any setback will be seen as proof of your inadequacy. But no matter what happens, you are not inadequate. What you are doing is right and proper for you. And just because there is no assurance of winning, you should not stop trying. If we refused to enter any race we weren't sure of winning, we would enter precious few races.

—Harold H. Benjamin

Awareness of one's inner healing potential provides an opportunity for sharing responsibility—not assuming all of it. These new [healing] techniques introduce the possibility of influence; they offer a golden opportunity to assist the treatment process and they provide a means of reclaiming some areas of expanded personal authority.

—Robert Chernin Cantor

There is only the fight to recover what has been lost
And found and lost again and again: and now, under
   conditions
That seem unpropitious. But perhaps neither gain nor loss.
For us, there is only the trying. The rest is not our business.

—T. S. Eliot

"Ten Percent Can Make All the Difference in the World"

One of the first things I discovered about Type C behavior was that it wasn't the sole cause of anyone's cancer. Nor was it the only reason a person succumbed to the disease. This laid to rest the oversimplified, misleading ideas bandied about in the pop-science press, such as "mental factors cause cancer," and "with the right attitude, anyone can beat cancer." My findings did not support those kinds of reductionistic conclusions, and I never found evidence for them in the medical literature. Rather, I saw that Type C behavior played absolutely no role in some people's cancers, a modest role in others', and a significant role in still others'. This explained why scientists had not found simple cause-and-effect relationships but *had* discovered strong correlations between mind states and cancer. Indeed, there is no causal connection, but rather a strong association with cancer, for many risk factors, from asbestos to dietary fat to electromagnetic fields.

In a recent interview, Ken Wilber, a leader in transpersonal psychology, clarified the mind's role in cancer with the story of a hypothetical patient. I'll call him Greg. Greg's survival, said Wilber, would be determined by many variables, including his genetic makeup and his diet. But his way of coping with the stress of cancer would also make a difference. If you broke down all the factors that would influence his recovery, psychological coping might contribute as much as 10 percent. Since Greg's doctor told him that he has a fifty-fifty chance of survival, how he copes could be a vital factor.

"In a tight election," Wilber said, "ten percent can make all the difference in the world."

Hypothetical Greg is quite similar to a vast number of real-life cancer patients. Often, a patient's odds for long-term survival are close, and any factor that weighs in his favor is worth considering. Even if the Type C pattern is a small contributor to malignant growth, it is, unlike one's genes, a factor that can be changed. One of the characteristics of healthy copers is that they can distinguish elements they can control from those they can't. This enables them to let go when it's appropriate, and seize control with passionate intensity when their efforts make a difference. Many cancer survivors know intuitively that their mind state *matters,* so they fight with everything they've got.

I like to use the image of the pie chart to visualize the many factors involved in each person's cancer risk and recovery. Each variable, such as genes, diet, and environment, is a slice of the pie. The mind-cancer researchers whose work I respect claim only that *psychological factors are one slice of the pie.* We can't say exactly what percentage of cancer risk or recovery is due to the mind, but for each person, the size will vary.

The pie analogy provides an alternative to the outmoded cause-and-effect thinking that has pervaded medical research. In our medical detective work, we're learning to apply a *systems* approach—one that searches for multiple factors that combine to cause disease. Once we adopt this view, we can readily grasp the dynamic role of the mind in malignancy. Type C behavior is not like some superpowerful virus that causes disease in every person unfortunate enough to have been invaded. Rather, it's like most other factors in illness: one piece of an intricate puzzle that makes sense only when all the pieces are properly put together.

To deal with these complexities, I embraced what is known as the *biopsychosocial* model of health and illness. Coined in the 1970s by George Engel, M.D., of the University of Rochester, this new paradigm referred to the interaction of biology, psychology, and social relationships involved in almost every disease. His idea was a radical revision of dated medical models that invoked "one cause, one cure" for every illness. Engel taught what many of us know intuitively: that our environment, our diet, our genes, our relation-ships, *and* our psychology combine, in unique blendings for each one of us, to create our state of health. Once we accept that diseases have multiple causes, we must develop therapies that address each of them. Engel's model was a framework enabling me to study the many causes of cancer and the varieties of treatment needed for a truly holistic medicine.

I conceived the Type C pattern both as a reflection of my own findings with patients and as a concise reflection of the shared characteristics found in patients in all the best studies conducted up to that time. I also developed methods for measuring and testing Type C behavior that made it possible for a rigorous scientific approach to the question *Is there a behavior pattern that really influences the growth and development of cancer?*

OUR CANCER DEFENSE SYSTEM

We have within us a remarkable anticancer network. This network is mainly comprised of immune system cells and substances, though it also involves hormones, enzymes, and certain products of the nervous system. The cancer defense system, as I will call it, operates to repair cell damage, prevents cells from becoming malignant, and detects cells that do become cancerous and liquidates them before they multiply. It can stop cancer cells from proliferating into full-blown tumors and it can slow or sometimes even halt the spread of an already existing tumor. Through these abilities, our cancer defense system acts as our own internal apparatus of cancer prevention and control.

What determines the strength of our cancer defense system? For the answer, I must return again to the biopsychosocial model. Many factors govern the readiness, sensitivity, and vigor of our immune defenses. Our genes are the first and foremost influence on immunity. Environmental agents affect immunity, and so do our dietary habits. Now research in the young field of psychoneuroim-munology teaches us that our behavior patterns and mind states also affect the immune system. We finally have scientific proof that the mind plays a part in the activity of our vital natural defenses.

How is the mind biologically linked to immunity? I will explore this mystery, and the new answers being developed in the 1990s, in

Chapter 9, "Type C and Mind-Body Science." In brief, the linkage involves brain chemicals called *neurotransmitters* and *neuropeptides.* These are literally the chemical carriers of emotion. Neurotransmitters are discharged by nerve cells, and when an emotion is aroused in us, they act on other cells throughout the brain and body, causing all sorts of physiologic changes. Neurotransmitters are the biochemical triggers of human thoughts and feelings.

The breakthrough in mind-body science came in the past decade, with the discovery that these same substances also help to regulate our immune defenses. *The chemical carriers of emotion, it turns out, are also agents of influence over our immune system.* Neurotransmitters act as messengers between the brain and the immune system, and the "messages" they carry will differ depending on how we think, feel, and act.

Our immune cells are the lead soldiers in our defense network, the ones that carry out the tasks of recognizing and destroying disease agents. Whether these soldier cells receive a "call to arms" message or a "cease and desist" message from neurotransmitters may depend, at least partially, on our state of mind. Through a complex chain of command, the nervous system—with our mind/ brain at the controls—transmits various orders to our soldier cells while they're out patrolling for dangerous interlopers, like bacteria, viruses, and cancer cells.

I concluded that our immune system was probably the main link between mind and cancer. If we could not cope effectively with the stress in our lives, then our immune defenses might get faulty, weak, or inappropriate signals from brain chemicals responsible for regulating their activity. After studying the melanoma patients at the clinic, I proceeded with a working hypothesis: the Type C coper is susceptible to a weakening of his immune defense against cancer.

COPING AND CANCER GROWTH

Melanoma is an aggressive and dangerous form of cancer. We all know that the earlier we see our doctors with a potential cancer, the better our chances for successful treatment. This could not be more true than in the case of melanoma, because patients who notice their tumor early and receive prompt treatment will probably be cured. Melanoma usually begins with a change in a mole, and if a person ignores or misses the change, the tumor has a chance to grow. Melanoma tumors will become thicker and begin to invade the lower layers of skin. With time, the danger increases that melanoma cells will enter the bloodstream or lymph system and travel throughout the body. This spreading of cancer cells, or *metastasis,* is the reason why melanoma is potentially so deadly.

Skin cancer specialists have a precise method for determining the prognosis of patients with melanoma. They surgically remove the tumor, measure its thickness, and ascertain the level to which it has invaded the skin. The thicker the tumor, the worse the prognosis.

This simple fact about melanoma supplied me with an opportunity to explore linkages between Type C behavior and the growth of cancer.

I initiated my first study in 1979, seeking an answer to the following question: did the melanoma patients who displayed Type C behavior have thicker, more aggressive tumors? If Type C patients had thicker tumors, then they also had less chance of complete recovery.

My colleagues and I selected fifty-nine patients from the UCSF Melanoma Clinic. The codirectors, Drs. Sagebiel and Blois, provided us with numbers indicating each patient's tumor thickness and level of invasion. We did not look at this data, however, until all of our interviews were completed. Within a month of their biopsies, we met with all our subjects. In an hour-long interview, we asked them a comprehensive set of questions about their emotional and behavioral responses to having cancer. How did they feel when they first noticed the tumor? When they were first told they had cancer? What were they doing to cope? How were they feeling, reacting, and acting? We also probed them for information about the stress in their lives, past and present. How had they handled severe stress? We asked them to recall the angriest, saddest, and most fearful times they could ever remember. What did they do when they were angry, sad, or anxious? I also gave them a series of standard psychological tests revealing moods and emotional states, and one questionnaire I developed to determine character style.

We videotaped all the interviews. Then we analyzed the tapes and gave our subjects a score in each of a long list of coping categories. Was the patient a denier? An optimist? A fighter? A person who put his faith in God or the doctors? An emotional expressor? An anxious Type A coper? A passive Type C coper? My methods would provide the answers.

TYPE C AND CANCER SEVERITY

I tallied the results of our research, looking for connections between psychological factors and the severity of each patient's cancer. Among the many psychological factors evaluated, four were significantly correlated with tumor growth:

1) **Nonverbal Type C behavior:** We had a special category for patients who were judged more "Type C" by their nonverbal behavior, including facial expressions and gestures. As a group, *these Type C copers had thicker tumors than the rest of the patient population.*

2) **Faith:** These were patients who said they coped with cancer by "placing my faith in God" or "placing my faith in the doctors." For purposes of brevity, I called this category "faith." *Patients who exhibited this kind of faith had thicker tumors.*

3) **Histrionic character style*:** These were patients who responded to stress in a histrionic manner, acting out their feelings in an overt, dramatic manner. As a group, the people with a histrionic style had *thinner, less dangerous tumors.*

4) **Narcissistic character style*:** This group exhibited narcissistic tendencies. They were self-centered and self-seeking in their behavior patterns. As a group, patients with a narcissistic style had *thinner, less dangerous tumors.*

As I conceived them, Nonverbal Type C and Faith represented essential facets of Type C behavior. Patients who exhibited these coping styles had thicker tumors, *thus confirming my hypothesis that Type C behavior would be associated with more advanced cancer and a worse prognosis.*

Patients who scored high in Faith said that their fate was in the hands of a higher authority, be it God, the doctor, or some other

*As determined by my questionnaire, the "Character Style Inventory."

entity. I realize that faith can mean something quite different, but here, the term was used strictly for people who felt that their destiny depended upon a person or force outside themselves. These patients were passive in the face of illness—a central feature of the Type C behavior pattern. I later called this quality "passive faith."

Both the Histrionic and Narcissistic character styles represented the exact *opposites* of Type C behavior. The Type C individual never acts out his anxiety or divulges his depression the way a histrionic person would. The Type C person is self-sacrificing, not self-centered. The histrionic and narcissistic patients had less dangerous tumors.

A few nonpsychological factors were also associated with tumor thickness. It was no surprise that patients who delayed seeking medical treatment for their lesions ended up with thicker tumors, since their cancers had time to grow before being removed by a doctor. My colleagues and I conducted an analysis of our data and found that, by and large, the Type C patients were not the same people who delayed seeking treatment. Therefore, patient delay was *not* the real, underlying reason for the Type C connection with tumor growth. Indeed, I found no other medical, behavioral, or demographic factor that either explained or eradicated the relationship between Type C behavior and tumor thickness.

TYPE C AND THE YOUTHFUL MIND

I found that the Type C connection was much stronger among younger patients. I split our population into two groups—those under fifty-five and those over fifty-five—and discovered a powerful relationship between Type C behavior and thick tumors in the under fifty-five group. The correlation was quite weak among the older patients.

Why was the Type C connection stronger in the under-fifty-five group? I've discussed this issue with Bernard H. Fox, Ph.D., a foremost expert on mind-cancer research with whom I have collaborated on several papers. He has found this same pattern in many other published studies on cancer and the mind. By way of explanation, Fox points out that parts of our immune system deteriorate with age—hence, in our later years our cancer defenses may lose their vigor. The elderly are also more vulnerable to the effects of carcinogens because of the long lag time between exposure and the development of cancer. Hence, contact with carcinogens that occurred in our youth or midlife may finally take their toll in our later years. (This may hold true for the skin cancer–causing effects of too much sun exposure.) When we're young, our cancer defenses ought to be intact, and we've had less long-term exposure to carcinogens. Therefore, Dr. Fox presumes—and I agree—that other risk factors play a greater role in our thirties, forties, and fifties. Among these other factors is Type C behavior.

This was an important insight. My study strongly affirmed the mind's role in cancer progression among relatively younger patients. (This doesn't include children and adolescents, in whom genetic and environmental factors seem predominant.) As Dr. Fox has emphasized, it's easy to understand why the elderly are more susceptible to cancer. It's much harder to understand why a middle-aged person succumbs—even if he or she has been exposed to environmental carcinogens. Many smokers escape tobacco-related disease until they reach old age. Why do some develop lung cancer in their forties? Why does one woman who has sunbathed since childhood get melanoma at fifty, while another woman with the same sun exposure gets it at eighty? What about the young woman with no family history of breast cancer who still contracts the disease? Finally, why does a middle-aged person *with no apparent risk factors* get cancer at all? We in medical science have never known the answer, though we do know that it happens all the time.

I had discovered that Type C behavior—and its psychological underpinnings—could play a *considerable* role in the progression of cancer in people in their third, fourth, and fifth decades of life.

THE UNSPOKEN LANGUAGE OF REPRESSION

Charles Darwin once wrote, "The movements of expression give vividness and energy to our spoken words. They reveal our thoughts and intentions to others more truly than do words, which may be falsified."

I believe that Darwin's insight explains why I found a strong relationship between advanced cancer and *nonverbal* Type C behavior.

On the one hand, I could intuitively grasp, plainly see, and well understand my subjects' behavior patterns. But I could not so easily capture them in the butterfly net of scientific measurement. Type C, it turns out, is a very slippery behavior to quantify. I couldn't ask the patients direct questions such as "Do you tend to hide your feelings from others?" and "Do you often behave nicely when you're really seething underneath?" I'd already figured out that Type C's hide their feelings unknowingly. Often, they have no idea what they're feeling underneath.

What I learned was that Type C behavior could be scientifically measured through probing one-on-one interviews. The interviews were designed to bring out the *context* of each person's behavior, the big picture that illuminated their real motivations, coping mechanisms, and veiled emotions. Jake, a fifty-year-old melanoma patient whom I interviewed, said that he wasn't frightened when he found himself in the midst of a raging forest fire. He wasn't upset when his doctors told him he had a life-threatening tumor. He wasn't angry when his son took his car without asking and got into an accident. Holding back one's feelings can be adaptive or it can be dysfunctional. Which it is depends upon the circumstances and the person's typical response pattern. Does he or she *always* hold back anger, or only in certain situations? The former is telltale of Type C; the latter is quite normal. Jake's typical response—regardless of the situation and despite intensely stressful triggers in his environment—was passive and emotionless.

But the interviews brought out much more than context. They also revealed the entire, rich dimension of body language. Dr. Ray Rosenman had already established that Type A people could be detected by their tense facial expressions, their aggressive hand movements, and their rapid and explosive speech patterns. I realized that a body language approach would be especially useful for Type C's, since by definition Type C involves the concealment of thoughts and emotions. Decades of experimental research has shown that the human face and body are like maps of the soul, areas where detectable traces can be found of hidden thoughts, feelings, and personality traits.

Martin, whom I introduced to you in "A Portrait of Type C Behavior," exemplified how nonverbal responses reveal more than words. Martin told me he wasn't angry or fearful about the spread of his cancer to his lymph nodes. But he smiled awkwardly when I asked if his recurrence frightened him. He squinted with bewilderment when I asked if he was angry. He laughed nervously at the mention of death. He literally shrugged his shoulders when I asked if he was concerned about his future. Everything was "fine," he said again and again.

Martin's nonverbal behavior told me that everything was not "fine." His anxiety was there, his sadness was there. But I could discern these cloaked feelings only by inference and, more concretely, by the physical expressions of discomfort that betrayed his words of stoic acceptance. Because we videotaped Martin's interview, my colleagues and I were able to review his body language with care and precision.

My main collaborator in this phase of research was Bruce Heller, Ph.D., then an intern in clinical psychology at the Langley Porter Psychiatric Institute. Heller had worked with Paul Ekman, Ph.D., director of the Human Interaction Laboratory at UCSF. Ekman is recognized as the world's leading expert on how human emotions are expressed on the face. He has refined the scientific reading of facial expressions, and he has trained psychologists to be able to tell whether subjects are telling the truth, deceiving others, or deceiving themselves.

Heller brought his expertise in face reading to our Type C research. In studying the videotapes, he noticed that Type C patients revealed hidden emotions in momentary flashes of facial expression. He used what Ekman calls "microfacial analysis" to pinpoint the precise configuration of facial muscles that—literally in the blink of an eye—told the truth about a patient's inner state.

Heller was particularly struck by Carolyn, an impoverished middle-aged woman from a rural area of California. Carolyn had never married, but had instead devoted her entire life to taking care of her large family. She first realized that something was wrong when a large scab on her upper arm kept bleeding profusely. She laughed about this during her interview. "I was bleeding all over the family's towels," she said. Her biggest worry was that she would have to wash them more often.

Heller asked Carolyn how she felt when first told by her doctor that it was cancer. She laughed again and replied, "Oh, fine, it really wasn't any bother to me. I just hoped they wouldn't be upset about it."

Heller wondered how Carolyn could so blithely dismiss the

reality of cancer. In search of some clues to her inner state, he reviewed her videotaped reaction in super-slow motion. What he saw startled him: right after her laugh—for a fraction of a second—her mouth stretched downward and dragged all the muscles of her face into a look of horror. Carolyn's expression was striking and undeniable—a fleeting revelation of feeling rising up onto her face but not into her consciousness.

Carolyn's momentary expression, and similar instances with other patients, provided more evidence that Type C people registered emotions—but below the level of awareness. They weren't purposely deceiving others; they were simply unconscious of the negative feelings they had repressed for years.

Microfacial analysis was only one tool we used for picking up Type C behavior. Heller and I found that Type C's had a body language that matched their behavioral qualities. In a given Type C patient, I could often detect his compliance, passivity, and nonexpression just by reading his face. Martin's facial movements were constricted. He spoke slowly, deliberately, and monotonously, as if each word and sentence had to be approved by some internal censor before being uttered. His energy level was "flat"—there were no highs, no lows. I soon discovered that Martin's body language resembled that of other Type C patients. As you might expect, Type A researchers have observed an opposite pattern in their subjects. Type A's functioned at a sky-high energy level, spoke in rushing bursts of words, and displayed facial expressions rife with anxiety.

Bruce Heller and I evaluated each patient's video by looking at body language to determine if he was more Type C, Type A, or somewhere in between—a balanced Type B. Using this method, we'd spot whether a patient was relatively passive (Type C) or active (Type A). Lethargic or hurried. Emotionally constricted or emotionally changeable. Bland or intense. Appeasing or hostile. Patient or impatient. Sad or angry. Smooth or jerky. Withdrawn or extended. Given up or struggling. Accepting or controlling. These were but a few of the Type C/Type A contrasts we observed and rated.

When my results showed that the nonverbal Type C's generally had thicker tumors, I was not surprised. For the methods I've just described revealed their behavior patterns more truly than did words, which, as Darwin pointed out, "may be falsified." These patients were not liars, but they were hiding from themselves. Their "movements of expression" told me more about their hidden selves than they would have been able to articulate.

MITCH'S FACE TELLS HIS STORY

Mitch, a forty-five-year-old auto worker, was one of the melanoma patients who displayed nonverbal Type C behavior. I asked him how he felt about his recent diagnosis. His first words to me were "I have no feeling at all. I just wonder what's happening."

At first, Mitch seemed almost jolly, with his portly presence and nonstop smile. As we began talking, I found him to be quite withdrawn. He was quiet, gentle, self-effacing, and he struggled to answer many of my questions. His wife was present, and she frequently responded to questions I put to him. As if by habit, Mitch turned to her when he was stumped by one of my more personal inquiries. Mitch relied on his wife to give words to his unformed thoughts. She also participated in his attempt to deny any discomfort about his illness. Their dependence on each other was all the more striking because they had no children, little extended family, and few close friends. They had no desire to tell anyone about Mitch's cancer—they would deal with it by themselves.

Two words spring to mind in trying to capture Mitch's qualities, as evidenced by his words, speech, face, and body. They are *constricted* and *selfless*.

Mitch's emotional expression was severely constricted. Most of our discussion was about charged topics—coping with cancer, mortality, the most stressful experiences in his life, etc. Throughout, Mitch kept smiling. I saw how forced the smile was—he spoke through his teeth, his words barely audible, and had little expression in his eyes. In his research, Paul Ekman has shown that a smile is genuine when the expression around our eyes changes naturally as the mouth curls upward. When the expression around our eyes is fixed, the smile is not genuine but strictly for the sake of social harmony. Mitch's smile remained plastered in place whether I asked him about his favorite hobbies or his prospects for survival.

Mitch told me that he wasn't upset about his cancer. He said he needed no special support. When I asked, "What would the part of your body with melanoma say if it could speak?" he replied, "Play it cool. Don't get excited. Sit back and see what happens."

When I reviewed Mitch's interview on tape, I noticed the momentary flashes of unconscious feeling that Bruce Heller had observed in many Type C patients. Mitch's facial mask was firmly set, as evidenced by his forced smile, his closed-mouth style of speech, the minimal movement of his head, and the squinty defensiveness in his eyes. When asked a disturbing question, Mitch's smile would broaden and he'd chuckle nervously. An instant later, his head would turn downward and he'd lose eye contact with me. When this happened, his social mask fell—for as long as a breath—and a forlorn expression showed itself; then he'd murmur a comment that revealed a sense of helplessness. Mitch said that the most depressing experience he could remember was his convalescence from a life-threatening bout of hepatitis. I asked about his thoughts at the time. "You wonder what's going to happen." He laughed. Then his face dropped and a fleeting sadness took over. His squinty look melted and his eyes showed fear. "Who knows if you'll be around tomorrow," he whispered. He chuckled again and quickly reconstituted his mask. This sequence repeated itself ten times in the hour and a half we spent together.

Mitch's words were generally optimistic. He believed he was going to be fine. But the truth I saw on tape was more complex, more layered. Mitch was pretending—for me, his wife, and himself—that everything was OK. But those breaks in his facade told me that Mitch was scared. What's more, he felt powerless to do more than "play it cool," "sit tight," and "wonder what's happening."

While we tend to associate selflessness with benevolence, Mitch's selflessness had more to do with reticence, denial of his own needs, and self-doubt. Perhaps the most striking sign of Mitch's selflessness was the fact that, in our lengthy interview, he almost never used the word *I*. He constantly referred to himself in the second person—"You just don't have enough energy." Often, he used no pronoun at all, as when I asked him if he'd ever seen a psychologist. "Not really. Worked with someone, took several classes," he said. "Saw a counselor. More a job-training type of thing. Sort of like this interview, not quite."

I went over Mitch's tape and found only one instance in which he used *I* repeatedly. I'd asked him what he said or did when he was depressed during his recuperation from hepatitis. "I don't know if I said much. I never do," he replied, laughing. Then his expression became forlorn again. "I never say much," he muttered. It was a rare moment of self-recognition, which, I believe, is why he finally resorted to using *I*. Throughout the rest of our session, Mitch was hiding himself and never used *I*.

Mitch's body language enabled me to rate him as a nonverbal Type C coper. And, like most of the Type C patients, Mitch's tumor was quite thick—considered a high risk for fatality. The Type C connection could not have been clearer than in the case of Mitch. I must stress, however, that every Type C person is unique and has a history of stressful life events that shaped his behavior. What made Mitch so selfless and constricted? Why, and how, had he developed such a stiff armor against unpleasant feelings? I wasn't able to find out. Mitch didn't reveal much about his family or his past. But there was one clue. It came in response to my question about anger. He answered by telling me a cryptic tale of a war experience. Mitch remained emotionally detached while describing this incident:

> During the Korean War, you lost a couple of good friends. So you're gonna get even. That was what you did. In those days, you would get it over with and get on. If you survive, fine. If you don't, I guess that was fine, too. You work with people for quite some time, you become good buddies, and you see them get wiped out. You're not angry at one particular person. You can't see who did that. You're angry at a whole group of people. At a time like that, your training takes over. You plan everything down to the *nth* degree because you know the same thing can happen to you. When that particular phase takes over, you begin to lose your real anger and you become like a machine. You don't have any thoughts except what you have to do. All you knew was a getting-even type of thing. You didn't lose control, because you knew you couldn't.

I tried unsuccessfully to elicit more details from Mitch about what happened when his friends were killed, or the actions he took in the aftermath of their death. But the contours of his story are those of trauma and the repression necessary to sublimate grief and rage into controlled action—action that probably produced even more trauma. All this suggests that Mitch's war experience helped to shape his Type C defense against strong emotions. It was a stoic defense that helped him survive the war and function later in life. Nevertheless, the roots of the Type C pattern invariably lie in childhood. I would never learn about that part of the origins of Mitch's behavior.

PASSIVE FAITH VS. ACTIVE FAITH

In order to find one's place in the infinity of being,
one must be able to both separate and unite.
—from the *I Ching*

I asked Mitch how he was coping with cancer. "I don't know," he replied. "I guess I have to put my faith in whatever the medical profession attempts to do to solve my problem—if it can be solved." Mitch's voice trailed off, revealing his sense of quiet futility. Later he came right out and said, "There's not much I can do about my cancer."

Mitch actually lacked faith in *his own power* to affect his recovery. His faith in the doctors was, more accurately, a belief that a group of faceless professionals would see him through the experience with their medical magic. The healing process was their business, not his. Mitch felt that they were the "experts" and he had no important role to play—except to wait and hope.

Both words—*faith* and *hope*—have an active and a passive definition. Active faith implies a strong bond between self and other: *I believe that I can do it, with the doctor's (God's) help.* Passive faith involves no such bond: *I just have to put my fate in the doctor's (God's) hands.* In this worldview, the power to heal belongs to an outside entity, and the individual is powerless. One is acted upon, one doesn't act in concert with an external power. Likewise, hope can be grounded in conviction and self-esteem or it can be based on relinquishing the self, as in *All I can do is pray.* When a cancer patient says that to me, there's usually an accompanying gesture. Whether it's a shrug of the shoulders, upturned palms, or raised eyebrows, the underlying message is always the same: "there's nothing *I* can do." While I see this passivity as a problem, I don't believe that prayer is by its nature passive. The power of prayer may be realized when the person feels that she is still the agent of her own healing.

My finding that Type C patients with passive faith had thicker tumors led me to consider the role of faith in recovery from physical illness. I believe the distinction between active and passive faith is crucial to mind-body health.

Active faith is rooted in a spirituality that embraces the oneness of self and external power, whatever form that power takes for the individual. This form of faith has its roots in both the great Asian spiritual disciplines as well as in Judeo-Christian traditions. Passive faith represents not only an abdication of self but of responsibility and power. It is the faith of powerlessness. Studies have shown that when we lose our sense of power in the face of stress, our immune systems are diminished.

Adherents of twelve-step programs for the treatment of addiction preach that surrender to a higher power is a healing stance. But they also attest to the unity of self and higher power, and to the need for the individual to take responsibility for his own recovery.

Gail Sheehy, in her book *Pathfinders,* drew this distinction: "Those who surrender unconditionally to God may be directed by the most spiritual sort of passion. . . . But there is another kind of surrender of will that is not associated with passion, or with pathfinding. That is when a person feels too tired, weak, or frightened to struggle any longer with the hard questions."

A person with active faith accepts herself, her responsibility for her wellness, and her power to get well. She experiences herself and her higher power as indivisible. Perhaps she can't articulate it, but she views self-realization as the highest expression of spirituality.

I interviewed several melanoma patients who were priests. One of them, Paul, had what I call active faith. Paul had always been a people-pleaser, loathe to reveal weakness or discontent in his relationships. But cancer had shaken him up, and he told me about his fear of death, and his anger with church members who "were acting as if I was going to die." Paul had great flexibility and insight into his feelings. He was familiar with transactional analysis, which posits the existence of both an inner child and adult. After his diagnosis, Paul said, "My [inner] child was frightened. Not in touch with reality. My adult was reasonable and rational but hadn't acknowledged the seriousness of the situation."

Paul drew on his faith but he was convinced that how he confronted cancer—what he thought, felt, and did about it—was critical.

LT: How did you react when you found out it was melanoma?
Paul: I knew that the worst was still ahead of me, and I was going to face it come hell or high water. After I got the biopsy results, I was alarmed. But now I'm ready to fight. I think I can whip it.
LT: What are you doing now to cope?
Paul: I pray. I believe in God. I believe in life after death. Naturally, I've been frightened. But I have a strong element of hope. I don't want to die right now. I'm using all my resources and faith and knowledge.

I have found that the most effective healing is that which embraces the natural back-and-forth shifting between surrender and control, between letting go and taking charge. You seek a spiritual union with an external force—often through surrender—as a way to nourish yourself, to strengthen yourself for the fight ahead. It doesn't matter whether that external force is a higher power, a doctor, a healer, a lover, a shrine, or a pet hamster. (If it's a doctor, that union can take the form of a "healing partnership," to coin a phrase from surgeon Bernie Siegel.) You let go to that force in order to be replenished, then take charge on the field of battle. In this ideal scenario, you don't see yourself as a passive recipient of healing powers. You see yourself as an active participant in your own recovery, with the help of someone—or something—in which you deeply believe.

THE MIND'S ROLE IN DISEASE PROGRESSION

The research I've described in this chapter illuminates the mind's role in the progression of an already-existing tumor. I wasn't the only one to make this discovery, and several investigators have since confirmed my findings.

In 1985, Mogens R. Jensen, Ph.D., then at Yale University, followed fifty-two women with breast cancer, in search of factors that influenced the spread of the disease. After two years, Jensen came upon a cluster of psychological traits in the women whose cancers had spread. The cluster included a repressive personality style, inability to express negative emotions, helplessness-hopelessness, chronic stress, and comforting daydreaming. (Jensen interpreted the daydreaming as an escape valve for people in denial about the seriousness of their condition.) These psychological factors played a significant role in disease progression, above and beyond the medical factors that doctors rely on to predict a patient's outcome.

Dr. Jensen's research provides more support for the Type C concept. Since Type C behavior is associated with disease progression, reversing the pattern offers cancer patients a chance to improve their outlook. (See Chapters 11, 12, and 13.) Changing Type C behavior may be the hypothetical 10 percent that makes "all the difference in the world." For some, it may be 50 percent; for others, only 2 percent. But for patients who find themselves in a "tight election," all swing votes are welcome.

It's important to recognize, however, that none of us is omnipotent. In the fight against cancer, we have to embrace not only our strengths but also our limitations. We can't wish or will cancer away—none of us is that powerful. But we do have a degree of leverage over cancer via the mind. The benefits of grasping that margin of psychological control are many, even for those who don't overcome their disease. Changing Type C behavior means self-renewal, emotional expression, and taking a stand on your own behalf. It entails meeting your own needs and learning how to ask others for support. Regardless of one's life span, these changes represent a form of psychological enlightenment that is inherently valuable. For those of you who are cancer patients, as long as you embark on a path of transformation *with hope but without illusions,* you won't blame yourself if your illness does not vanish forever. You'll never regret having taken the path of change.

CHAPTER 5

Express Yourself Completely
then keep quiet
Be like the forces of nature
when it blows, there is only wind;
when it rains, there is only rain;
when the clouds pass, the sun shines through.

> —*Tao-te-ching,* Lao-tzu

One cannot fight for health when one is split off from
one's feelings. The despair that underlies many cancer
cases erodes a person's energy unless it is brought to the
surface and expressed.

> —*Alexander Lowen*

He who does not perceive emotional expression as
renunciation, that is, who affirms and does not fear it,
will not need to use either a physical or a psychic illness
to drain off his emotional life. The utilization of the rich
scale of emotions of the human psychic life, with its
capacity for feeling pleasures and pain in small doses, is
the best guarantee for remaining well and happy.

> —*Otto Rank*

Emotions and the Mind-Body Bridge

Max's face, like an open book, spoke volumes about what he'd been through since his doctor told him he had cancer. As he recounted his recent experiences, his expression showed shock, surprise, dread, heartache, contemplation, hope, and even full-fledged optimism.

When he first found out it was melanoma, he felt horrible. "It was like being hit by a truck," he said. But he read about melanoma, talked out all his concerns with his doctor, told friends, expressed his fears to his wife, and soon, the shock wore off. He described how he was coping:

> The main thing is to talk about it. To surface the feelings so that they don't get lost. When I feel paranoid, to talk about the fear, to cry, to laugh, to get the feelings out as much as possible. And I try to relax. I don't want to bury myself in my work just to forget about it. I try to grasp opportunities to sit down, calm myself, and release some of the tension.

Max brought his wife, Andrea, along for his interview with me. Her mother had died of melanoma. That was one of the reasons it had been so hard for them. Max and Andrea told me how they shared everything with each other and with their friends. They didn't do this to advertise their problems, they said. They did it because it made them feel better.

"I like the attention I get because of this situation," Max said. "I know that sounds strange. And I feel funny about it. But I can't deny that I enjoy the concern. It makes me feel warm. I feel gratitude for the friendships."

Now, weeks since his diagnosis, Max was still scared. But he wasn't depressed. He had great energy. He was buoyed by the tremendous love and support from his wife, friends, and family. I had an image of Max floating on that love and support, as if he were bobbing along on a life raft on dangerous seas. Max knew that the life raft would carry him to calmer waters. "I'm feeling very positive now. Even though there's a chance this will recur, I believe I'm going to live a full life."

After Max and his wife left the interview room, another melanoma patient named William entered. Here's how our conversation began:

LT: How did you react when your doctor told you you had melanoma?
William: It didn't shake me up. It really didn't faze me. Why should I sit here and worry? I'm not going to let it ruin my life. Really, it's no worse than having a wart cut off.
LT: Is there anything that makes you nervous about melanoma?
William: The only thing I'm worried about is doctor bills.
LT: Nothing else?
William: I get tired of people talking about it. Like my family. Why should they worry when I'm not worried?
LT: Did your doctor say anything to you about your chances?
William: No. I don't think I have anything, really. I don't think there's any cancer. I don't think anything is spreading. I'm not worried about it.
LT: How are you coping with this situation?
William: I don't think about it. Praying doesn't hurt.
LT: Do you pray?
William: A little. Mainly, I keep busy.

Max and William were the same age, thirty-four, but they could not have been more different. Max *had* to express his anguished feelings to others. William denied feeling distress over his illness and denied the need for communication. Max had a wide circle of friends and family. William was single, lived with his mother, and had few friends. Max was profoundly concerned about the impact melanoma might have on his health, his family, and his life span. William said that melanoma had no impact on his life, other than unwanted bills. Max was optimistic about his recovery. William had so thoroughly denied the import of his illness that the question of his optimism, or pessimism, was moot.

Max's way and William's way are just two different means of coping. Each of these men was dealing with cancer the best way he knew how. But Max's capacity to let his feelings surface, and the social support he procured, gave him hope and energy. Although William said he was unaffected, he seemed uncomfortable and quietly anxious. William's nonexpression prevented him from facing his illness and getting support. It short-circuited his ability to develop true optimism.

I knew that Max's emotional expression represented a healthy psychological adaptation to a terribly stressful life event. But did Max's coping style give him a better chance for full *biological* recovery? On the other hand, did William's Type C style dampen his *biological* cancer-fighting ability? These were the questions with which I was confronted.

THE TOXIC CORE OF TYPE C

For twenty years, Type A researchers searched for one core factor that explained the relationship between Type A behavior and coronary risk. Recently, leading investigators claim to have discovered that core factor. They've found that *hostility* is the one variable strongly correlated with heart disease and death from heart attacks. While other Type A traits such as impatience or competitiveness often coexist with hostility, they are not the crux of the matter.

After my first study, I began to suspect that there was a core factor in Type C behavior—*nonexpression of emotions.* I found most of the Type C melanoma patients to be pleasant, passive, and self-sacrificing. But I found *all* of them to be nonexpressive.

Redford Williams, M.D., a leading Type A researcher, has referred to hostility as the "toxic" core of Type A behavior, the element that quite literally damages the heart. I saw nonexpression as the toxic core of Type C, the element that quite literally damages the immune system.

To test my theory, I studied a new group of fifty-eight melanoma patients. I conducted the same tests and interviews as before, but this time I went to the heart of the issue of emotional expression. I used new strategies to discover the extent to which each patient expressed his or her feelings—especially the negative ones.

In looking for signs of emotional expression, I never expected the patients I interviewed to erupt into sobs or throw a tantrum. I asked myself, What is the norm of expression? I consulted prior research on this issue, and relied on my clinical experience as a psychologist to make determinations in each individual case. I also recruited psychologist Neil A. Fiore, Ph.D., an expert on cancer and coping, to use his own rating system to validate my judgments of each person. Ultimately, I considered a person expressive when he communicated his feelings in a simple and straightforward manner, accented by subtle facial changes or gestures. That was sufficient.

THE LOST VOICE

In order to be accurate and specific in my reading of a patient's expressiveness, I had to break down his emotional responses into three dimensions: bodily sensations, thoughts, and actions. I would ask each patient to recount an event that evoked a particular feeling, including sadness, fear, anger, and happiness. Then I'd find out what he felt physically at the time, what he thought, and what actions he took based on this feeling. The results were like an X ray of the person's psychological structure for processing emotion.

Alice was among the first melanoma patients upon whom I conducted this "X ray." She was sixty years old and had a lovely disposition and quiet sense of dignity. But I got the impression that she was lonely and afraid. She had recently lost her husband of forty years and soon after was diagnosed with melanoma. She told me she coped by keeping busy with housework. She made no mention of seeking the support of friends and family. Here is the part of our conversation that dealt directly with emotional expression:

LT: Tell me the time you were most angry.

Alice: [Long pause.] Gee, I really can't. I can't really describe any particular time when I was most angry.

LT: Can you recall a time when you were just angry?

Alice: I guess when a person is younger, you probably take everyday things a little more seriously. Then you get older and some of those things don't bother you as much. I don't know if you grow callous as you get older, or what. But I know that there used to be things that irritated or upset me, and now I wouldn't take them seriously. Why make yourself unhappy over something that really isn't that important? I guess I do get irritated a little, sometimes.

LT: Can you think of a time when you were irritated?

Alice: I suppose when my son stays out late, I get worried about him.

LT: Tell me a little more about that.

Alice: Well, one time I told him to be home at midnight and he didn't get back till after 1 A.M. I was getting a little concerned about him so I got into the car and tried to find him. Then I saw him walking down the street with one of his girl-friends.

LT: When you were irritated with him, can you recall any bodily sensations?

Alice: No, I really don't. A little tense, maybe. I was tense because he wasn't home when he was supposed to be home.

LT: What were your thoughts at the time?

Alice: I knew he had a rowdy friend, kind of a bad seed. I thought he might have been seeing him, and that this kid had influenced him to stay out drinking and cavorting. That turned out wrong—he was with his girlfriend.

LT: What did you say or do when you finally saw him?

Alice: I told him, you were supposed to have been home at a certain time and you weren't. I said, I might not let you use the car next weekend.

LT: Can you tell me a time when you were the most happy?

Alice: I've had a few of those. Graduating from school, getting married, having children. With your first, you anticipate a great deal because you don't know what to expect. But you're always very anxious about your first pregnancy.

LT: When you were carrying your first child, and feeling that happiness and anticipation, can you recall any physical sensations?

Alice: I don't know about physical sensations. I did keep getting bigger. [Laughs.] I was happy to be having a child. I think any woman kind of looks forward to having children. At least one, anyway. I worked most of the time while I was pregnant. They used to kid me at the office where I worked—you're getting so big you won't be able to get out from behind your desk.

LT: What were your thoughts during the time you were happily expecting?

Alice: I was thinking of having the child and hoping it was a healthy and normal child.

Alice couldn't think of an incident in which she felt anger, so we settled on "irritated." But she was unable to clearly describe her physical and emotional experience of irritation. She was "worried," "a little concerned," and "a little tense, maybe." I had no sense that she was truly aggravated by her son's behavior. Alice's facial expression showed that she didn't have an emotional grasp of the moments she was describing. Her face did not change configuration, and the usual signs of anger—a slight widening of the eyes, a subtle tightening of the muscles of the jaw and mouth—were not there. In fact, when she talked of her son's transgression, she seemed bemused, not annoyed.

When I asked Alice about a happy time, she spoke of the birth of her children with few signs of excitement. I'm sure that Alice was happy about the birth of her first child, but her joy did not come across in words or expressions. The entire time she spoke about giving birth, her face actually showed *worry*. I found it interesting that Alice said "you're always very anxious about your first pregnancy" after I had asked her to report a happy feeling.

Alice had a hard time articulating emotional thoughts and sensations, and a hard time distinguishing one emotion from another. These facts enabled me to assign her to the category "nonexpressor." Although I don't like categories, the regimen of scientific method compels me to put people in them. Otherwise, I wouldn't be able to find out if people like Alice suffer physically from the long-term effects of their behavior patterns. Alice, and the patients like her, never *chose* to be nonexpressors. They stopped expressing emotions at an early age in order to foster security in their social environment. Of course, there is a price exacted for this trade-off. Somewhere along the way, Alice had lost her emotional voice.

Other patients seemed to have blotted out emotional memories altogether. Jennie, a thirty-five-year-old patient, told me that her recent divorce was the most stressful time in her life. Here is part of our conversation:

LT: Can you tell me the time you remember feeling the most angry?

Jennie: Probably not. That was one of my problems—I never expressed anger. I guess when I was breaking up with my husband, I probably expressed anger for the first time in my life. It wasn't as great as it should have been—it wasn't very great anger. It wasn't as though I had bottled it up for forty years and all of a sudden it came out. It was very minor at the time.

LT: Do you remember . . .

Jennie: I can't remember any specific time, but I'll try. I hardly remember what it was all about.

LT: Do you recall any physical sensations at the time you were angry?

Jennie: No.

LT: Do you remember your thoughts at the time?

Jennie: No. I don't even remember the event, really.

LT: Did you take any actions, do anything in particular?

Jennie: I really couldn't say.

Jennie couldn't recall her angry feelings *even though the breakup of her marriage occurred less than one year before.*

Jennie's blocked memory had nothing to do with mental aptitude—I found her to be very intelligent. She worked as a consultant for an advertising firm and had recently started a new relationship. Jennie couldn't remember what happened because she had sidestepped the emotional issues involved in the breakup of her marriage.

At first, I was surprised that Jennie admitted harboring anger—earlier in the interview, she denied feeling mad at her ex-husband at the time of the divorce. Like many Type C people,

Jennie had psychological defenses that could peel off like the layers of an onion. After relaxing with me, she changed her view—yes, she *had* been angry with him. Jennie had enough flexibility to acknowledge that anger to him and to me. But she still couldn't remember her sensations, thoughts, or actions. I am certain that, with more time and trust and focus—as in psychotherapy—Jennie could recover these memories. Any person who can admit, as Jennie did, that nonexpression is a "problem," can regain the capacity to recognize and express feelings.

At the time of our interview, though, Jennie was a nonexpressor. I saw in her frozen smile an intense desire to please others and keep up a likable front. Her gestures and words made it clear that Jennie was still struggling to give voice to her needs and her frustration.

EXPRESSORS: THE EXCEPTIONS

I asked David, a twenty-nine-year-old career counselor, how he reacted after his doctor told him he had melanoma. Here is his response:

> I was shocked, wiped out, and utterly scared. When I first saw my wife that night, I cried. I was frightened—and mad. So many family members had gotten cancer. None of them had melanoma, but they had other cancers—intestinal, lymph node cancers. Two uncles, and two of my grandparents. It wasn't fair to me or to the whole family. I felt violated by this cancer. I really hate it. My wife and I went up to our bedroom and just laid down together. We both cried. I held her. The closeness is what I needed—sympathy, I guess. To have someone really there. I stayed up the rest of that evening. I got most of the emotion out that night. The next day was hard. I couldn't talk to people about it for a few days. But the following weekend, my parents came up for a visit and I told them. I felt better once I could talk to them about it. Since then, I have been able to tell others, and I don't feel quite as bad. One good thing has come out of all this. What really touched me was the concern and compassion from my close friends. That

has reassured and reaffirmed what I may have taken for granted.

David, like Max, was exceptional. Few of the melanoma patients were able to admit and express *any* negative feelings in the aftermath of their diagnoses of cancer. David, on the other hand, ran the gamut from anger to sadness to fear. His words alone explain better than I ever could the value of emotional expression. Because David was able to feel his distress, he also experienced the need for loving support. Type C patients who can't feel their distress don't think they need help. If nothing is wrong, why seek support? David accepted the reality of his illness, felt the negative feelings, and *therefore was compelled to get his needs met.* He needed that closeness with his wife. Then, in a few days, he was able to tell the important people in his life, and felt better for having done so. If David had never confided in them, he would have never reaped the rewards: "the concern and compassion from my close friends."

The support he got enabled him to reduce his distress in a real way—through human contact. Type C patients who deny distress often isolate themselves from others. The distress lingers on indefinitely, under the surface, where it can wreak psychic and perhaps immunological damage.

The contrast between David and the Type C patients was night-and-day. Yet he wasn't at the other extreme, a Type A person boiling over with anxiety and rage. David was not even effusive—he didn't wear his feelings on his sleeve. He was simply aware of his feelings, able to acknowledge them, and able to express them when it was necessary and appropriate. The watchword of healthy expression is *balance.*

David told me that he sometimes supressed emotions. He remembered one such instance, when he visited his mother, who was about to have cancer surgery, in the hospital. The sight of his mother, who looked "worse than I'd ever seen her," shocked him.

"I didn't say that much," David confided. "It was more than I could handle, and I didn't want to upset her. I went in with my dad, held her hand, and reassured her. Maybe that was a way of reassuring myself."

Because David had awareness, he was able to make conscious decisions about how, when, and where to express his feelings. He chose not to show his shock to his mother, with good reason. Extreme Type C's are not free to make such choices, because their feelings are unavailable to them. The repressed emotions show up in other ways—in compulsions, depressions, fantasies, or physical symptoms.

I've told you how Type C patients answered my litmus question: What would your cancer say if it could speak? David's response was "It would say 'ouch.' I take a personal affront at this cancer. I feel violated, assaulted. Maybe it would feel the same way. I'm very p.o.'d and I hope it would be too." No other patient responded to that question with such clarity and intensity.

David's ability to cope through emotional expression was not a new trend brought on by his diagnosis of cancer. As with the Type C patients, David's coping style had been established much earlier. Here's another part of my conversation with him:

> **LT:** Can you tell me the saddest time you can recall?
>
> **David:** The saddest time I can remember was after the death of my grandmother. I had never experienced a death in the family before. And until the age of five, my father was in the service so I lived with my grandmother. Later, I saw her fairly often— we were very close.
>
> **LT:** How did your body feel when you were sad about her death?
>
> **David:** Like something was caught in my throat. My throat hurt, like I was trying to cry but it wouldn't come out.
>
> **LT:** What did you do?
>
> **David:** Well, eventually it did come out. I went back to Montana, where she lived—where I used to live, too—to be with the rest of the family. That's when I finally broke down and cried. I got the emotions out and felt relieved.
>
> **LT:** What were your thoughts at that time?
>
> **David:** It was hard to believe she was gone. It was just hard to take it in.

David's expressiveness was evident in each of his responses. First, he chose to remember a genuinely sad event. He lucidly described physical sensations associated with grief and sadness. What did he do to cope? He shared his grief with his family. And his nonverbal responses fit hand-in-glove with his verbal ones. David made eye contact with me, spoke with vigor, and the subtle expressions on his face and in his eyes told the story as poignantly as his words. He didn't gush or even cry; he simply spoke his heart.

As I said, expressors like David were exceptions. More common were the emotionally flexible Type C patients, habitual nonexpressors who nonetheless showed some capacity to recognize and communicate their feelings. I hypothesized that each patient's degree of expression, or nonexpression, would make a real difference to his recovery. And I would look for that difference on the *cellular level*.

EMOTIONAL EXPRESSION AND CANCER DEFENSE

For every patient in my new study, I conducted the same "X ray" of emotional expression. This enabled me not only to tell whether a patient was an expressor, like Max and David, or a nonexpressor, like Alice and Jennie. It also gave me a sensitive readout on the *intensity* of each one's pattern.

Then, in my search for mind-body connections, I looked at three indicators of the patient's cancer growth and cancer defense system. As in the previous study, I utilized tumor thickness. This time, I added a new litmus test of tumor growth: the rate of cell division of cancer cells (called "mitotic rate"). Cell pathologists know that a high rate of division means the tumor is growing rapidly.

Finally, I applied a crucial test of each patient's cancer defenses. Through Dr. Sagebiel, I obtained a count of the number of lymphocytes that had invaded their tumors. Lymphocytes are white blood cells of the immune system capable of destroying cancer cells. Immunologists have found that patients with more lymphocytes infiltrating their tumor have a better prognosis. The greater number of lymphocytes indicates that the body's defense is more active, keeping tumor cell growth in check and protecting the individual from the spread of cancer.

Among the fifty-eight patients studied, I found striking connections between emotional expression and these three indicators of tumor growth and tumor defense. They are as follows:

- The more emotionally expressive patients had thinner tumors and more slowly dividing cancer cells.
- The more emotionally expressive patients had a much higher number of lymphocytes invading the base of the tumor. In other words, their cancer defense systems were operating more effectively.
- By contrast, the less expressive patients had thicker tumors and more rapidly dividing cancer cells. They also had tumors that more deeply invaded the skin.
- The less expressive patients had relatively fewer lymphocytes invading the base of the tumor. In other words, their cancer defense systems were operating less efficiently.

Here was sound evidence that expressing emotions was associated with a strong cancer defense system, while inhibiting emotions was associated with weaker defenses.

My belief that nonexpression was the toxic core of the Type C behavior pattern was bolstered by these strong connections between emotional expression, cancer growth, and cancer defense.

Many immunologists view cancer development as an internal battle between the "host" (the organism afflicted with cancer) and a piece of tissue made up of cells gone awry. Whether the host or the mutinous cells gain control of the organism depends on the balance of power between host and tumor. Let's take the example of melanoma. At some point in the growth of a melanoma, it is surgically removed. The future of the host may depend on how well its immune defenses have contained the growth of the tumor up until that point. If immune cells travel to the area, and stop the cancer cells from deeply invading the skin, then the host is likely to win the battle. Tumor cells will have been prevented from migrating into the bloodstream—the first step toward a lethal recurrence. If the host has not responded vigorously, the lesion has a chance to grow and spread before it's surgically removed. In that case, surgery may not cure—the unleashed cells can form a new tumor months or years later, in an organ where surgery is difficult or impossible.

What I had discovered was a link between emotional expression and our capacity to sway the balance of power in the fight against cancer. On all counts, patients who could express emotions had the advantage: thinner, slower-growing tumors and more immune cells in the area of the tumor. On all counts, patients who could not express emotions had a disadvantage: thicker, faster-growing tumors and fewer immune cells in the area of the tumor.

I wouldn't argue that emotional expression is the make-or-break issue with regard to cancer survival. But it should be considered alongside other factors that determine survival, such as genetic heritage, diet, adhering to good medical treatment, and other lifestyle practices.

THE IMMUNOLOGICAL BRIDGE

I've often been asked, If mind and cancer are linked, what is the biological pathway between them? Psychosomatic researchers have long speculated that the immune system is the bridge, but too few studies provided evidence to support this view. My findings showed not only that immune functions are affected by the mind, but that immune cells that *specifically target tumors* are influenced by the mind.

Critics of mind-cancer research assert that it's not enough to show that the mind alters immunity. I often hear them say, in so many words, "The fact that emotions affect one subset of immune cells may not have the slightest impact on a person's health." What my study showed was that psychological factors affect an immune cell reaction with definite clinical significance to the cancer patient. For the person with melanoma, it matters whether he has many lymphocytes at the site of his tumor. His future recovery may hinge—at least to some extent—on whether these cells are present and doing their job to control cancer.

I'm not the only researcher who has shown that the mind can regulate our anticancer forces. In 1981, Sandra M. Levy, Ph.D., a leading investigator of behavior and cancer, joined with her colleagues at the National Cancer Institute to study patients in the early stages of breast cancer. They were able to gauge the strength of the women's "natural killer cells." These killer cells are essentially preprogrammed to wipe out cancer cells in the body. Levy discovered that patients who had no problems "adjusting" to cancer, made no complaints, were listless and apathetic, and had poor social support had *weaker* killer cell activity. Patients who complained more, had difficulties "adjusting" to cancer, and had good social support had *stronger* killer cells.

In a seeming paradox, patients who have problems "adjusting to cancer" are often psychologically and physically the strongest. Levy's study is not the only one to come to this conclusion. I've seen cancer patients who were enraged, struggling, and scared whom I considered to be in the throes of a healthy coping process. What is sometimes called "adjustment" may really be Type C nonexpression.

As with my findings, Levy's immune measures appeared to have real clinical significance for the patient. The women with more vigorous killer cells had fewer cancerous lymph nodes—the key to a good prognosis in breast cancer. Those with weaker killer cells had more cancerous lymph nodes. For these women, the activity of their killer cells represented, potentially, a life-and-death difference.

Levy's listless, apathetic, acquiescent breast cancer patients reminded me of my Type C melanoma patients. Even though she'd studied a different type of cancer, her test results mirrored mine: the Type C–like individuals had weaker cancer defenses, signs of advancing tumor growth, and a relatively worse prognosis.

The immune system is the main bridge in the mind-cancer connection, as I will explain fully in Chapter 9. We are beginning to explore that bridge, to discover its complex architecture. With evermore precise instruments—both psychological and immunological—I believe we will delineate its structure in fine detail. For now, we have evidence that the bridge extends from the highest centers of emotional processing to the lowest levels of cellular activity.

CHAPTER 6

. . . let me speak to you regarding the things of which
you must most beware. To get angry and shout at times
pleases me, for this will keep up your natural heat; but
what displeases me is your being grieved and taking all
matters to heart. For it is this, as the whole of physic
teaches, which destroys our body more than any
other cause.

> —*Maestro Lorenzo Sassoli, in a letter written
> by the physician in 1402*

Facts . . . in respect to the agency of the mind in the
disease (cancer) are frequently observed. I have myself
met with cases in which the connection appeared so clear
that . . . questioning its reality would have seemed a
struggle against reasoning.

> —*Walter Hyde Walsh, M.D., 1846*

What is the matter with us is primarily chagrin. Then the
microbes pounce. One ought to be tough and selfish: and
one is never tough enough, and never selfish in the proper
self-preserving way. Then one is laid low.

> —*D. H. Lawrence, letter to Ottoline Morrell
> May 24, 1928*

Is Type C a Risk Factor?

For centuries a body of folklore has been passed down that mental states can lead to cancer. It began with Galen, ancient Greece's most respected physician and a seminal figure in the history of medicine. Galen noted that breast cancer occurred far more often in women who had a "melancholic" rather than a "sanguine" temperament. He offered this insight in the second century.

We've come a long way since Galen. Yet, despite all our medical, psychological, and technical sophistication, we still have no consensus as to whether the mind contributes in any way to the onset of malignant disease. My research shed light on emotional factors in the *progression* of cancer—but not the *causes*. I devote this chapter to clarifying what may be the most controversial issue in the mind-body field.

When I first tackled this question, I sat down and thoroughly reviewed the existing medical literature. Most of the early reports were from physicians who wrote in the eighteenth through the mid-twentieth centuries. They stressed the role of "mental misery," "habitual gloominess," "depressing emotions," and "deferred hope" in the development of cancer.

But I noticed an interesting turn of events in the early to mid-twentieth century. The mind-cancer investigators became more sophisticated in their psychological evaluation of cancer patients.

With this refinement came a change in emphasis. Put simply, the focus shifted from depression to repression. In upcoming chapters, I'll explain how depression and repression may *both* be involved in cancer. For the moment, let it be said that half a century ago, a handful of prescient minds grasped the role of emotional inhibition in cancer.

In a 1931 paper excavated by Lawrence LeShan, Ph.D., the French physician Dr. E. Foque described his theory of the multiple causes of cancer. Based on his long experience treating patients, he came to accept mental factors as "secondary causes in the activation of human cancers." But Foque was quite specific in his description of the psychological states associated with cancer. LeShan wrote:

> He found, clearly apparent in many of his patients (one third of those with cancer of the stomach and one fifth of those with cancer of the breast), "great crises, grave depressive afflictions, profound mourning, and all the sad emotions which have prolonged repercussions. . . . you can see in the patients prolonged and silent sorrow *without the release of sobs and tears."* [Italics mine.]

In 1952, researchers Bacon, Rennecker, and Cutler reported on the psychiatric case histories of forty women with breast cancer. They summarized their findings as follows:

> Thirty-five of the women had a "masochistic character structure," and thirty "had no techniques for discharging anger directly or in a sublimated fashion." Other consistent characteristics were "an unresolved hostile conflict with the mother, handled through denial and unrealistic sacrifice," and delay in securing treatment.

J. M. Trunnel also in 1952 delivered a report to the American Cancer Society on his study of patients with prostate cancer. He observed that the average prostate cancer patient was ". . . unusually tractable, nice, eager to please, and in general, of a remarkably unaggressive nature."

In 1954, researcher Eugene M. Blumberg and his colleagues studied a group of cancer patients with different types of cancer. In the journal *Psychosomatic Medicine,* the researchers described the majority of their patients—and particularly those with rapid tumor growth—in psychological terms:

> They were . . . consistently serious, over-cooperative, over-nice, over-anxious, painfully sensitive, passive, apologetic personalities, and, as far as could be ascertained from family, friends, and previous records, they had suffered from this lack of self-expression and self-realization all their lives.

Dr. Byron Butler studied a group of patients with malignant tumors as part of his study of hypnosis in the treatment of cancer pain. In the conclusions of his 1954 paper, he wrote:

> There may be a "cancer personality." From a very intensive study of these cases, either an inhibited individual with repressed anger, hatred and jealousy, or a "good" person consumed with self-pity may be the prototype.

These reports, and many others like them, have a great deal in common. They all come from reliable sources: doctors trained in clinical observation. But they are just that—clinical observations. They are not scientific studies in today's sense, with reliable measures and careful calculations of statistical significance. Nevertheless, they are striking both because the observations are so similar, and because they so accurately presage the Type C concept.

Beginning in the early 1960s, various investigators began scientific research of behavior and cancer. Dr. David Kissen at the University of Glasgow, Dr. Sandra Levy of the National Cancer Institute, and Dr. Leonard Derogatis of Johns Hopkins Medical Center, among many others, conducted well-designed studies on cancer and the mind. But their research, like mine, revealed psychological factors in the *progression* of cancer, not its causes.

The vexing question—Is Type C a cancer risk factor?—can be answered definitively only by *prospective* studies, the gold standard of mind-body-cancer research. (These are long-term follow-ups of healthy individuals, to determine whether certain factors are linked to later development of disease.) Few of these large-scale projects have been carried out, but the ones that have are worthy of serious attention. I'll describe their compelling findings at the end of this chapter. The difficulty with prospective studies is that they require hundreds, if not thousands, of subjects, enormous sums of money, and a period longer than ten years before results are available. For researchers with less funding and patience, other methods have to suffice. Using these alternate methods, I and other investigators have sought preliminary answers to the most fascinating and perplexing question in mind-body science.

DOES TYPE C BEHAVIOR PRECEDE CANCER?

Critics of mind-body research argue that cancer patients might repress their feelings in *response* to a dreaded diagnosis of cancer. If the critics were right, that explains why investigators keep finding repression in people with cancer. The same patients might not display repression prior to their diagnosis. The critics ask, "How could repression help *cause* cancer if it wasn't present beforehand?"

In fact, there is substantial evidence that repression and other psychological states *do* precede cancer. I've found this evidence in the mind-body literature and in my own research experience.

Recently, I had a rare opportunity to test my belief. I was given direct access to twenty-two-year-old audiotaped interviews of healthy people from the renowned Western Collaborative Group Study (WCGS). The WCGS began in 1961, when more than thirty-five hundred people were evaluated and followed for years. This landmark study first revealed the Type A behavior pattern as a true risk factor for heart disease. Compared with "healthy" Type B's, the Type A subjects had triple the risk of developing heart disease later in life. In 1988, I attended meetings at SRI International, a research concern in California, to find out whether the same tapes could be used to rate Type C behavior. If so, the tapes could be used to determine who developed cancer in the intervening years.

As a preliminary test, I was given fifteen seven-minute audiotapes. I was told only that there were cancer patients among them—not how many or what kinds of cancers they had. After listening carefully to the tapes, I was quite certain that one man had developed malignant melanoma. His responses were identical to those of the Type C melanoma patients I had encountered. At the next meeting at SRI, I stated this rather risky prediction. My colleagues and I looked eagerly toward the participant who held the folder with the subjects' medical records. He told us that, in fact, this man had contracted melanoma years after his interview was recorded.

Several other taped subjects displayed Type C behavior, but not as clearly. I thought they had developed cancer, though I was unsure of the type. As it happened, I did somewhat better than chance in guessing correctly which men later developed lung or prostate cancer. The fact that I fared better in guessing the melanoma patient underscores a long-held theory: the mind affects some cancers more than others. Because Type C behavior mainly influences our immune defenses, it stands to reason that Type C will have more impact on cancers that we can resist immunologically. Our immune defenses are better able to control some cancers than others. For example, the role of immune containment has been more well established in melanoma, colon cancer, and breast cancer. There is less evidence of immune control over lung and prostate cancers. Also, in the case of lung and prostate cancers, other factors such as smoking and a high-fat diet could supercede psychological factors.

My "dry run" merely hinted at the potential utility of the Type C profile for predicting health outcomes years in advance. I await the possibility of further analysis of the audiotapes from the WCGS. While these tapes are not ideal for picking up Type C (video is far superior), the good results obtained with only very brief audiotapes tells me that words and voice may be sufficient.

I don't mean to leave the impression that my predictions make me a medical clairvoyant. What they suggest is that anyone, with the proper training or experience, could spot Type C behavior and make such predictions.

Empirically-minded scientists (and I count myself as one) often give short shrift to clinical experience. In my view, clinical experience should inform and enrich our efforts to study mind and body in a rigorous scientific manner. And in my clinical experience, I found that the Type C pattern was set in place years before onset of the disease. My interviews with scores of cancer patients confirmed that Type C was not a surprising new development in the life of the individual. In the face of life-threatening illness, these patients relied on the same resources—and defenses—as they always had.

Consider the words of Tina, a fifty-year-old melanoma patient. I asked if she used any special coping strategies in her bout with cancer:

No, this is no different from the way I've coped with any number of things in my life. I'm considered a strong person. I am tough. I am not emotional. I don't cry. I haven't cried. As a psychologist, you can interpret this any way you wish. But I've been this way for a long, long time. This is my image. This is what I am. This is how people see me.

I believed Tina, just as I believed the other patients who described their past patterns. As I've said, the Type C patients weren't liars. On the contrary, I found them to be remarkably truthful. To whatever extent they were able, they reported accurately on their behavior. They only deceived themselves about layers of emotion and experience which had been lost to them over the course of decades. Tina couldn't tell me about the frustrations and fears she had banished from her conscious mind. But Tina *could* describe her Type C coping with absolute veracity.

PRE-CANCER STATES OF MIND

Here's the problem: unless one follows a big population of healthy people for a decade or more, how does one "catch" a person before he contracts cancer? How does one study the mind of the individual prior to his bout with malignancy?

While working at King's College Hospital in London, psychiatrist Steven Greer, M.D., came up with a creative solution. He interviewed and tested 160 women who came to the hospital with breast lumps, before anyone—patients or doctors—knew whether they had cancer. Greer also interviewed the patients' spouses or close relatives to corroborate his psychological findings. All the patients faced the same stress of waiting for a biopsy result. After the biopsies were completed, Greer looked for differences between the sixty-nine women who had cancer and the rest who had benign tumors.

As a whole, the breast cancer patients and the benign group did not differ in terms of age, class, social adjustment, stress levels, and personality types. But one discrepant finding stuck out like a red flag: there were extraordinary differences between the two groups in terms of expression of emotions.

Close to 50 percent of the cancer patients were found in their interviews to be *"extreme* suppressors of anger." These were women who "had never or not more than twice during their adult lives openly shown anger." (Greer's patients remind me of my melanoma patients, for whom anger was the phantom emotion.) By comparison, only 15 percent of Greer's benign group had such a background of suppressing anger. This difference—one in two as opposed to one in seven—was extremely significant.

Greer's breast cancer patients also tended to suppress other "negative" emotions. Over half of them were extreme suppressors of sadness and anxiety, compared with 30 percent of the control patients.

In his report, Greer referred to the pattern of nonexpression among his cancer patients: "We were able to establish by careful questioning of patients and their close relatives that the pattern had at least persisted throughout adult life, and often since childhood. Consequently, it seems probable that these patterns predate the onset of cancer."

Greer's study design is not considered foolproof. There has been some question as to whether biochemical factors accompanying the presence of a tumor could change a person's mental state. However, to date, there is not one solid piece of evidence that tumor-associated chemicals could somehow cause a person to suppress her anger.

I've also found confirming evidence in mid-1980s research by German scientists. Dr. Horst Scherg and Dr. Michael Wirsching conducted separate studies in which, like Steven Greer, they tested women with breast lumps before it was known whether they had cancer. Scherg's cancer patients expressed less anxiety, showed less Type A behavior, and were more committed to social and religious norms. They "put off their own wishes in favor of more socially desirable behavior." Wirsching reported that "adequate expression of feelings was not observed in *any* of the women with cancer," compared with 50 percent of the controls who lacked expression. "All of these women," he wrote, referring to the cancer patients, "tended to an extreme degree to avoid trouble and conflict."

But what if Type C is a lifelong style among all sorts of people?

What if this pattern was found in a majority of healthy people, or people who contracted other diseases? That would surely disprove any causal role of Type C behavior in cancer. Type C would simply be an epidemic behavior, rampant in the general population. The fact that these investigators did *not* find the same pattern in their benign control groups argues against this interpretation. In my next study, I found a new way to show that Type C behavior is strongly tied to cancer susceptibility.

REPRESSIVE COPING: THE MIND-BODY SPLIT

I learned a lot about Type C from a handful of patients who had the uncanny ability to articulate the nuances of their behavior. These insightful patients were in the throes of a life transformation, sometimes brought on by their diagnosis and sometimes brought on by changes in their lives before they got cancer.

Bob, a middle-aged social worker, was one of these extraordinary patients. Based on our interview, it was clear that Bob had always been a Type C coper, but he had been changed by the experience of cancer and was openly confronting the issues it brought up for him. I asked if he'd ever sought psychotherapy.

"It would be out of character for me to seek psychotherapy," he answered. "First, because sharing my feelings has not been characteristic of me. It is *becoming* characteristic. But I have been very private in the expression of my emotions. I have not been particularly aware of my feelings. But I have been *very* aware of other people's feelings. And I think that's why I'm in the line of work I'm in."

When I asked Bob about anger, at first he responded the same way as other Type C patients. He could not recall a single memory of anger. Unlike the others, though, Bob went on to explore this peculiarity. My question stirred in him a series of deep questions he had about himself. "One of the reasons I'm having trouble here is that expression and awareness of aggression and anger has been peripheral for me," he mused. "It's not been OK. So there are no clear unambiguous feelings of anger."

I encouraged Bob to take more time, until he turned up a memory. He recalled a time when his supervisor at work pooh-poohed his recommendations regarding a particular client. Bob remembered thinking, I know this client, I've worked with her for years. Why should he know better than me? To make matters worse, the supervisor interrupted Bob several times—as though he couldn't have cared less about Bob's point of view. But Bob let it go and followed his orders—orders he felt were dead wrong. Through all this, Bob acted not the least bit perturbed.

I asked Bob if he felt any physical sensations when talking with the supervisor. "Yes, tightness," Bob recalled, "tightness in my shoulders, back, chest, and stomach."

"What did you do?" I asked.

"I tightened up more," he said. "I tightened up and searched for control. In these situations, I tend to become less aware of things that go on around me. I even start to get tunnel vision. The more I'm under stress—and that is often when I'm trying to keep my anger under control—the more I begin to lose contact with my environment."

Bob had cut to the heart of the problem of repressive (Type C) coping. When repressors find themselves in the midst of an anger-producing situation, their struggle to maintain rigid control simply intensifies their stress. The answer for Bob would not have been to explode; he would have risked losing his job. But he could have told his boss to stop interrupting him, and asserted his knowledge of his client.

If you can find a productive outlet for anger, you not only squarely address a problem, you also reduce your own tension. I often make this analogy: when you turn the heat up on an open pot of water, you get steam. When you turn the heat up on a pressure cooker, you get trouble.

Comedian Robert Klein has a wonderful routine that could serve as an analogy for the stress-increasing effect of repressive coping. He tells of sitting helplessly in the dentist's chair, an air pump hanging from the corner of his mouth and thick wads of cotton stuffed in his cheeks. As it happens, his dentist is a meddler and a chatterbox. In between rounds of drilling, he makes disparaging comments like "I hear your mother is having an affair with the superintendent." Or—this during the height of Watergate—"Gee, that Nixon is getting a raw deal, isn't he?" (offending Klein's political sympathies). All Klein can do is emit high-pitched, muffled moans of protest. The dentist can't make out what he's saying—he assumes it's just oral discomfort. So he continues jabbering and

Klein can only moan louder. He's been rendered verbally impotent, which causes his frustration level to skyrocket.

The cotton, air pump, and hovering drill are impediments that prevent Klein from having an outburst. Similarly, the repressive coper has built-in psychological impediments that make his anger impossible, creating a bottleneck of inner tension. The only difference is that Klein would like to explode, while the repressive coper has blocked his anger for so long he's no longer aware of it. Certainly, in the course of daily events, we must regulate our expression of anger. But if we blot out anger entirely, the bottleneck never clears and access to our feelings becomes impossible.

Along with my colleague, psychologist Andrew Kneier, I set up an experiment to study repressive coping. We compared the coping style of cancer patients, heart disease patients, and healthy people. Kneier and I chose these three groups in order to scientifically test the validity of my coping continuum—which indicates that Type C and Type A (heart disease–prone) behaviors are opposite extremes. We'd also find out whether Type C behavior was more characteristic of cancer patients than of heart patients or healthy people.

We recruited the three groups from the University of California medical clinics—twenty cancer (melanoma) patients, twenty patients with cardiovascular disease, and twenty people with no health problems. During the experiment, each person was shown fifty slides flashing anxiety-provoking statements. The statements were designed to disturb the person, i.e., "you've done nothing worthwhile," "no one loves you," and "you're furious inside." Different statements were meant to provoke anger, sadness, anxiety, threats to self-esteem, or threats to interpersonal needs.

We hooked up each subject to a machine that registers the skin conductance response (SCR). SCR is a reading of nervous system arousal, a physiological sign of the person's emotional response. Each time a slide was flashed, the SCR reading revealed the intensity of each person's *inner* reaction. At the same time, we asked the group members to mark a scale indicating how "bothered" they were by each statement.

The repressive copers were those subjects who repeatedly said they were *not* bothered but whose SCR readings told a different story—their bodies registered high anxiety, anger, fear, sadness, or stress.

As we predicted, the cancer patients had the highest Repressive Coping scores, the heart patients had the lowest, and the healthy subjects were right in the middle. The differences between the cancer patients and the heart patients were statistically significant. Whereas the cancer patients reported far less upset than their bodies registered, the heart patients reported much more upset than their bodies registered. This confirmed my hypothesis that cancer patients are mainly repressors, heart patients are "hot reactors," and healthy individuals occupy a moderate middle ground.

All our patients had been diagnosed, on average, a year and a half earlier. They were beyond the initial shock and distress of a heart attack or cancer diagnosis, and had returned, more or less, to their "normal" state of mind. Hence, repressive coping was not just a response to cancer; it was indeed a long-held pattern.

The experiment enabled us to capture those fleeting moments when a person's nervous system reacts strongly, but he has little conscious emotional response. I call this the "mind-body split," and although we all experience it from time to time, for repressive copers it is a continuing malady. I was often amazed when cancer patients handed in written forms indicating how "unbothered" they were by certain slides, when their SCR readings had skyrocketed during those very slides.

Now I had experimental data showing physiologically what I had already seen behaviorally. In my view, the procedure was a way to capture scientifically little moments just like ones I'd observed in my interviews with patients. Consider how Sandy, one of many nurses I interviewed, reacted to having cancer. She claimed to be intellectually engaged but emotionally unaffected. "I've always handled things that way," she said. Sandy's prognosis was fairly good, but she knew that melanoma was still a very dangerous and tricky disease. I wondered how, with her medical knowledge, she was not the least bit anxious. Here was her answer:

I have been involved in a lot of medical situations through my work that I consider so much more serious, so much more tragic and hopeless and heartbreaking than anything I could ever go through, that what I have by comparison is trivial. I have watched people bleed to death; I have mopped the blood up off the floor so the doctors wouldn't slip on it while they tried to stop the bleeding. I have seen stabbing victims wheeled in with the knife still sticking out of their back. What I have is child's play compared to what you see on a daily basis if you work in intensive care medical situations.

Reading this, perhaps you are convinced by her argument! Sandy got so caught up in her description of medical horrors that for one moment I thought, maybe she's right. But of course, this is testimony only to how effective her powers of rationalization were. Melanoma isn't "child's play." It's a frightening illness, and no amount of focusing on the catastrophes of others would change that fact. Sandy *was* able to lower her sense of dread. This psychological defense mechanism—a sophisticated form of denial—can work, up to a point. The problem is that it doesn't actually get rid of anxiety—only *awareness* of anxiety. Sandy's underlying tension was apparent in her tremulous voice and the worry in her face. By the end of our interview, she admitted to a chronic headache, which had only gotten worse since her diagnosis. These signs were exactly like the SCR readings in my experiment—telltale hints of anxiety that belied Sandy's statements of calm control.

The answer for Sandy would not have been to dwell on her condition. That kind of preoccupation can lead to panic or depression. But if Sandy had admitted her fears—even just for brief moments—she might have asked for, and gotten, the support I knew she needed. As it was, Sandy strenuously denied needing any support during her illness.

The observations and research I've cited indicate that the Type C pattern precedes cancer. Though this finding is highly suggestive, it still doesn't prove that Type C is a real cancer risk factor. To do that, researchers must evaluate people when they are physically healthy, and follow them for at least a decade to see who contracts the disease.

THE GOLD STANDARD OF MIND-CANCER RESEARCH

When scientists study the behavior, habits, and life-style of healthy people before they get sick, they're engaging in a relatively foolproof approach to discovering risk factors in disease. The Type A connection was considered fairly indisputable once the findings from the Western Collaborative Group Study (WCGS) were known. Thirty-five hundred people with no signs of heart disease were tracked for over a decade. When first evaluated, the subjects weren't reacting to an illness or an experimental situation—their behavior patterns were studied in their natural state. When the researchers discovered that Type A's had a threefold risk of later heart disease, critics could not charge experimental bias of any kind.

The search for factors that contribute to a person getting cancer requires prospective studies like the WCGS's. They remain the gold standard for proving any causal link between mind and cancer.

Not many people are aware that several prospective studies have demonstrated psychological risk factors in cancer. In my experience, few in the mind-body field are even aware of these studies. The following chart provides an overview of the key prospective studies:

Prospective Studies of Mind and Cancer

George Kaplan and Peggy Reynolds

SUBJECTS: 6,848 healthy people in a California Department of Health Services Study (Alameda County)

YEARS FOLLOWED: 17

FINDINGS: An increased risk for cancer incidence and death among individuals who were "socially isolated."

Ronald Grossarth-Maticek

SUBJECTS: 1,353 healthy inhabitants of a Yugoslav village

YEARS FOLLOWED: 10

FINDINGS: The people who contracted cancer were those who had shown evidence of "rational and anti-emotional behavior." Grossarth-Maticek found similar patterns in two later studies conducted in Heidelberg, Germany. Grossarth-Maticek's methods are controversial, and they are currently under review by recognized statisticians.

Richard B. Shekelle and Colleagues

SUBJECTS: 2,010 middle-aged male workers at a Chicago Western Electric plant

YEARS FOLLOWED: 17

FINDINGS: The men who, on original psychological tests, were found to be depressed, had twice as high a risk of death from cancer.

Patrick J. Dattore and Colleagues

SUBJECTS: 200 disease-free veterans who had been psychologically tested upon entry into a VA hospital. Records of 75 who went on to contract cancer were compared with 125 who remained healthy or developed other diseases.

YEARS FOLLOWED: 10

FINDINGS: The cancer patients were far *less depressed* and significantly *more repressed* than the control subjects.

Dr. Caroline B. Thomas and Colleagues

SUBJECTS: 1,300 medical students at Johns Hopkins University

YEARS FOLLOWED: Several intervals, up to 40 years

FINDINGS: As I've reported in Chapter 3, thirty years later Thomas found that the cancer patients were people who'd experienced a lack of closeness to their parents in childhood. But there were other fascinating findings. They had also reported the least demonstrativity—or open expression of love—in their families. Dr. Pirkko Graves analyzed the students' original Rorschach tests, and found that—of all members of the sick and healthy groups—the cancer patients had the poorest "relationship potential." This was defined as the capacity to accept negative and positive emotions in oneself and others in close relationships. In 1987, Dr. Graves and Dr. John W. Shaffer reviewed the original personality tests for 972 of the students. Those who'd been "loners," and who suppressed their emotions "beneath a bland exterior," had the highest risk of cancer. The "loners" were *sixteen* times more likely to develop cancer than those who "gave vent to their emotions."

I believe that Drs. Kaplan and Reynolds tapped one aspect of the Type C phenomenon: I found many melanoma patients who fit their description of people who were "socially isolated." Such individuals—like Mitch, the selfless, constricted fellow whom I introduced in Chapter 4—kept their needs to themselves, told no one about their illness, and had a limited network of support. Other Type C patients were quite gregarious, had many friends and relatives, and were constantly involved in social activities. I distinguished their Type C behavior by the fact that they were nonexpressors and compulsive care-givers. They were out in the world tending to others but asking for little in return. So I found no hard-and-fast rule regarding social isolation. Or, more accurately, I found a split in my population between loners and sociable types.

Dr. Grossarth-Maticek's findings are compelling but, until the controversy over his methods is resolved, I cannot say whether his research adds significantly to our understanding of the mind-cancer relationship.

At first glance, Dr. Shekelle's discovery of an association between depression and death from cancer appears inconsistent with the Type C concept. I believe, however, that many Type C's do suffer from a silent, hidden form of depression, more accurately termed *hopelessness*. As I will elaborate in Chapter 8, this hopelessness rarely becomes apparent until some jarringly stressful event prompts it to the surface. For many people, a cancer diagnosis is just such an event—for the first time, the Type C person can no longer maintain the facade that everything is just fine. He may feel despair in the face of a stressor with which he cannot cope. But the key point is this: the Type C person is not likely to acknowledge depression until his facade is either worn down or broken apart by stress. That's why I would not expect depression to be observed in Type C people years *before* they contracted cancer. And, with the exception of Shekelle's study, none of the major prospective studies have made such an observation.

Why, then, did Dr. Shekelle make this observation? There are several explanations, but here is one: Shekelle found a link between depression and death from cancer, not onset of cancer. As I've argued, these are two quite distinct issues. Perhaps the men who showed early evidence of depression were those who—once cancer struck—were selectively more prone to hopelessness. Hopeless reactions have been tied to early death from cancer. This could explain why depression didn't affect the risk of *getting* cancer, only the risk of *succumbing* to it.

I consider the research of Drs. Dattore and Thomas to be compelling evidence that Type C is a cancer risk factor. Dattore's study is relatively small, but his methods were sound and he forged a strong link between repression (not depression) and later cancer. Thomas's study of medical students is highly regarded, and the recent follow-up discoveries by Graves and Shaffer cut to the heart of the Type C concept. The cancer-prone individuals were loners who hid their feelings and had trouble accepting positive and negative emotions in relationships. The people with the lowest risk of cancer were those who *vented* emotions.

Thomas began her pioneering study in search of psychological factors in cardiovascular disease. She never expected to unearth a cancer connection. She recently wrote, "Forty years ago, the idea that psychological and behavioral patterns could contribute in important ways to the occurrence of cancer seemed absurd. . . . However, such a link became more and more apparent. . . ." Thomas described her cumulative results as ". . . objective evidence to the effect that certain characteristics of the youthful mind are associated with the later occurrence of cancer."

Finally, the highly intriguing results of a seventeen-year-long prospective study of a group of residents of Tecumseh, Michigan, called "The Life Change Event Study," were just published. The lead investigator, Dr. Mara Julius of the University of Michigan School of Public Health, reported on the relationship between psychosocial factors and death from various causes for the 85 subjects out of a total population of 696 who had died. Suppression of anger was a significant predictor of death from both heart disease *and cancer,* independent of all other risk factors (age, smoking, weight, etc.). It remains unclear why this association was not found among the men, but the Type C connection among women was undeniable.

The decades-long debate over psychological risk factors has yielded more heat than light. Critics charge that there is no reliable data; adherents point to one or two studies as positive proof. With regard to the scientific evidence, I take a position somewhere in the middle. It is folly to ignore the positive data, and equally wrongheaded to assume that the studies thus far conducted eliminate all doubts about the role of the mind in cancer's causes. Based on my work and all available evidence, I believe that Type C behavior is a modest but important risk factor for cancer. Nevertheless, more long-term studies, using today's sophisticated methods for measuring behavior, are certainly needed to confirm my belief.

CHAPTER 7

Alfred Amkraut and I found that mice which
spontaneously developed fighting behavior had greater
immune resistance to virus-induced tumors. It pays to get
mad, even if you are a mouse!

—*George F. Solomon, M.D.*

Then I rose up like fire, and fire-like roared
What, all is only beginning not ending now?

—*Robert Browning*

I wanted no elegies. "Sing no sad songs for me." I wasn't
dead yet. True, I was scraping the bottom. Yet even in
the darkest days I never stopped feeling I could somehow
start the arc of health moving upward again. I felt it in a
tropism of conviction that seemed to come from wherever
the springs of the life force rise and flow.

—*Max Lerner*

Fighting Spirit and Survival

The will to live. Grit. Determination. Faith in one's own healing capacities. Fighting spirit. These are qualities that many people intuitively believe can help us overcome serious illnesses such as cancer. Growing up, we learn that the same qualities usually get results in the outside world—whether our goal is being admitted to a top university, obtaining a long-sought job, establishing a relationship we've coveted, or creating the perfect paragraph, drawing, or melody. Desire itself drives the behavior that brings us what we want, and circumstances outside our control often fall in line, we discover, if we simply put our minds, hearts, and energies wholly into the endeavor. How do these characteristics apply to the "inside" world of physical health? We know that recovery from illness can hinge on certain external actions we take, such as seeking the best medical treatment and complying with our doctor's orders. But can desire translate into internal, biological actions that foster healing within our bodies? Does a fighting spirit carry weight in the unseen battlefield of our bloodstream, lymph system, tissues, and cells? Is there scientific evidence that such evanescent states of mind have an effect on the body, even on surviving cancer?

The answer is yes. Several strong lines of evidence all point toward the survival value of a fighting spirit. We've also learned that the shadow side of fighting spirit—namely, hopelessness—can diminish our healing abilities and reduce our chances of recovery from cancer.

What is fighting spirit? It's hard to define and even harder to measure. I'll return to this conundrum, but fighting spirit is perhaps best defined by patients themselves, through their stories.

When Mae, a woman in her mid-fifties, came to the melanoma clinic, a CAT scan showed that her disease had spread to her liver. She was not expected to live more than six months. I interviewed Mae two weeks after she received the bad news. I was surprised by her fighting spirit, until I spent more time with her. After she told me her life story, I understood how this unique person had arrived at a point where she could face down cancer.

Mae was raised in a farm family that always had to struggle to make ends meet. She now lived in the California countryside, and was still struggling. Her hardships had been more than economic, and she'd endured more than her share of losses. Despite a lifetime of suffering, Mae had a spunkiness and spirit that reminded me of a character from a John Steinbeck novel.

Her husband, John, had died a year and a half earlier. Mae noticed the strange-looking mole on her shoulder a few months later, but was so stressed by John's death that she chose to ignore it. Cancer ran in her family, and her fear of the disease fed her fierce denial. In retrospect, she realized that she had been broke, scared, and unable to cope with the prospect of being sick. Now, one year later, Mae had come to the melanoma clinic to deal with her illness. A bit of her background will explain how she found the strength to both accept and fight her cancer.

Mae's life history was one of rebounding from loss, of being battered but not spiritually broken. It began when she was a young child, and her fourteen-year-old brother was dying of bone cancer. She had several brothers, but he'd been the one to whom she felt close, the "gentle one" who always had his arm around her. He had a leg amputated and the spread of the disease caused him to lose his senses one at a time. Mae remembered reading to him even after he'd lost his hearing, because it was still "a way to communicate." Mae's memory of his death was vivid: she was alone with her mother in their farmhouse in North Dakota, with no telephone, and the temperature was twenty degrees below zero. Her mother noticed that the boy had stopped breathing. Before dashing out to the nearest phone, two miles away, the mother told Mae to get into bed with her brother. She instructed her to hold her brother tight and keep his eyes closed, because he was tired. Mae didn't understand that her brother had died until days later at the funeral. That was her seventh birthday.

At the age of nine, her maternal grandmother, to whom she was very close, also died of cancer. Mae and her mother tended to her needs during her final days. It was another tough loss because Mae closely identified with her grandma, who seemed hard and self-possessed to others but showed her tender side to Mae. "I think that's where I learned it, if you want to know the truth," she said.

The worst loss was the slow death of her mother from stomach cancer, when Mae was fourteen. For eighteen months, Mae took care of her. She even administered shots of morphine when her mother's pain became overwhelming. Mae saw that as her most traumatic experience, one she began to understand and accept only decades later.

Five years before I interviewed her, Mae was working for a poverty program. There she met an elderly woman, Connie, whom she helped with a claim against a local property owner. They became fast friends. Later, when Mae heard nothing from Connie for seven months, she called to touch base. Connie explained that she had cancer and had been ashamed to call. She'd been alone, with little help from her distant family. Hearing Mae's warm voice again, Connie felt comfortable making a request. She asked Mae to spend time with her, help her with chores, and stand by to monitor her medical care. Mae couldn't refuse. While taking care of Connie, Mae said she "fell in love with the old lady."

"It was like a reincarnation of my mother," she remarked. "I think it balled up all these childhood losses into the present."

Mae went through this experience with the support of her husband, John, who was also her best friend. She'd return home from a day spent with Connie, and John intuitively understood what was happening. "We'd go to bed, he'd turn out the light and say, 'How was Connie?' Then I'd cry a little and tell him how it was," she said. "He knew I was reliving my experience with my mother through Connie."

All John could do was wait for the "crash" he saw coming and be there to cushion her fall. It came early one morning with a phone call informing her of Connie's death. Even though she expected it, Mae felt a sudden emotional shock and sobbed uncontrollably. "I don't know how much of it was for Connie, and what part of it was back there for Mama."

Mae said her "reliving" of her mother's death through Connie had a healing effect on her spirit. The emotional reparation was possible only because she could come home to her husband, let down her guard, and grieve.

When I asked Mae what was the saddest event of her life, she didn't say the loss of her mother or Connie. It was the more recent death of John, from hardening of the arteries.

> When he died, I collapsed. The pain was too great. It wouldn't have hurt me to have died, too. John was the only person that I'd ever let see through my outside shell real good. And I couldn't run any kind of bluff on him. None. I'd get up on my high horse and start my lecturing, and he'd just look at me and grin and wink. That would blow me right out of the saddle. How can you lecture and preach when somebody knows you don't really mean it? You don't pick that kind off of every cabbage patch. You don't get a man who's never been married to take a woman with five kids—and he helps you raise them. Those children never thought of him as a stepfather. He's Dad. I was a very fortunate woman. I was with John for ten years, and it was the best ten years a woman could ever have. Even with his illness, he was still a pillar of strength. Only thing was, I couldn't run him! He'd call me "sarge" if I got too bossy.

Mae was tough, self-protective, though not one to lose her temper in anger. She coped with her traumas by taking care of other people's needs and keeping her own pains inside. For a long time, this helped her retain her psychological integrity and sense of dignity. Later, through her relationship with her husband, she was able to express those pains, let down her defenses, and allow herself to be nurtured. This transformation led to emotional growth and the happiest years of her life. But when she lost John—the one person with whom she could be herself—she finally lost hope. For the first time, Mae wasn't sure she wanted to go on living. Only a few months later, the melanoma lesion appeared. This sequence follows closely the life history pattern described by many psychological cancer researchers—most notably Lawrence LeShan—who showed that the loss of a crucial role or relationship often precedes cancer by a matter of months.

But Mae was by disposition a fighter. Through her experience with Connie, she had also learned how to grieve. John had helped her with that, and a year after his death, she emerged from the fog of hopelessness. She realized that she wanted to live for her children, grandchildren, and herself. I asked Mae what she thought was the best way to cope with cancer, and how she was dealing with her illness:

> I can't say that the best way to handle it is with a stiff back and a stiff upper lip, 'cause I don't think it's possible. Who has the intestinal fortitude for that? I know I don't.
>
> You see, I think your chances of recovery from cancer are a lot in your mind. It's true of any ailment, really. If you think, "Oh, God, I've had it," then you won't make it. You've got a "die button" in there, and if you push it too hard, it works! I haven't read anything or studied anything to prove this, but I've seen people not appearing to be terminally ill, and they end up that way because they just gave up.
>
> I can't say that I know they're gonna cure me. I hope and pray they do, because I'm just reaching the point where I can reap a little from all those hard years. I'd sure hate to get cheated out of that. But I'd be a liar if I said I wasn't scared.
>
> Listen, I'm determined to go all the way with this. I'm in the ball game till they strike me out. I have so many things that I still want to do, that I believe they're gonna take it off, and this old gal's gonna live to a ripe old age. I'm just now getting a crop of grandkids, and that's what I've been spending this whole life to get to—those beautiful kids I can spoil and then send home.

Mae was uneducated, had never read about the mind-body connection, but had an intuitive grasp of the mind's role in recovery. (In fact, Bernie Siegel, in his book *Love, Medicine, and Miracles,* published years later, used the same metaphor of a "die button" for hopelessness.) She lived another four years—miraculous, by medical standards—before finally succumbing to the metastatic tumor in her liver. Mae's fighting spirit had seen her through. She had desperately wanted more time with her children and grandchildren, and despite the overwhelming odds against her, she got the time and was able to reap some joy after so many hard years.

In the case of Mae, it's possible that her giving up after the death of her husband weakened her defenses and contributed to her melanoma. However—and this is crucial—her reaction to having melanoma turned things around. By the time she went to have her mole checked, her postbereavement despair had lifted. After her physician diagnosed cancer, she was ready and determined to beat her illness. I find it hard to believe she'd have won those extra years without a fight.

Cancer patients who become overwhelmed by hopelessness need the most caring support systems. For them, more than quality of life is at stake—life itself may hang in the balance. Mae's story underlines a point I will reiterate: regardless of past traumas, despite feelings of hopelessness, and even in the face of poor prognosis, people with cancer can develop a fighting spirit and boost their chances for recovery.

FIGHTING SPIRIT VS. DESPAIR

Many books on the mind-body connection tell stories of patients with fighting spirit who've beaten the odds. Hard-nosed scientists and skeptics cry, "But those are just anecdotes!" And they are right. While I believe that stories like that of Mae's are more than flukes, they still don't prove that fighting spirit can extend one's life span. More questions arise when skeptics point out that some patients with fighting spirit *don't* beat the odds.

If mental factors were the sole determinant of cancer growth, then every patient with fighting spirit would beat cancer, and every patient who gave up would succumb. We know that doesn't happen. However, if the mind-body connection is an aspect of cancer recovery, then the survival value of fighting spirit should show up in properly designed studies.

And it has. British psychiatrist Steven Greer demonstrated the role of fighting spirit in recovery—and the relationship of hopelessness to cancer death—in a ground-breaking study of women with breast cancer. In 1974, Greer and his colleagues Tina Morris and Keith W. Pettingale began their research at King's College Hospital Medical School in London. They began with a group of sixty-nine women, all of whom had early breast cancer and had been treated by simple mastectomy. Three months after surgery, Greer conducted one-on-one interviews with each patient. He and his team obtained a wide range of data, but they focused intensively on one question: how was the patient adjusting—mentally and emotionally—to the diagnosis of breast cancer?

Greer found that his patients' coping styles could be grouped into four categories:

1) **Fighting spirit:** The patient fully accepts the diagnosis of cancer, adopts an optimistic attitude, seeks information about cancer, and is determined to fight the disease. Example: "I won't let cancer beat me, I'm trying everything to get better. . . ."

2) **Denial:** The patient either rejects the diagnosis of cancer or denies or minimizes its seriousness. Example: "The doctors just took my breast off as a precaution. . . ."

3) **Stoic acceptance:** The patient accepts the diagnosis, does not seek further information, and adopts a fatalistic attitude. Example: "I know what it is, I know it's cancer, but I've got to carry on as normal, there's nothing I can do. . . ."

4) **Helplessness/hopelessness:** The patient is engulfed by knowledge of the diagnosis; her daily life is disrupted by preoccupation with cancer and dying. Example: "There's nothing they can do, I'm finished. . . ."

Greer and his team came up with a remarkable set of findings regarding mental adjustment to cancer. After five years, the patients with fighting spirit had by far the best outcome: 80 percent were alive and well. Deniers also fared well—70 percent were alive and well. Those who were stoic or helpless/hopeless had a much less favorable outcome. Only 37 percent of the stoic acceptors were alive and free of disease, while only 20 percent from the helpless/hopeless group had no evidence of disease. Grouped together, *the fighters and deniers were more than twice as likely to be alive and well five years later than those who were stoic or hopeless.*

But would these findings hold up over time? To find out, Greer continued to track these patients. At both ten and fifteen years from the outset of the study, Greer's results held strong. The fighters and deniers remained more than twice as likely to be alive than the stoic and helpless/hopeless patients.

(Greer has developed a new questionnaire, called the MAC— for Mental Adjustment to Cancer—to measure fighting spirit, denial, stoic acceptance, hopelessness, and other coping responses. Over the past five years, his group has administered the MAC to six hundred patients. Greer and his associates will follow the patients for many years to see if their previous results are repeated.)

How do Greer's findings relate to the Type C pattern? Patients with fighting spirit show the opposite of Type C behavior. They are active, not passive. They are aggressive in taking charge of their medical care. They stand up for themselves with doctors, nurses, and family members. They know how to go about meeting their psychological, spiritual, and physical needs. Greer's fighters reminded me of my exceptional patients who were emotional expressors.

At first glance, the fact that deniers fared well was surprising. But the reason appears to be Greer's particular definition of denial. I spoke with Greer about this issue, and he clarified his view: "These were patients who said, 'Look, there might have been a few cancer cells there, I don't know, but as far as I'm concerned, I don't want to know about it. I just want to get on with my life.' " Greer saw a certain energy and adaptability in the deniers. (His stoic acceptors were the ones, he said, who showed the most repression.) Recently, he renamed the deniers "positive avoiders."

"These patients 'positively avoid' in order to lead a normal life." Greer remarked, "so they are different from those with 'fighting spirit,' who try to get all the information they can to fight the disease. But they are similar, in that both seem to be saying, 'We are going to go on.' "

Greer's deniers resembled my Type C patients with flexibility. These were people who couldn't squarely face their illness or openly express their feelings, but they had—or developed—indirect channels for emotional and creative energies. They got on with life and continued to function reasonably well. I'll explore the dynamics of denial shortly.

Greer's stoics were the most like my Type C patients. These individuals accepted their cancer but were passive and unemotional in response to the diagnosis. Close beneath their calm veneer lay a sense of profound powerlessness: they felt there was nothing they could do to bring about their recovery.

Like Greer, I, too, had come across melanoma patients who felt hopeless and helpless. These were patients who appeared to have suffered a collapse of their Type C coping style. Their attempts to repress negative emotions had become dysfunctional in the face of cancer, a stressor too great for them to completely deny. They became bereft and surrendered to feelings of hopelessness—the most precarious state for mind and body.

I realized that my melanoma patients had responded to cancer along the same lines that Dr. Greer had so astutely drawn. But could I reproduce his findings in my population? To find out, I collaborated with researcher Ralph J. DiClemente, Ph.D., in a new investigation of all the subjects from my first two studies. After three years, twenty-five out of the total 117 melanoma patients had either died or suffered recurrences. We reviewed all our videotaped interviews with a fresh eye, to discover whether each patient had been a fighter, denier, stoic, or hopeless/helpless responder.

Using this method, we unearthed strong relationships between mental adjustment and survival. Of fifty-three women, seven had either died or suffered recurrences, and the remaining forty-six were alive and healthy. We found that five of the seven women whose disease progressed had been stoic acceptors. Stated differently, *71 percent of the women who died or relapsed were stoic—Type C—in their adjustment to cancer.*

We also discovered that, among our group of sixty-four men, those who were hopeless/helpless had a significantly greater likelihood of death or relapse, independent of all the other medical or demographic factors.

Our findings—that stoic women and hopeless/helpless men had a greater risk of succumbing to cancer—confirmed central aspects of Steven Greer's pioneering research on the mind's role in recovery. Put another way, Type C behavior and to an even greater extent the breakdown of Type C coping into hopelessness, can diminish our cancer-fighting abilities.

"TOO MEAN TO DIE"

Fighting spirit doesn't depend on getting good news from the doctor. Steven Greer told me that a few of the fighters from his original study later suffered relapses. These patients were told by their doctors that they had little hope of recovery. Despite the bleak prognosis, they held fast to the same fierce determination they had in their first bout with the disease. They seemed indomitable.

Greer feels that these patients were not indulging in false hope or delusional thinking. Rather, they had decided—quite rationally—to ignore the statistics, to live life to the fullest, and to take whatever medical steps were available to beat their illness.

Clark, a young man in one of my studies, demonstrated some of that indomitability. He was a physical therapist, a bright, active fellow with a love for mountain climbing. One day he noticed some bumps on the back of his neck. He thought they were calcifications, and went to his doctor to have them removed. When Clark was told it was cancer, he felt utter disbelief. Here he was, he thought, in the prime of his health. Why this? Why now?

The mystery deepened when the doctors had trouble determining what kind of cancer Clark had. They thought it was lymphoma, or one of several types of head-and-neck cancer. Then Clark remembered that four years earlier he'd had a mole removed. He hadn't thought of it before because the pathologist's report at the time was negative—no cancer. With that clue, his current doctors discovered that he actually had a recurrence of melanoma, which had spread to his lymph glands. The shock of this was bad enough, and Clark was angry because the pathologist had misread his slide—an atrocious error, in terms of Clark's well-being. But that wasn't the last error made in Clark's case.

Clark told me about the emotional roller coaster he'd been on since hearing the news. He cried a lot. He was furious this should happen to him when he had so much to look forward to. And he was angry at his treatment by the medical personnel.

"I really got mad," Clark explained, "when some nurse called me at six o'clock—at dinnertime—to tell me that I have even-money odds to live two years. Or maybe less. How could they say that? I could outlive them all. Who knows?"

Clark knew that he needed hope. He'd come to the melanoma

clinic for a second opinion, looking for doctors he could trust. "If someone is giving me information about my life, I want to feel that they're telling me the truth. I'm not looking for false hope, but I'm not interested in doomsday talk, either. I want to know that I have a good chance. If I know that, then I *will* have a good chance."

Clark's prognosis was guarded, but he got a clearer perspective and a great deal more compassion from his doctors at the clinic. He was faced with several treatment options, and he made his choice on this basis: "It has to be something I can really believe in. Something where I am participating in helping myself. If something's going on in my body, I need to know that I have control over what happens, with a little help from the doctors."

Clark chose a course of chemotherapy, and he was as active a participant as I have met. In his mind, the drugs were not being shot into him, he was receiving and using them for his well-being. That sense of choice and involvement may be one reason why visualization techniques are useful—they foster belief in one's own healing powers in tandem with one's medical therapy. (Visualization, also known as *guided imagery,* is a method whereby the patient relaxes and imagines chemotherapy—and/or his own immune system—destroying and mopping up cancer cells in his body.) Clark had that belief, without the use of guided imagery.

When I first interviewed him, Clark said, "I have the feeling that I have enough strength in my body to get rid of it. It's going to go away. I don't know how, but I really do believe it. That I can beat the thing."

With his medical treatment, and his fighting spirit, Clark did "beat the thing." Medical reports indicate that five years later, he was alive and well. Undoubtedly, he's been climbing in the Sierras, his favorite activity in the world, enjoying his victory over cancer and the "doomsday talk."

Clark's story reminds me of another tale told by the late Norman Cousins, author of *Anatomy of an Illness* and a leading light in mind-body research. Several years ago in Los Angeles, he attended a self-help health group comprised of many cancer patients. There he met a statuesque woman who reminded him of an older Grace Kelly. He was struck not only by her beauty but by her grace and composure. The woman recounted to Cousins how she was diagnosed with cancer years earlier. Her doctor had told her—in these exact words—that she had six months to live. Cousins asked her how she had responded. "I told him," the woman said, " 'go fuck yourself.' "

Six and a half years had passed since the day she had so vehemently rejected her doctor's grim pronouncement.

Both Clark's story and Cousins's anecdote illustrate an essential of fighting spirit: cancer patients don't have to accept a gloomy prognosis as a death sentence. While patients have a right to expect the truth from their doctors, they don't have to put their faith in a doctor who, by attitude and disposition, makes them feel helpless and hopeless.

Fighters are often (though not always) the "difficult" patients—the ones who bitch, agonize, and give their doctors a hard time. This is best expressed by the adage, apparently coined by nurses in cancer wards, that certain patients are either "too good to live" or "too mean to die."

The cancer nurses have been proved right in a handful of scientific studies. Psychologist Leonard Derogatis, Ph.D., at Johns Hopkins University followed thirty-five women with advanced breast cancer. Compared with the women who died, those who survived longer than one year had been rated by their doctors as "poorly adjusted." They expressed more anger, anxiety, and distress. "The patients who survived longer appeared more capable of externalizing their negative feelings," wrote Derogatis, ". . . and did not appear to suffer any self-image loss as a result of communicating in this fashion." The survivors weren't despondent, they were just mad—and scared—and not about to hide that from the world.

Rarely, a fighter can be so ornery that he alienates family members or medical personnel. More often, however, the fighter is simply fierce in his determination. He wants fair treatment and some measure of control over his fate. He asks questions and demands answers. This may explain why some doctors withhold their support for an attitude of fighting spirit. In their view, such patients—whether they're truly ornery or just querulous—make their supremely stressful job even more difficult. And yet, the fact that complaining patients tend to outlast their passive counterparts has been demonstrated in several investigations.

Kathleen M. Stavraky, Ph.D., a researcher at the Ontario Cancer Foundation Clinic, conducted a fascinating study of more than two hundred patients with different types of malignancy. She found that the long-survivors were angrier but without loss of emotional control. The average survivor, wrote Stavraky, was "a well-integrated person with considerable underlying hostility or aggressiveness, however he might appear on the surface." These patients demonstrated "the antithesis of the 'hopelessness' or 'giving up' reaction." Stavraky seems to have tapped the same quality as Dr. Greer: fighting spirit.

We must recognize that patients who go through periods of being ornery are, in fact, struggling to cope with their illness. The healthy aspect of the fighting style is implied by Derogatis, whose complaining patients didn't "suffer any self-image loss," and by Stavraky, whose aggressive survivors never lost "emotional control." These patients weren't mentally ill or hysterical. Nor did they display the constant hot-tempered outbursts often seen in Type A people. Their aggressiveness was both well founded and well focused. In ways we scientists have yet to fully understand, the fighter's intrepid feistiness makes existence awfully difficult for his or her developing tumor. Perhaps Albert Schweitzer put it best when he said, "Serious illness doesn't bother me for long because I am too inhospitable a host."

DENIAL: AN EARLY STAGE OF HEALING?

Richard, one of my melanoma patients, said, "I keep busy and try not to think about this problem. I had the thing removed and as far as I'm concerned, that's that." Richard's emotional window was not open enough to accept the reality of cancer, so he used denial to function and stave off despair.

Elisabeth Kübler-Ross, the renowned doctor, psychiatrist, and thanatologist whose books include *On Death and Dying* and *AIDS,* has deepened our understanding of how patients and their families deal with terminal illness. Kübler-Ross has shown that denial is a normal early stage in a process of coping with the eventuality of death. It's the first reaction in a healthy progression toward acceptance. Lawrence LeShan has likened denial to the formation of a scab above a wound: it protects the person from infection and is part of the healing process. As the underlying tissue regenerates, the scab shrinks and eventually falls off. Denial protects the person's psyche from being overwhelmed. When he or she recovers from the initial distress, denial wanes and is slowly replaced by healthy acceptance.

When patients are diagnosed with early cancers—as in Dr. Greer's study and my own—the prognosis ranges from good to bad, and death is not a certain outcome. But such a diagnosis still carries with it the *possibility* of death, a different yet equally stressful state of affairs. The not-knowing, the uncertainty, can be even more unbearable than knowing one has a terminal illness. Thus, denial as a way of coping with early cancer can be part of a healthy process of accepting one's illness and one's mortality, just as it is for patients who are terminal.

However, Kübler-Ross reminds us that some terminal patients get "stuck" in denial and are never able to face the prospect or reality of death. In my experience, certain Type C patients appeared to be stuck in denial.

For cancer patients, being stuck in denial is a double-edged sword: it helps some patients to stay functional, while it hurts others who will be unprepared for later events in the course of cancer. Psychologist Richard S. Lazarus, a leading authority on stress and coping, has shown that denial has both costs and benefits. "We must face the seeming paradox that illusion or self-deception can be both adaptationally sound and capable of eliciting a heavy price," he wrote. Then he asked the key question, "What kinds and degrees of self-deceptions are damaging or constructive, and under what conditions?"

The answer, argues Lazarus, depends on the individual, with her unique background and characteristics. Some patients stuck in denial fare well emotionally and physically. Death, the feared end result of cancer, does not cloud their horizon—as long as they stay well. In these cases, the person's coping mechanism helps her to get on with life unperturbed. Over the long-term, however, a heavy price could be exacted. If her cancer spreads, she'll have to abandon her "business as usual" approach. The rug is pulled out from under her, leaving her with fears and feelings she's unable to process. The longer a person maintains denial, the more the costs rise and the benefits subside. Research dating back to the 1950s offers confirmation that excessive denial and defensiveness do not bode well for recovery. Dr. Bruno Klopfer, a leading expert on Rorschach testing, found that cancer patients who were more deeply invested in their "ego defenses" had faster-growing tumors. The patients who were less defensive had slower-growing tumors and less recurrence.

I advise the family and friends of cancer patients to respect their loved one's denial. When they provide steady emotional support, the patient's denial will usually shift through many stages toward acceptance. This is the healthiest path. Over the long haul, the softening of denial frees the patient to express emotions and get her needs met. This will enable her to handle a later recurrence without lapsing into despair. As Norman Cousins has said, "Don't deny the diagnosis. Just defy the verdict."

HOPELESSNESS: THE COLLAPSE OF COPING

Everyone and every family hit with cancer knows the profound sorrow caused by this disease. I felt some of that sorrow when I found out that Harry died, one year after I first met him at the melanoma clinic. He was only twenty-eight, recently married, and had just had his first child. I remembered him well, and my memory was enhanced when I went back and once again watched the videotape of our interview together.

One month after his diagnosis, Harry looked and sounded as if his world had been turned upside down. He was fatalistic about his chances. "I don't know what I can do about it," he whispered. His face was etched in sadness, the kind of sadness that is unrelieved because there is no release in tears. His forehead was knotted with worry and confusion. My impression of Harry was of someone so weighed down by psychic pain that it was hard for him to breathe.

Harry said he was scared, upset, "sorry for himself." While he admitted these feelings, he hadn't expressed them—a crucial distinction. He hadn't cried, he wasn't overtly angry, and he had no fighting spirit. Every time he told me he felt bad, it was modulated, qualified, and muffled in tone. He acknowledged fear, but I saw that fear had him by the throat. He ruminated about his cancer, and was unable to work or sleep normally.

In a word, Harry felt hopeless. He was overwhelmed by negative emotions that he was unable to express, causing him to feel confused and powerless. Harry differed from the Type C patients whose coping style, whatever its shortcomings, was "working." Harry was a Type C person whose psychological defenses had fallen apart under the strain of his cancer diagnosis.

Harry's case shows that hopelessness can be a dangerous state of affairs for mind and body. But my view of Harry provided something new: a glimpse of *how* and *why* patients become hopeless. In search of greater understanding, I went back and reviewed all the data on twenty deceased or relapsed patients. For the purpose of comparison, I matched each one of them to another patient in my population who was alive and free of disease. Each match was exactly the same in terms of age, sex, stage of disease, tumor thickness, cell type, and tumor location. So I had two groups, twenty each, the same in every way, except one group had remained healthy while the other had succumbed to melanoma.

One remarkable difference emerged between the two groups. It came from the patients' responses to the psychological questionnaires I had given them. *Those who had died or relapsed scored higher than their disease-free counterparts on every single measure of negative emotions or distress.* Compared with the healthy patients, the poor-outcome group was more tense, depressed, distressed, angry, and fatigued. The healthy group scored higher in only one category: vigor, a positive mood state.

Type C copers don't admit or express negative emotions. Why did the relapsers acknowledge negative feelings? Were they not Type C?

I suspected that the relapsers were caught in the same trap as Harry. On written tests, Harry marked down that he was angry and sad. But he couldn't express these turbulent feelings to me or his loved ones—that was clear from our interview. My hunch that the relapsed patients would follow this pattern turned out to be right. I went back and reviewed the emotional expression ratings for all twenty who had died or suffered recurrences. I discovered a striking discrepancy: on questionnaires, these patients said they were angry or sad; in our interviews, *they had not expressed these same feelings.*

This seeming contradiction actually hit upon a complex truth about many suffering cancer patients. Characteristically, such an individual always had trouble expressing strong emotion. Since his diagnosis, the person could no longer deny the fear and sadness—and sometimes, even the anger—that had leaked into his consciousness. But the emotions had no place to go. He couldn't voice them to trusted friends or family.

The simple reason for his trouble with expression was that he never learned how. His early caretakers taught him a variety of ways to *avoid* expression. Worse still, his parents may have instilled what family therapist John Bradshaw calls "toxic shame," making him believe that his feelings were bad, indulgent, manipulative, or signs of weakness. How could a person with this background be expected to suddenly share his fear, anger, and sadness? He can't, and that's why he needs special knowledge and empathic support to be able to do so.

I once told a cancer patient to *own* his sadness and fear; otherwise, his sadness and fear would own him. The relapsed patients were gripped by feelings they couldn't fully accept in themselves or confide in others. My findings led me to believe that a new therapeutic approach was needed to help cancer patients live through despair. Telling people to have a "positive attitude" isn't enough. If Type C behavior sets the stage for hopelessness, then we—the patient, doctor, and psychological helper—must endeavor to change Type C behavior.

A recently diagnosed patient who begins to feel distress is at a critical juncture. At that very moment, I believe the person may be able to work through his despair by expressing emotion. I see signs of hope in the very dissolution of the Type C style, though I know that this crucial time must be handled with the utmost care and compassion. In the next chapter I will describe how patients can seize this moment to effect a radical change from their old pattern.

Compared with their healthy counterparts, the relapsed patients also lacked energy, drive, determination, and fighting spirit. When I pieced together all these findings, I came to an inevitable conclusion: like Harry, these were people beset by hopelessness.

Another angle on this discovery involves the toxic effect of impacted negative emotions. It's utterly natural for someone recently diagnosed with cancer to go through stages of shock, fear, anxiety, sadness, and anger. Repressing these natural reactions makes it impossible to work through and transcend them. The result is a kind of toxic build-up in mind and body—the beginnings of chronic hopelessness. When the cancer patient can confide these feelings to others, he not only lifts a heavy weight from his shoulders, he finds himself less alone. Emotional expression can prevent a lapse into total despair. This seeming paradox—that expressing negative feelings prevents negative health consequences—is one of the hardest realities for many people to face. On the surface, it contradicts the superficial doctrine laid forth by many a New Age and holistic advocate—that negative emotions are "bad" for your health. I am reminded of the wise comment of my colleague Dr. Rachel Naomi Remen: *The only bad emotion is a stuck emotion.* My research lends scientific credibility to Dr. Remen's simple statement, one which cancer patients and any person with serious illness can take to heart.

HOPELESSNESS: THE THREAT TO MIND-BODY HEALTH

While hopelessness and depression may overlap, they are not the same. Depression is a mental state characterized by feelings of melancholy and an inability to function normally. In extreme forms of clinical depression, a person withdraws completely from the stream of life. Of course, there are degrees of depression, and it's normal to get depressed in the wake of a severe loss or stress. There's no reason for a depressed cancer patient to feel that his mind state will "hurt his chances." According to Kübler-Ross, depression is an expected stage in the process of accepting severe illness or impending death. Depression is often derivative of sadness—a person is depressed until he can integrate his sadness and live through, or change, the conditions that make him sad.

Hopelessness is both a mind state and, if you will, a nonbelief system. A person who feels hopeless may go about business as usual, but inside he has given up on life's possibilities. He finds that his needs—psychological, spiritual, creative—have been frustrated and, in his view, will remain that way into the distant future. What is significant is not that he feels trapped, unfulfilled, and abandoned; it's that he feels trapped, unfulfilled, abandoned and *has no faith that things can ever change.*

The cancer patient is prone to two shades of hopelessness. She may suddenly look back on her life and realize "I've never had a full sense of meaning and joy in my work and relationships, and I never will." The other shade relates to the fight against cancer. The person says, "There's nothing I can do to help myself get better. I'm never going to recover."

For three decades, mind-body scientists have documented that *chronic hopelessness*—different from depression—can be damaging to our health and, specifically, to recovery from cancer.

Drs. A. H. Schmale and Howard Iker from the University of Rochester studied a group of sixty-eight women before a biopsy to determine cervical cancer. The researchers were able to predict which patients had cancer with 73 percent accuracy. The single factor upon which they made their predictions was the presence of hopelessness. Karl Goodkin, M.D., and his colleagues at the University of Miami evaluated seventy-three women awaiting workup for an abnormal Pap smear. They discovered that patients with advanced disease had more life stress, *and* had reacted to that stress with hopelessness.

Hopelessness has been studied in animals as well. How, you may ask, can we tell if an animal feels hopeless? While animal researchers can't exactly re-create this peculiarly human state of mind, they *can* create a close analogue: helplessness. The loss of control mirrors and overlaps the human experience of the loss of hope. To induce helplessness, researchers place mice in experimental situations in which they are unable to remove a source of stress—usually a shock delivered to their tails. In dozens of such studies, the helpless mice have been shown to suffer severe damage to their immune systems. Tumors implanted in these mice grow faster and cause death more rapidly. To the extent that we can translate from mouse to man—and most mind-body scientists think we can—the lesson is simple: when we lose control over our inner and outer environments, our disease-fighting abilities are impaired.

I observed this loss of control in melanoma patients who were felled by their disease. James was one. He told me bluntly, "I have no leverage over my chances." James was a young married man, though he and his wife had recently separated and been reunited. He wouldn't talk about his marital problems. He didn't have many friends and was not very happy in his job. Now he was confused, and I felt his anguish. I sensed that underneath his stoic front, James felt cheated by life, and cancer was the final insult.

Had this disease frightened or enraged him? "I'm not a person who gets angry," replied James. "When I'm mad, I become silent. I never explode." When I asked him how he was dealing with his illness, he said, "I don't know if I'm coping," and "I feel like I'm in suspended animation." I saw in James the tragic progression of someone who never expressed anger and sadness, to someone now helpless in the shadow of cancer.

I understood why James could not handle his bout with melanoma. Nonexpression breeds loneliness and powerlessness. Of course, James was not to blame for his difficulties or his decline. His inhibitions originated long before he was a freely acting and choosing adult. They began when he was an impressionable child who altered his responses to meet the demands of his environment. Now James had no conscious grasp of the forces that had shaped his behavior. To quote R. D. Laing, first we forget, and then we "forget that we have forgotten."

THE DOWN CURVE

I've studied cancer patients whose hopelessness was just a stage. From time to time, they felt like giving up. They were exhausted, fed up, and tired of fighting. This lasted for a day or several days or perhaps a few weeks, but it never persisted. Their hopelessness was a period of surrender before they once again rediscovered their will to live. It was the down curve in a natural cyclic progression. They'd soon see the up side again.

I tell such patients not to worry: their hopelessness is not a "bad sign." However, chronic hopelessness, the kind I've been talking about until now, *is* something to be concerned about. The person who gives up and *stays* given up can lose his psychological ground and physical resistance. This is no reason for panic (which never helps), but it is a reason for action.

Chronic hopelessness is an alarm bell. It's a symptom, like cracks in the side of a building, that a structural defect threatens the integrity of the whole. If you recognize chronic hopelessness in yourself, or others with cancer, you can repair the underlying defect that threatens your health and well-being. The defect is not a character flaw; it's a block to full expression of your needs and your individuality. Don't deny your hopelessness; that will keep it frozen in mind and body. Recognizing it, and addressing its root causes, can actually spur recovery—both emotional and physical. Your old structure may be verging on collapse, but you can rebuild a new, more flexible structure. Mae, the fighter I introduced at the beginning of this chapter, fell into hopelessness when her husband died, but she rebounded and found her will to live. As with any alarm, there's time to reverse the threat before irrevocable damage occurs.

THE DISGUISED IMPULSE TO LIVE

For some patients, hopelessness is actually a cover for something deeper, something far from bleak. One melanoma patient, Roger (introduced in Chapter 2), brought this home to me with great force. Roger was forty, married, and had been a public health official his entire working life. He'd seen his share of illness. This was his second bout with malignancy—eight years earlier he had colon cancer, which was treated successfully with surgery and radiation. Two years before, Roger had been in a motorcycle accident, and his neck injury—due in part to the fact that he wore no helmet—left him with chronic pain. Roger couldn't resume his favorite activities, such as weight lifting and competitive swimming. He was frustrated and depressed by his physical condition. Yet he said he never got mad and rarely experienced sadness.

That's Roger's background—here's how he responded to cancer. In our interview, Roger made all of the following statements:

"After the diagnosis, I felt a sudden hopeless despair. It was an instantaneous depression."

"I thought it must have metastasized all over my body and I was a dead duck."

"I'm sort of resigned."

"I'm not a very optimistic person. I anticipate the worst."

"I don't want any sympathy calls from friends. I just want to be left alone."

"I wish I knew why I was susceptible. Some people have natural immunity. I guess I just don't. This is going to be my fate."

"I've had a lot of very black thoughts."

"Why me *twice*?"

"I don't want to go through a lot of futile, hopeless suffering."

"I've considered suicide."

"I figure I'm just lucky to be born. I'm ready to go. Cancer is going to get me."

I hadn't heard such a barrage of despairing statements from any other patient. I had no doubt that Roger felt hopeless, and that his mind-set was an obstacle to his recovery. However, even in the most hopeless patient, there lies a disguised impulse to live. If I spent enough time with a patient like Roger, I usually came upon that life impulse.

In Roger's case, the clue was in his anxious readiness to leave this world. Essentially, he was saying, "I can't take this anymore. I want to throw in the towel." But I discovered the deeper message in Roger's seeming death wish, when I asked him about sadness. The only time he felt deeply sad was when his father died, twelve years earlier. As a young child, he looked up to his father, who was also a public health official.

But Roger knew that all had not been roses in his childhood. He was an only child who felt distant from both his parents. His mother was cold, his father hard to reach. "We weren't close," Roger said of his father. "Everything was on a businesslike basis instead of a personal basis—not what you'd associate with father and son." When his father died, Roger realized that he never really *had* his father.

After his father's death, Roger told his wife his wish—one he'd never voiced before: he wished he'd been able to find common ground with his father. "I still think about him," he sighed. "There's such a void. I see his image every day of my life, even though he died nine years ago."

Then, Roger revealed to me a truth he himself didn't seem to grasp. "Lately I've been thinking," he mused, "if there's a great public health department in the sky, maybe I'll see him there. Then I'll get to say those things I never had a chance to say."

It struck me that Roger's readiness to die was actually a veiled wish to reconnect with his father. While the "great public health department in the sky" was a fanciful wish, it reflected all of Roger's thwarted hopes to resolve this relationship. Roger had never grieved over the loss of his father—or the loss of the relationship he yearned for but never had. He was haunted by these unfinished feelings.

In Roger's fantasy, he'd meet his father in another world and speak his heart. I don't think Roger wanted to die—I think he wanted to make his emotional life whole. In that sense, his death wish was really a life wish.

And, for all his frank statements of despair, Roger had the quality I spoke about in Chapter 3—emotional flexibility. He was able to talk about his yearnings, his desire for closeness with his parents. His eyes sparkled, and his face was mobile with expression. These, too, were signs of Roger's latent life impulse.

Roger was one of my research participants, not one of my patients. Therefore I was not in a position to advise him. Had I been, I would have illuminated for him the hidden messages he transmitted—his call for help and his wish for change. Then I would have helped him work through his grief, his anger, and his unspoken love.

I never saw Roger again, so I don't know how he worked through his despair. I do know, from medical records, that Roger was alive and free of cancer four years later.

SPONTANEOUS REMISSIONS: CLUES TO SURVIVAL

Hidden clues to the mind's role in recovery can be found in extraordinary cases of men and women whose cancers disappear for no known reason. The medical literature is replete with such cases, called "spontaneous remissions." The sudden tumor regressions occur even though no reliable treatment has been applied. Some of these fortunate patients even had terminal cancer. Brendan O'Regan, Ph.D., a neurochemist and vice president of the Institute of Noetic Sciences in California, has compiled the world's largest data base of spontaneous remissions, covering thirty-five hundred cases.

O'Regan calls this area of investigation "a gold mine." He is searching for psychological and physical factors that might explain why people overcome cancer without effective therapy. Already, O'Regan sees patterns emerging that confirm the mind-body connection. "They point to the extraordinary self-repair capacities in these people," he says. "And they plead for an answer to the question, How can you turn them on?"

One person who has a tentative answer is psychiatrist Charles Weinstock, M.D. For a decade, he led the New York Psychosomatic Study Group, a gathering of psychotherapists and doctors who compiled and studied cases of spontaneous remission. Weinstock claims that, in almost every case, the person underwent a major life change of significant proportions. "Within a short period before the remission, ranging from days to a few months, there was an important change, such as a marriage, an ordination, the birth of a grandchild, or removal of a relationship that was unwanted. There was a psychosocial rehabilitation of one sort or another, and then the cancer was healed."

Weinstock documented many of these cases—all substantiated by other physicians—in several published papers. One middle-aged woman with lung cancer was given no real hope of recovery and rejected treatment altogether. She was a frustrated musician whose career was blocked, she felt, by her much-hated husband. He was an unemployed drug abuser, financially and psychologically dependent on his wife. The woman felt hopeless about her life before her diagnosis. Afterward, she simply went home to die. Her condition continued to deteriorate until, one day, her husband suffered a sudden stroke and died. Soon thereafter, her health improved rapidly. Within a month, X rays confirmed the complete regression of the tumors in her lung.

Weinstock also reported the case of a homeless woman who had wandered all over New Jersey for years. She was diagnosed with terminal cancer and, with no hope for physical recovery, was sent to a psychiatric hospital. According to case reports, this nomadic woman thrived in the supportive atmosphere of staff and patients at this particular hospital. She had finally found a home. Some time later, her cancer disappeared.

Weinstock's interest in the field began when he read a paper on the subject, which spurred a personal memory of his wife's aunt who, he realized, had undergone spontaneous remission. She was an unmarried, lonely forty-year-old woman when she contracted colon cancer. Her life until then had consisted of taking care of her mother. The cancer, which had spread throughout her abdomen, was discovered when doctors performed an exploratory operation. The surgeon closed her up and sent her home, though he didn't tell her he'd found cancer—a common practice in the 1930s. She was expected to die within weeks or months. However, an interested suitor had just entered the picture, causing her spirits and physical condition to take a sudden turn for the better. Wedding plans proceeded apace as her health continued to improve. She recovered fully, enjoyed a happy marriage, and lived several decades longer.

Almost every case of spontaneous remission reported by Weinstock involved a renewal of hope. Whether the hope stemmed from a new relationship, the sudden blossoming of a stagnant career, or the realization of creative dreams, all these circumstances gave the patient something to fight for and live for.

WHAT IS FIGHTING SPIRIT?

While hope is a basic element of fighting spirit, there are other ingredients: assertiveness, emotional expression, and a strong raison d'être. But there is an intangible aspect to this quality that can't be captured by the language of science. Rollo May, in his book *Freedom and Destiny,* used these words to describe spirit, which could well be applied to fighting spirit:

> Spirit is that which gives vivacity, energy, liveliness, courage, and ardor to life. We speak of the Spartans fighting at Thermopylae "with great spirit." When one is "high-spirited," one is lively, active in the sense that Spinoza meant when he described the free person as active and not passive. Or one has "lost all spirit," meaning that the person is in deep despondency and at the point of giving up life entirely. We borrow from the French phrase "esprit de corps," implying the confidence that comes from participating in the spirit of everyone else in one's group. Spirit increases as it is shared, and decreases as one's freedom is blocked off. Spirit has its psychological roots in each individual's inner freedom.

May hits upon an essential aspect of fighting spirit when he says it "increases as it is shared and decreases as one's freedom is blocked off." I'll translate this wisdom for cancer patients: you can mount a strong resistance to cancer by seeking the support of your family, friends, and other patients. And your fight will be bolstered when you exercise freedom to express your needs and creative impulses.

Is fighting spirit synonymous with the capacity to express anger? Not exactly. Some nonexpressors of anger have fighting spirit, and some expressors don't. Fighting spirit involves other factors, such as hopefulness and resilience. However, most fighters can contact their anger, and they certainly can stand up for themselves. I recently came across a wonderful passage on how anger can spur recovery, in a book by psychologist Robert Chernin Cantor, Ph.D., called *And a Time to Live:*

> A vivid description of how anger can literally sustain life is contained in the documented account of a shipwrecked family's struggle to survive. During the seventh day on a life raft in the mid-Pacific with little water and their morale at a low ebb, they finally sighted a cargo ship and began to celebrate their anticipated rescue. The father set off hand flares when the ship was within three miles of them. It seemed unimaginable to him that some crewman could fail to see his distress signals spiraling through the sky. But the ship sailed slowly by and disappeared over the horizon. "I surveyed the empty flare cartons bitterly . . . and something happened to me in that instant that for me changed the whole aspect of our predicament. If those poor bloody seamen couldn't rescue us then we would have to make it on our own and to hell with them. . . . I felt a strength flooding through me, lifting me from the depression of disappointment to a state of almost cheerful abandon. I felt the bitter aggression of the predator fill my mind." (From Dougal Robertson, *Survive the Savage Sea.*) The family did survive. They stayed afloat and lived off the sea for thirty-eight long days and were finally rescued. The turning away from despair and the emergence of a cunning instinct for survival would not have been possible without the father's passionate anger. Honest anger in the service of physical or spiritual self-preservation is never petty or ugly.

The line, "I felt the bitter aggression of the predator fill my mind," captures how the primordial survival instinct can well up inside a person whose life is suddenly threatened. This powerful impulse plays a role in recovery for some cancer patients. Yet the more one tries to pin down fighting spirit, the more elusive it seems. Anger is part but not all; the will to live is part but not all; hope is part but not all; a sense of control is part but not all.

In a surprising and important study, Dr. Sandra Levy demonstrated the role of positive emotions in recovery. Beginning in 1981, Levy followed the progress of thirty-six women who had suffered a recurrence of breast cancer. Seven years later, two thirds of the women had died. Levy discovered that the other one third—the survivors—had something in common: at the beginning of her study, *they had expressed more joy.* This one variable—joy—was a more powerful predictor of survival than several medical factors that doctors rely on to determine prognosis.

Levy assumed that the joyful women had more hope and optimism. On the other hand, I've cited studies showing that angry, complaining patients were the ones to wage a successful battle against their illness. What's going on here? Don't these studies seem to contradict each other?

They do not, and the beauty of fighting spirit is that it embodies the seemingly opposite—but truly complementary—qualities that many cancer survivors possess. Healthy coping can't be reduced to one narrow emotion or manifest attitude. The attempt to do so only diminishes the psychological depth of mind-cancer research. The profile of the survivor reflects the complexity of the human animal. Dr. Steven Greer believes that fighters are optimistic, joyous, *and* they assert their needs with unerring conviction. The term itself—*fighting spirit*—captures this yin-yang interrelation of opposites: *fight* represents the aggressive, "take charge" side; *spirit* the hopeful, life-affirming side.

When I break these qualities down I find both anger and joy, strength and the capacity to admit need. One thread running through all the survivor studies is expression—expression of positive *and* negative emotions.

Marco, a thirty-five-year-old melanoma patient, personified all the seeming contradictions of fighting spirit. When I met him, Marco struck me instantly as energetic, vivacious, "spirited." Here was an upbeat, smiling young man—but he wasn't taking his cancer in stride. I asked him about his diagnosis. "I almost fainted," he said. "I've never been that afraid before."

Marco had been through a stressful five years, with two moves, two job changes, and a divorce. But he'd settled into a new job and a relationship with a young woman who accompanied him to the interview. Marco spoke enthusiastically about the job and lovingly about his mate. He felt hopeful about his new life, and was furious that cancer should now threaten to obliterate his hard-won happiness. "I was bitter at first. But now I feel, I'm *not* gonna die from this," he said passionately. "If I could speak to my cancer, I'd say, 'To hell with you.' " Marco described himself as "not having much anger" in his character, but his anger was clearly mobilized for his fight against cancer.

Marco's primary drive, he said, was to stay alive and to live fully. I asked him how he planned to do that. "First, I want to take control of the medical situation," he replied. "I'm not going to take anything for granted. My attitude is, I will persevere." Marco had what Norman Cousins called "blazing determination."

I asked him whom he could rely on for help, and he talked about his family's support. "But I'm not putting all my faith in the doctors. I have to have faith in myself."

Although he'd read nothing on the subject, Marco said he believed in the mind's power to affect recovery. His mother's positive approach, he said, had enabled her to overcome colon cancer. He also talked of his grandmother, who sank into a dark depression after losing her husband of forty years. She developed cancer and gave up hope completely. "That's what killed her," he said.

Marco spoke about his hopes and dreams. His anger was his rallying cry, but his love of life was the real motivator in his fight against cancer. He expressed his outrage, his faith in himself, his need for support, his fear, and his joy—all in one sitting. Everything he said made sense, and everything sprang from his desire for a full life. Marco suffered a recurrence a year after we spoke, but he persevered again. He is alive and well today, enjoying the life he dreamed about nine years ago.

CHAPTER 8

For what wears out the life of mortal men?
'Tis that from change to change their being rolls;
'Tis that repeated shocks, again, again,
Exhaust the energy of strongest souls
And numb the elastic powers.

—*Matthew Arnold*

People are constantly seeking a way to comprehend what
is happening to them; this *ongoing process* of construing
reality is a constantly changing one, depending on many
factors within and outside of the person. Thus, when we
consider denial, or any other kind of self-deception or
illusion, we are dealing with flux, and we must always be
aware of the slippery nature of the event we are trying to
understand.

—*Richard S. Lazarus*

I know of no formula that will predict whether a person
will be broken by a traumatic event or energized and
transformed by it. I can simply tell you that all of us need
to be aware that trauma has a twofold potential: it can be
the catalyst for creative change or the cause of self-
destruction. It depends on your courage to embrace the
unresolved pain you repressed at the time the trauma
happened and the meaning you chose to give it.

—*John Bradshaw*

The Type C Drama

We all live out our own dramas, from scripts first written for us when we're so young that we become unwitting actors reading lines and following stage directions. Through the normal course of development, we gain increasingly greater control over our life scripts. Our brains and bodies develop. We move toward autonomy from our families. We find ourselves facing crises and pivotal moments of decision that force changes in our script and alter the direction of our story. Certainly, we're never all-powerful directors of our drama. Too many plot developments are beyond our purview. But, as we leave childhood behind, we become protagonists instead of puppets. We begin to write and direct our own lines, discover our own character, and make choices that drive and shape our story.

After years of studying Type C cancer patients, I saw that they were engaged in a life drama based on a powerful early script. And, although Type C can be a rigid behavior, it does not remain static through the years. My own studies made clear that it was a fluctuating behavior, one that shifted with the vicissitudes of time. I realized that, as a scientist, I must account for these changes. (I had to develop what social scientists call a "process model.") When I began to view Type C as an ongoing drama, the heretofore mysterious aspects of cancer and the mind suddenly came into sharper focus.

One reason Type C behavior blocks growth is that it impedes the natural process whereby the individual secures increasing control over his life. Very often, tumultuous changes occur later in life for Type C's than for others who make the passage from dependence to independence in incremental steps over decades. The Type C person's individuality is severely stifled until she is finally confronted with extreme circumstances—like an illness—that put her at a crossroads. That's the moment in the drama when something has to give.

As in any drama, this one unfolds over the years with a certain structure—there is a beginning, middle, and end. But there are also twists, turns, climaxes, and surprise endings. And the foundation of the story—the source of the protagonist's actions and motivations—are embedded in the first act.

The poet Robert Bly touched on the beginnings of Type C with his metaphor of an "invisible bag" that we drag behind us, containing parts of ourselves denied since infancy:

> When we were one or two years old we had what we might visualize as a 360-degree personality. Energy radiated out from all parts of our body and all parts of our psyche. A child running is a living globe of energy. We had a ball of energy, all right; but one day we noticed that our parents didn't like certain parts of that ball. They said things like: "Can't you be still?" Or "It isn't nice to try and kill your brother." Behind us we have an invisible bag, and the part of us our parents don't like, we, to keep our parents' love, put in the bag.

The entire Type C drama covers the long arc of a lifetime of bag-stuffing and the knowing and unknowing attempts we make to retrieve the lost parts of ourselves. The plot is studded with moments of crisis, when growth requires that we reopen the bag and confront old wounds and fears that made us use the bag in the first place. If we can, we may uncover resources we never knew we had, strengths and creative energies bound in the bag with repressed emotions. The tension of this drama derives from the question, Can we summon the courage to change?

Viewing Type C as a drama helped me do justice to the rich complexity of human behavior in the face of turmoil and flux. And turmoil and flux are what we all face daily. It also enabled me to make sense of seeming conflicts among the mind-cancer studies. For example, scientists have found one set of psychological factors in studies of cancer risk, and a different set in studies of cancer survival. My point is that these factors are entirely distinct, reflecting periods in the Type C drama that are far apart in terms of time, plot, and character development.

George was a middle-aged patient in my study who had worked for the San Francisco social services department for twenty years. He had an admirable commitment to helping others. In his spare time, George's great love was classical music. When he got pink-slipped, he fell into a dark depression. He found work as an administrative assistant, but it was a disheartening comedown. George never got angry—before, during, or after his firing. At the time, he had rationalized it. It was no one's fault, he thought.

One year later, George was diagnosed with melanoma. The reality of his illness jogged something loose in him; it angered him. Why, he thought, should I be victimized by this illness? Not only was George furious at the bad cards he'd been dealt, he was frustrated with the direction his life had taken. George realized that he'd expended too much energy on others and too little on himself. He wanted more out of life. So he started to attend music school at night to get his degree, the first step in his dream to teach musicology. Although he continued his office job part-time, he was beginning to live out his desires.

Five years later, George was alive and well—for all intents and purposes, cured. George's denial of his deeper frustrations set the stage for his despair once he was fired. His hopelessness may have influenced, to some degree, the onset of his cancer. *But everything changed once he got cancer.* The diagnosis had a specific and powerful effect on George. He felt he had to transform his life, and he did. I believe that his anger and his conviction helped him to survive. The mental factor that contributed to his cancer (hopelessness) was entirely different from the ones that contributed to his recovery (anger, conviction, and the desire to make life changes).

Not all cancer patients react the way George did. An unknowable mix of elements, including one's unique life history, genetic background, social influences, and personality all come together to determine how one responds to the life climax of a cancer diagnosis.

THE FIRST ACT

How and why does a person develop Type C behavior? What drives an individual to continue this style of coping—no matter how inadequate—for years? We don't know all the answers. There may be a genetic component to this behavior that is as yet undiscovered. But, as I've emphasized, Type C behavior certainly originates in the family. The child is taught to cope with stress and trauma by controlling his emotions, appeasing his parents, by being polite and respectful at all times—in other words, by toeing the line.

For the infant or child conditioned to behave this way, there is little choice involved. He may lose his parent's approval or be actively punished unless he keeps up his "good" behavior, which, in these instances, means no anger or unpleasantness. The Type C facade is put in place early—even before brain development is complete—so the pattern has deep roots.

The child who sticks to the Type C pattern from an early age has made a trade-off. He puts the so-called negative parts of himself into the bag, where they can't be seen by the world. Soon, the bag is so deep and its contents so scary that even he can't get to them. But the bag-stuffing has accomplished its goal: he's kept harmony in the family.

We know from developmental psychology that infancy and early childhood is a time when powerful imprints are laid down, shaping the person's behavior for decades. Early experiences are so potent because the child is completely dependent on his family for his survival needs—feeding, safety, touch, and affection. He lacks the resources to meet these needs on his own. In essence, the young child will respond in any way possible to secure fulfillment of his primal needs. The "choices" he makes to adopt certain need-filling behaviors (like Type C) are made on the lowest levels of consciousness; they aren't rational or intentional. *That is why the Type C individual can never be blamed for his behavior pattern, for its tenacity, or for any negative health consequences that result.* By driving home this point, I'm able to help my therapy patients to stop blaming themselves for patterns they developed as dependent children. Once they understand that they had no alternative, and find compassion for the children they once were, their self-blame vanishes.

Parents are not to blame, either. When people in psychotherapy change their Type C behavior, they uncover legitimate anger toward parents who stifled their development. But that's not the same thing as blame, and it doesn't preclude the possibility of forgiveness. Therapy patients come to understand that their parents were passing along roles they donned when *they* were dependent children. Type C behavior is a multigenerational legacy. By the time parents are engaged in child rearing, they've long since lost touch with the origins of their behavior. They simply don't understand that they're robbing their child of wholeness. As literary critic Randall Jarrell once remarked, "One of the most obvious facts about grownups to a child, is that they have forgotten what it is like to be a child."

THE GOAL: HOMEOSTASIS

So the Type C person trades expression and individuality for family harmony. Another word sums up what the child gets from this transaction, at least temporarily: *homeostasis.* Walter B. Cannon, the renowned Harvard physiologist, used *homeostasis* to mean, roughly, "staying power." This power is based on the organism's ability to maintain its balance despite inner and outer changes. The child is cooperative, unassertive, and appeasing because this enables him to avoid conflict—and to foster homeostasis with his social environment. Being the nice child keeps his parents' wrath (or anxiety or disapproval) at bay. He's found something that works!

His approach not only reduces discord, it protects him from his own emotions. The child "bags" his anger and sadness because they also threaten his psychological balance. Were they to emerge, he'd lose the inner security he worked so hard to gain from his environment. Suddenly, he could find himself in the deep waters of familial and social rejection: "Why are you so angry?" "You're usually so nice—what's wrong with you?" "Why are you crying?—I thought you were the strong one." By keeping up the good front, the child not only avoids these reactions, he escapes feeling hurt, confused, and abandoned.

The Type C person learns that he can win approval, no matter how limited or superficial, by maintaining his behavior. He develops into a people-pleaser, avoiding fights on the job or in his family.

Often, he becomes the model worker, or a model citizen involved in community activities. (Certainly, these are real and admirable achievements.) The Type C individual usually garners sufficient self-esteem from the acceptance and social rewards to feel psychologically balanced—safe—over the course of many years.

However, as I've said, all this comes with a hefty price tag. The person who blocks expression of needs and feelings for years will suffer a host of harmful consequences. Whoever loses touch with primary emotions also loses touch with physical sensations. The biochemical processes of repression appear to carry with them an almost systemic numbness. When you can't feel anger or fear or sadness, eventually you have a hard time feeling anything. The insensate person may not know when he's exhausted or when his body is in pain. He also can't experience pleasure as readily— whether it's sexual pleasure, emotional joy, or sensual delight. He doesn't stop to smell the flowers, because the scent doesn't even register.

As the child matures through adolescence into young adulthood, the numbness limits his experience. It also leads to self-destructive behaviors. When a person loses inner signals of pain or fatigue, he's in a particularly precarious state. He may continue to work, to please, to placate, to struggle, long after his physical resources have been depleted. And, of course, he loses touch with his psychological needs. Loneliness, fear, and anger tell us something is wrong in our environment and demands rectification. If these emotions don't reach the structures of consciousness within our brain, we lose the crucial information value they carry, such as, "I need help," "This relationship isn't working," "I must not let them walk all over me." The very pattern that fostered homeostasis in childhood will, sooner or later, threaten the delicate balance by robbing a person of his inner voice and ability to act on his own behalf.

HOPELESS ASSUMPTIONS

She may not be aware of them, but the Type C coper holds certain underlying assumptions. They come with her from childhood. Among them:

It is useless to express my needs.
My needs cannot or will not be met by my environment.
If I express my real emotions I will be rejected.
My creative impulses are not all right if they don't meet with
   approval from those upon whom I depend.

These assumptions lead the individual to harbor what I call "hidden hopelessness." Underneath, she believes she will never be fully accepted by others—too many parts of herself are "bad," "unacceptable." Her deepest needs will never really be met.

The hopelessness remains hidden because it belies her mask of normalcy and self-sufficiency. The Type C person is caught in a wicked bind: She must tell her family and friends "I'm fine," because she fears rejection for revealing her fears or disappointments. However, she can never change the underlying despair until she's able to acknowledge the truth of her situation. Considering what she's been taught her entire life, the actual cure for her ills seems out of the question. She *can't* ask for help, she *can't* admit failure, she *can't* be depressed, she *can't* get angry on her own behalf.

In early childhood, the Type C coper stumbles, unconsciously, on what she believes is the solution to her bind. She will keep her unhappiness a secret even to herself. This reduces her inner tension—for a time. That time can be until adolescence, when powerful emotions erupt into consciousness and alter the Type C pattern. Or that time can extend fully into adulthood if the person remains insulated from her feelings and her hidden hopelessness. To return to Robert Bly's metaphor, when bag-stuffing never ceases, the bag gets fatter and fatter with rejected parts of the self. Finally, all that's left of the real person is "a thin slice." Still, it's remarkable how many people seem to get by with that thin slice. For extended periods, they handle everyday stresses well and remain unperturbed that parts of themselves are "missing." I call them "functional" Type C's. And I don't mean that perjoratively. Some Type C individuals may never change, and they're better off with some method of coping than none at all. But any person who moves from repressive coping toward a more flexible, expressive style will awaken to the lost parts of herself. In so doing, she gives herself a chance for levels of mind-body health she never knew were possible.

A FRAGILE ACCOMMODATION TO THE WORLD

There's another reason why functional Type C's stand to benefit from change. It has to do with prevention. *The Type C style is a fragile accommodation to the world.* Eventually, the accumulated strains and exigencies of life take a toll on the person who can't feel physical and emotional pain. The greater the stress, the more the person represses; the more he represses, the greater the stress. (I've called Type C a pressure-cooker defense because stress-related emotions are held in, creating even more tension.) This buildup of tension eventually causes small fissures in his wall of repression. The hidden hopelessness may seep through, causing the person to become confused or depressed. Often, this depression isn't linked to a specific event—it's the cumulative burden of unexpressed needs and feelings.

Moreover, specific events that to some would be minor can deliver a shattering message to the Type C person. Another of his underlying assumptions is that his "good" behavior will help him win the love, goodwill, respect, and tranquility the world promises him in return. A series of events that subvert this assumption, that tell him there is no ultimate justice, no guaranteed payoff, can leave the person helpless and hopeless. (This echoes the valuable concepts developed by Harry Kushner in his book *When Bad Things Happen to Good People.*) I came across a passage by Karen Horney, in her book *Neurosis and Human Growth,* in which she describes this plot turn in the Type C drama:

> His claims are based less on a "naive" belief in his greatness than. . . . on a "deal" he has secretly made with life. Because he is fair, just, dutiful, he is entitled to fair treatment by others and by life in general. This conviction of an infallible justice operating in life gives him a feeling of mastery. . . . Conversely, any misfortune befalling him—such as the loss of a child, an accident, the infidelity of his wife, the loss of a job—may bring this seemingly well-balanced person to the verge of collapse. He not only resents ill fortune as unfair but, over and beyond this, is shaken by it to the foundations of his psychic existence. It invalidates his whole accounting system and conjures up the ghastly prospect of helplessness.

The undermining of his psychic foundations may happen consciously or unconsciously and may or may not be caused by an actual loss in his life. Nevertheless, a profound loss occurs within his self. The person loses his old way of life—the coping style he's clung to for years. This is as real a loss as the death of a dear friend, though far more difficult to prove or quantify. (That's one reason why some studies show a correlation between life traumas and cancer, and other studies don't. Overwhelming stress may stem from obvious external crises or internal, existential crises.)

Take the case of Jessica, whose story I told in Chapter 1. Jessica lost her job two years before the onset of her illness. Technically speaking, this was not an earthshaking trauma—she swiftly went out and got another job. However, the circumstances that brought about her dismissal carried with them a disturbing message that, I believe, cut her to the quick. She'd been a superb worker and had cultivated a friendly relationship with her much-admired boss. When the boss's wife falsely accused Jessica of trying to seduce him, the boss fired her. It was the height of injustice, as undeserved as if she'd been sent to jail for a crime she never committed. Her unfailingly good behavior had not caused the boss to do the right thing— he had other priorities, such as pleasing his wife. And Jessica's good-girl persona prevented her from standing up for herself, from fighting for her job and her integrity. She was not incensed by the experience; rather, she was deeply wounded. As I read her behavior, Jessica interpreted the event in a defeatist way: "This approach to handling my life's problems has failed, and I have nothing to replace it with."

THE BUILDUP OF STRESS

As time marches on, the Type C person's stresses build up like so many heavy weights on her shoulders. Inevitably, situations arise that stretch the limits of Type C coping, unless the person has etched out a niche that is hermetically sealed from the difficult or unpleasant aspects of living in the world. The great psychoanalyst Carl Jung was once quoted as telling a patient whose only son had just drowned while sailing off the coast of Maine, "Nobody, as long as he moves about among the chaotic currents of life, is without trouble."

A series of stressors may culminate in one event—a financial downfall, a divorce, the death of a loved one. Often, this is the straw that breaks the person's Type C style, at which point emotional and physical breakdowns become a real possibility. That's why I call Type C a fragile accommodation to the world.

Type C is so fragile because, ultimately, nonexpression is an unrealistic and untenable stance. If a person can't grieve or assert his needs, he can't cope healthfully with the inevitable losses he will suffer during his lifetime. The psychological balance achieved in childhood now teeters on the edge, and biological balance is severely strained. As I've shown, the person's immune defenses suffer from an overload of repressive coping. This represents—potentially—the first stage of cancer promotion.

Consider the case of Leonard, the rabbi I told you about in Chapter 2. Here was a man with reserves of great compassion, but I believe he suffered by not allowing himself to express any personal discontent. In the months before he developed cancer, his hopes of building his own temple evaporated, and his beloved father passed away. Suddenly, the world was no longer good to him, despite how good he'd been to the world. This was exemplified by a strange, even eerie circumstance surrounding the death of his eighty-five-year-old father. Leonard and the rest of his family had spent a year planning and building a new house for him—the realization of his lifelong dream. He derived great pleasure from this activity and eagerly anticipated his father's happiness. Tragically, Leonard told me, his father died the very night before he was to move into this new home. He called the experience "traumatic."

Certainly, anyone would have been depressed by these circumstances. But Leonard never allowed himself to give in to his emotions or ask for nurturance. "I was the one who took the brunt of the stress for the family," he said.

Leonard's cancer was diagnosed six months after his father's death. It's possible that the buildup of stressful circumstances had taxed his Type C coping style to the hilt, thus weakening his cancer defense. (In the next chapter, I'll explain exactly how Type C can diminish immunity.) And the tragic irony of his father's death right after the completion of his new home had shaken Leonard's underlying faith in a just and ordered universe.

I have tried to show that "loss" can play a part in cancer development, but that loss can be defined in many ways. In the

1950s and 1960s, Dr. William A. Greene demonstrated that the loss of a significant person or goal often predated development of lymphoma or leukemia. He even studied twins, one of whom developed leukemia, and discovered that the sibling with cancer had been subject to major emotional loss or stress to which the healthy twin had not been exposed. Greene's work showed that actual loss may well precipitate cancer development. My work and observations indicate that actual loss, an accumulation of stress, or even just the quiet inner sense of loss experienced when a person's way of coping no longer seems to work, are all conditions which may herald the onset of illness.

THE BREAKING POINT

Now we come to the climax of the Type C drama. The actual diagnosis of cancer is the pivotal moment, the apex in a series of minor or perhaps major events.

I call it the "breaking point." Few situations are as difficult, challenging, and potentially shattering as a diagnosis of cancer. Very often, the Type C person's reaction to his diagnosis is the moment of truth regarding the usefulness and meaning of his lifelong behavior pattern. How he interprets this moment of truth, and what he does about it, may influence his recovery from cancer. It will certainly alter the course of his mental and emotional life. For those able to see the breaking point as a positive turning point, it can mark the beginning of a hard but ultimately joyous process of self-renewal.

The breaking point is invariably stressful. For Type C's it is especially difficult, because their tendency has always been to put on a happy face. How does one put a happy face on cancer? Every Type C patient I've known or studied has had to grapple with that question. And every patient had his own solution. Although I discovered a wide variety of responses, I found that each person had taken, broadly speaking, one of three paths. They are:

1) The path of transformation
2) The path of entrenchment
3) The path of resignation

The path of transformation holds the greatest hope for psychological and physical recovery; the path of entrenchment yields decidedly mixed results; while the path of resignation can lead to decline. I will elaborate on these paths shortly.

How critical is the breaking point? In 1985, I conducted a study with my colleague David M. Sweet that confirmed its significance.

We administered a series of psychological tests to a new population of 261 melanoma patients who'd come to the UCSF clinic. The tests enabled us to place each patient in one of four categories: low anxious, high anxious, repressors, and defensive high-anxious. Put simply, the low anxious people said "I feel fine," and by all accounts, they could be believed. The high anxious people said "I'm anxious," and by all accounts, they too could be believed. The repressors said "I feel fine," but they could not necessarily be believed because they *habitually* put the best face on their feelings. The defensive high-anxious group were also people who kept up a facade but said they were anxious anyway.

You may ask, If the defensive high-anxious person keeps up a nice front, why would he admit anxiety? The answer comes from one of the originators of the tests we applied in this study, Gary Schwartz, Ph.D., formerly at Yale University and now at the University of Arizona. "The defensive high-anxious group," wrote Schwartz, "may represent repressors whose coping mechanisms are failing and have become ineffective." In other words, they were just like the Type C copers I've described whose defenses were collapsing. Their anxiety had broken through into consciousness but couldn't be fully expressed or resolved.

David Sweet and I obtained measures of tumor thickness for all the melanoma patients. *We found that the defensive high-anxious group had significantly thicker tumors than the rest of the sample.*

Stated differently, the patients with a faltering Type C style had an especially poor prognosis. This study confirmed what I had already seen clinically and shown empirically. These were patients who could no longer hold back the tide of negative emotions. But they still clung to their old defenses—the very ones impeding their ability to integrate and express emotions. Like Harry and James, whom I introduced in the last chapter, they were stuck in a no-man's land between feeling and nonfeeling. They had no new coping structure to replace the old one verging on collapse.

As far back as 1954, researchers Blumberg, West, and Ellis

described this psychological state of affairs. They found that cancer patients whose disease progressed rapidly showed "high defensiveness or a strong tendency to present the appearance of serenity in the presence of deep inner distress." As recently as 1987, Hoyle Leigh, M.D., head of the department of psychiatry at the Yale University School of Medicine, showed that people who succumbed to cancer were those who suffered a "massive defensive failure." Their inner distress, it seemed, had broken through their fragile defenses.

We've seen how some patients react to the breaking point by breaking down. While the breaking point is a precarious juncture, it is also a chance for growth and change. How you perceive this transitional moment will make a difference. You can notice the "cracks" in your psychological armor, panic, and fall into hopeless despair. Or, you can view the cracks as an opportunity to let out some feeling, and to rebuild your coping structure into something more pliant, expressive, and adaptable. Indeed, the patient who sees cancer as a positive turning point can experience a brilliantly revived sense of life's possibilities. I don't know how many cancer patients have told me that their illness was "the best thing that happened to me."

THE THREE PATHS

In every drama, the climax catapults the story to an inevitable denouement. In the drama of the Type C individual, the diagnosis leads inevitably to three possible conclusions—the three paths. Again, they are:

The Path of Transformation. The person begins to develop a more stable, functional, and flexible coping style. She might say, "The manner in which I've handled stress is no longer working. I must move toward a new, more life-affirming way." She begins to express her needs and feelings more openly. She may develop a fighting spirit in her confrontation with cancer.

The Path of Entrenchment. The individual continues to cope by repressing feelings, albeit with a great deal more strain on her system. She might say, "I don't need any help, I'll be all right. It's in the hands of the doctors. There's no point in getting worked up over this." She maintains her Type C style without falling apart, but her inner tension and loneliness increase. From a psychological standpoint, the path of entrenchment can "work" over time, keeping the person functioning reasonably well (as with Steven Greer's deniers). For some, however, the path of entrenchment can take its toll as the person struggles to keep the Type C facade over feelings of profound frustration, sadness, and anger (as with Steven Greer's stoics).

The Path of Resignation. The person's Type C approach breaks down, exposing the chronic but hidden hopelessness, which now becomes conscious and overwhelming. She might say, "I don't know what to do or where to turn. I have no control over this—it's useless." The person gives up hope of recovery, and gives up hope of a fulfilling life.

These three paths have profound ramifications for the cancer patient. The psychological results are self-evident. The biological results may be predicted, based on the substantial data I've presented thus far. Here is a schematic representation of the Type C person as he or she approaches the breaking point, and the potential paths that follow:

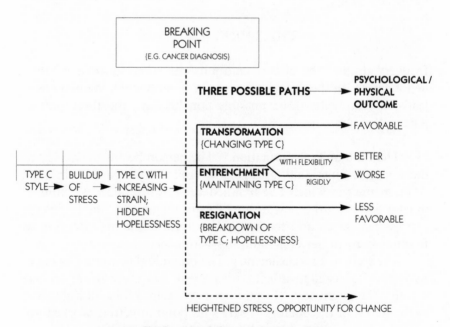

FIGURE 1. **The Breaking Point and the Three Paths**

THE TYPE C DRAMA   •   163

The path of entrenchment is the middle ground. It was the road taken by Type C's who couldn't find their way toward transformation but who still managed to keep their heads above water. It's as if they took refuge in the Type C bunker, continuing their old pattern come hell or high water. For some, this was an acceptable path that enabled them to maintain mind-body balance. In my experience, Type C's who had emotional flexibility and social support stayed the course, avoided a coping collapse, and recovered from their disease. In these instances, the worst that can be said is that the person missed an opportunity for growth. The best that can be said is that he retained his psychological integrity and got well.

Other Type C's who took the path of entrenchment lacked social support and were rigidly unable to express emotion. Their despair never broke through and showed itself openly as hopelessness, but I could sense it under the surface. For these patients, entrenchment was a tenuous solution at best. I knew that sooner or later, battening down the hatches would no longer work. With more life stress or health setbacks, the person would become vulnerable to a breakdown of his coping mechanism. My research findings and those of Steven Greer confirmed that such patients did not fare well in their chances for long-term survival.

Somewhere down the path of entrenchment lies a fork in the road. For flexible patients, the fork leads one way—toward relative psychological stability and physical recovery, if not change. For those who remain emotionally trapped and socially isolated, the fork leads the other way, toward mind-body imbalance and decline.

Of course, the path of transformation holds the promise of mind-body health, emotional growth, and physical recovery. But it's not enough to tell a cancer patient, "You can *decide* to take the path of transformation." He will need guidance to find his way. Certainly, how he perceives the breaking point is crucial. If he sees it as a death sentence, he's likely to give up right away. Though I encourage my patients to reframe their experience of cancer from "death sentence" to "opportunity," that's still not enough. Some patients can't budge from their view of cancer as a total catastrophe, because they see themselves in an inescapable trap. That trap is more than a cage of false perceptions and "negative attitudes." It's an emotional trap—the one set in place in early childhood. These individuals are locked into despair because they can't contact needs and feelings that form the wellspring of a fighting spirit.

Therefore, patients and their families have to work on several levels to get out of the trap. As I'll explain in Chapters 11 and 14, the levels of change are cognitive, behavioral, and emotional. While all three levels are vital, I've found that the emotional level is often the linchpin. When I can help a Type C patient to contact and communicate his feelings, the transformation has already begun. Toward this end, one of the first things I try to do is free him from the painfully oppressive obligation to appear strong, content, and happy in the aftermath of his diagnosis. The cancer patient who keeps up a false front in the name of "positive attitude" is doing himself a disservice. He's cutting himself off from emotions—fear, anger, sadness—that are necessary in the healing process.

Patients who work through these feelings come out the other end alive, energized, and ready to fight for life. Patients who accept their fear and grief become more willing and able to ask for support. Not only does emotional expression lift a great burden from mind and body, it's the conduit for human connections that heal the spirit.

And, as my research has shown, emotional expression is directly correlated with a stronger immune defense against cancer.

After the breaking point of a cancer diagnosis, psychological interventions—like therapy or group support—can help the person to modify long-standing behavior patterns. There is no simple road map for transformation, but one fact is clear: the cancer patient who commits himself to change, and who finds guidance along the way, has turned the "dreaded" disease into a most unexpected chance for psychological awakening.

I have described three resolutions to the drama, the ones I've most often observed. In the following sections, I'll present three case studies exemplifying these paths of transformation, entrenchment, and resignation.

THE PATH OF TRANSFORMATION

Gary, an auto mechanic, came to the melanoma clinic with a very thick tumor. He was a high risk candidate for the lethal spread of his cancer. It was one more terrible stressor in what had been several years of catastrophic stress. He was only thirty-one years old.

Four years earlier, both his mother and his best friend died of cancer within a ten-month period. His father, an alcoholic who physically and emotionally abused Gary throughout his childhood, died of congestive heart failure. Gary himself had been addicted to drugs and alcohol over the years and, by his own admission, had been involved with an unsavory crowd of people. In the prior five years, two of his other friends had died of drug-related causes.

By all expectations, Gary would now be an emotional wreck. He wasn't. He had a tenacious resilience, which came partly from denial mechanisms that got him through his traumas, and partly from a brave willingness to gradually shed the very defenses he had once erected to keep himself sane.

In my interview with Gary, he talked about the effect cancer was having on his life. "It scared the hell out of me," he said about the diagnosis he'd received a month before. "I was frightened and confused. I still am. What if I die? I cry about it. But I deal with it step-by-step. It's made me look at myself a lot more intensely. Now, I feel like I've finally swallowed this pill, I've accepted this reality."

Gary was articulate, honest, and self-possessed. He wasn't stuck in one emotion, he was moving through his emotions. "I can deal with this," he remarked. "I'm upset, but I'm not gonna fall apart. I still have a number of friends I can lean on when I need to." He'd come a long way from his earlier behavior patterns.

Gary's family had been dysfunctional, and he remembered his early life as sheer chaos. His parents fought constantly and violently, culminating in their divorce when he was nine. He and his siblings weren't spared the rod and lived in abject fear of their father. His father's alcoholic rages and his mother's "nervous breakdowns" dominated his world. Gary had no illusions that he came from a loving, supportive environment.

Gary said he had coped with his family life "through a series of intricate psychological games." He'd undergone short-term therapy after the deaths of his mother and best friend, at which time he gained his first insights into his childhood. He now planned to reenter therapy to finish the unfinished business of the past and cope with the uncertain territory of his present and future.

But Gary already knew that he'd dealt with his father's violent drunkenness by suppressing even a whisper of negative emotion—there was no room for his feelings in that early atmosphere of terror. Later in life, he became involved in self-destructive activities:

excessive drinking binges, drug abuse, and dangerous stock-car racing. Why do I do all these crazy, risk-oriented things? he asked himself. He'd learned in therapy that he'd turned his anger against himself, while unconsciously acting-out in nose-thumbing gestures of rebellion. "For the longest time," Gary said, "I couldn't even translate the feeling of anger. Slowly, over the last few years, I've been able to get angry when I have to. I use it to protect myself, and I need that now. My anger doesn't have to be like my father's anger, which bulldozed everybody."

He recognized the sick patterns in his family. While I sensed vestiges of denial in him, Gary embraced the reality of his problems and was seeking help. He was working on his addiction problems, which had diminished. He saw his illness as a spur to face his difficulties and find himself.

"My life has changed and I'll never be the same again. It's jolted me out of my old ways. I know that this is going to change my behavior, and I'm looking forward to the changes. I feel that my life is more valuable now—there's less room for bullshit."

Gary had a term for cancer that was as apt as anything I had ever heard from my professional colleagues. He called it a "positive disruption."

Emotionally, Gary said his biggest difficulty was the wall of protection he built around himself, a serious roadblock against close relationships. He moved from one romantic involvement to another and struggled with intimacy in his friendships. This is where his illness was having the most profound effect.

Without doubt, Gary saw cancer as a turning point in his emotional and social life. "A lot of my relationships have been unproductive," he confessed. "Several romances have broken up because I was confused about commitment. I've had a lot of superficial drinking friends. The type where you go out and get rip-roaring drunk. For weeks, I've been reevaluating. I'm learning what kind of friends I want and recognizing the value of people in my life. I want more serious, committed relationships."

After his brief stint in therapy years earlier, Gary had begun to understand how denial and repression had affected his quality of life. Now his illness precipitated an even deeper motivation to change. He talked about years of physical problems he had had— sore throats, boils on his neck, swollen glands. "How do you visual-

THE TYPE C DRAMA • 167

ize your neck area?" I asked him. He said he felt a powerful stricture inside his throat. He described his vocal cords as being "like a vaginal opening closed shut." There were feelings, he said, that wanted to burst through this opening.

"I have always tended to hide bad feelings—sadness, depression. That's the way I was brought up. I'm trying to get over that," he said.

"How will you?" I asked.

"I'm going to have to work on it and get help. I think you have to develop a sense of freedom, to play with things like that."

Gary's story illuminates as well as any study that how one responds to stress, and not stress itself, is the crux of the matter. He'd lived through heinous early-life experiences, a series of profound recent losses in rapid succession, and his own addictions and daredevil stunts. As I sat there with Gary, I saw and heard exactly how he'd managed to roll with the punches and bounce back. He did it by facing reality—both inner and outer—squarely. Gary's capacity for self-examination and expression was seeing him through, and he was stronger for it.

There was another crucial ingredient that helped Gary: he never blamed himself for his behavior or his cancer. Here was a young man who could have blamed himself for his father's violence, his mother's psychological leave of absence, the broken relationships, the loss of friends, his own destructive behavior; instead, his belief was, "I don't see this as God's way of punishing me for being a bad person. I have no guilt or shame about this cancer." Unlike Gary, many people with similar backgrounds see their illness as just desserts.

To Gary, cancer was not a symbol of failure, it was a catalyst—a call to action. In Chapter 10, "Blaming the Victim and Other Traps," I'll explore ways to avoid the guilt trap as Gary had done.

Gary described himself as someone who would always "do stuff people asked me to do even if I didn't want to." Now he was learning to express his wants and needs more. Having cancer stimulated him to do—in his terms—an "emotional spring cleaning." He was ready to deal with the nagging depression he'd lived with since the deaths of his mother and best friend. He was ready to overcome his fear of intimacy. He'd begun to accept his grief and anger.

Although Gary came to the melanoma clinic with a very severe cancer, he recovered fully. My last medical report had him alive and well six years later.

THE PATH OF ENTRENCHMENT

Erica, a nurse who'd seen her share of medical catastrophes, said she wasn't frightened or perturbed by her diagnosis of malignant melanoma. "All things considered, this is not a dire situation," she said. Her prognosis was good—about an 80 percent likelihood of five-year survival. She had to admit, though, that she wondered about "that other twenty percent," and "the prospects of survival at six or even ten years."

Despite Erica's moments of doubt, she seemed remarkably free of anxiety. I interviewed many nurses with melanoma, and she was one of several who said "I've seen so much worse." This defense mechanism served primarily to blot out her anxiety, not reduce it. Erica's hidden fears had a subconscious effect, one I detected through the course of our lengthy interview.

Erica said she was "strong," "positive," and "controlled." She always reacted to stress rationally, never by getting upset or enraged. "I don't cry. The last time was three or four years ago, when I had a few bad fights with my daughter." She denied negative emotions fiercely and was more concerned with her family's needs than her own. "I've always been this way," she said.

Erica, now fifty-six, was divorced ten years earlier, and had single-handedly raised her four children. The divorce was traumatic, since her husband left abruptly and offered no support. "I went from twenty years as the affluent wife of a neurosurgeon to the beleaguered mother on food stamps." She was proud of her accomplishments of the past decade: becoming a nurse and rearing her children into healthy adults despite the hard times.

The prospect of death concerned her but caused little distress. "For the first time I can sit back and say, the people who have depended on me in the past don't need me anymore," explained Erica. "All I have to think about is myself, so I'm relieved about the timing. The thought of death is less serious to me." Now that her caretaker role was complete, Erica seemed to feel less passionate about what life had to offer.

Her biggest fear was not death but infirmity resulting from a spread of her cancer. "I will take my own life before I will allow my kids to take care of me when there's no hope. I don't want to be a burden to my family."

Erica revealed the reasons behind this blunt and rather startling statement. When she was in her mid-twenties, her then-fifty-year-old father developed throat cancer. She nursed him during his final months, and recalled this as one of the worst times of her life. The cancer had spread to his lungs and brain. "He wasn't in great pain, but he regressed to his childhood. He thought he was a kid again. He thought he was back in his family home, in Arkansas. He asked us to bring him his rifle so he could go out hunting. My father was a business executive who lived in the city and hadn't gone hunting since he was a kid. To see a strong man deteriorate like that was more than I could overcome. I don't want to see anyone in that condition. That's why I could never subject my children to that ordeal. No one deserves that."

Erica was deeply disturbed by the experience of her father's decline, as anyone would be. But she focused on his loss of strength and stature, the aspect of his deterioration she found most terrifying. She hated seeing her father stripped of his facade, his inner child revealed—just as she hated to have anyone see her own weakness or dependency.

There was another reason—which I read between the lines—for her ardent wish that her children not become her caretakers. She saw them in her position with her father, a position she hated not so much because he was weakened, but because, in truth, she couldn't stand him.

Erica's mother had emphysema and was hospitalized throughout most of her childhood. She was raised by her father, who she said was "an overbearing, authoritarian, unreasonable person." He had absurdly high expectations of his daughter and criticized her angrily when she didn't live up to them. Erica tried to be the perfect daughter, which was the origin of her Type C mask of relentlessly good, selfless behavior.

Underneath, her father frightened and angered her. She recalled how she felt when, as a young teenager, he would come home from work in a surly mood: "I was always wondering what the next confrontation would be." What did she do with her fear and anger?

"I was very passive and restrained, because he was a violent, dynamic, hot-tempered person. There would have been no point in challenging him."

Erica kept her rage inside and tried to live up to his desires. It was no wonder that, years later, she resented tending to his every need.

Old feelings kept emerging during the course of my interview with Erica. She recalled the time when her brother-in-law and nephew had been killed in the crash of a small commuter plane. Erica's sister was left all alone. "That tragedy was just unbearable. I am ready to cry now, and this happened fifteen years ago."

She was clearly shaken by the memory, which carried with it several strands of meaning.

> **LT:** How did your body feel then, when you were depressed over the loss?
>
> **Erica:** Choked up. I'm gulping now and the tears are just ready to spill. Because I cannot deal with this. It was unreal. How can these things happen to young, healthy, happy, good people? How could my sister survive the loss of her husband and child? I know how I would have felt, and yet she's gone on, remarried, raised another man's family. She overcame.
>
> **LT:** What would it take for you to overcome the pain of those losses?
>
> **Erica:** I don't suppose I ever will. I guess what you mean is being able to talk about it without getting emotional again. Time should heal things, but every time I think or talk about this it's as if it happened yesterday. I feel the same sorrow. I don't suppose that my sister does that. Time stands still when I think about this. Maybe it's a recollection of a very happy time in my life. My marriage was good and my kids were little; we had good friends and good times. That tragedy just ended it. My marriage split soon afterward. The good times were over. I tell my sister that it's hard to be around her at times. We don't talk or see each other as often as we used to. We'll hang on the phone for an hour or two. But we don't talk about the past.

Erica had enough flexibility to be in touch with the profound loss she'd experienced fifteen years earlier. At the same time, her stoic front prevented her from fully grieving over her losses—the reason she could never shake the effect of these memories.

In the time I spent with her, Erica was a study in contradictions. She insisted that she was coping with cancer in her usual manner—intellectually. She wasn't upset; she was reading up on melanoma. But Erica was practically brimming over with unexpressed and unresolved emotions about her father, her ex-husband, her deceased family members, her past life, and her children. Without direct access to these feelings, she lacked the capacity for complete and joyful experience of the moment.

Perhaps this is why the possibility of death caused her little strife. While I sensed tremendous intelligence, vigor, and depth of feeling in Erica, she had channeled these considerable energies into her caretaking roles of daughter, wife, mother, and nurse. Now she was left with a great deal of unfinished business and without a solid identity outside her old roles.

The diagnosis of melanoma had thrown a wrench in Erica's normal pattern, stirring these buried emotions and memories. As they came closer to the surface, I sensed all that Erica had lost in her "bag." Not only had the sorrow of her many losses continued to haunt her, she also never found a way to resolve her rage toward her coldhearted father. Instead, she kept struggling to live up to his image of absolute moral rectitude.

I learned these things about Erica only because she was reaching down into the bag, trying to recover parts of herself lost during her journey. She was halfway there, on the verge of self-discovery. This created a great deal of tension, because—at the same time—she clung to her stolid front of self-containment as if it were an old familiar friend. But Erica had insight into this very contradiction.

As so often happens, the unexpressed emotions found form in bodily symptoms. She had an incessant cough for many years that troubled her greatly. Since her diagnosis, the cough had worsened. At the end of our interview, she said, "In all this talk about being tough and not crying, I'm not denying that I'm reacting to this whole thing. I am. I know I am. I have terrible allergies. I suspect that my cough has been aggravated by the stress. When I'm coughing I'm worried that there's something going on in my chest, like the spread of cancer, and I have a lot of anxiety about that. [Her father's cancer had spread to his lung; her mother had emphysema.] This is not something I talk about to anyone. So while you don't respond in an overt emotional way, your body reacts. This is probably more damaging to me than if I would just go and scream and pound the walls."

Erica continued to rely on Type C coping, but she had flexibility. She was in touch with a sense of loss from her past. And she had the love and support of her children and several close friends, even if she was averse to asking for such support. I believe these qualities and relationships made a difference in her recovery. I followed Erica's medical progress for four years, at the end of which she was alive and well.

THE PATH OF RESIGNATION

Marjorie's story is a tragic one. But bear with me, because I hope you'll find in her story the same kernel of inspiration that I found. She had the Type C background but was on her way toward change when she lost her footing. Based on my knowing her, I'm convinced that she would be ecstatic if she learned that her experience helped others find their way out of the trap of resignation.

Marjorie had been stressed out for three long years. Her job as a social worker was hard enough. Then her husband was in an industrial accident, which resulted in serious brain injury. This left him with neurological deficits and major depression. She now had two full-time jobs: the one in which she took care of indigent people and the one in which she took care of her disabled husband and her four-year-old daughter. She became pregnant. After six months of carrying the baby, she had a miscarriage, which caused her to become acutely depressed. Soon she became pregnant again, and gave birth to her son. But the problems in her marriage got worse and her responsibilities—in work and in her family—piled up like so many unpaid bills. For several months, she felt like a burnout victim, a ghost of her former self. People told her, "You look sick. Are you all right?" She looked at herself in the mirror once, and thought, I look like death warmed over.

Then she noticed the golf ball–sized lymph node in her groin.

Marjorie, now thirty, had had a melanoma removed nine years earlier. She thought the cancer had been cured. Usually, a person who is alive and well after five years can rest easy. But after all these years Marjorie's melanoma had spread. Statistically speaking, her prognosis was not good. She went forward with a combination of conventional and alternative treatments.

Her life, and now her cancer, had become too much for her to bear. Marjorie was very bright and struggled to regain her old energy and interest in life. But she was losing the struggle. She told me about her despair. She had devoted several years to taking care of her sick husband, but now, in her time of need, she felt no support from him.

"I understand his problems," she said. "But I just wish he could be more understanding and helpful. It makes me mad, it hurts my feelings. I think, Oh, God, this is when I really need a guy who could take care of things. But still, I'm handling everything, running the whole house, everything for him. He has lots of doctor's appointments, a lawsuit pending on his accident, and I go through all this with him. It seems like he's just not interested in my problem. I'll say something to him about my illness, and he won't have the faintest idea what I'm talking about."

She didn't blame her husband; she understood his limitations. But it was clear that she had no safe harbor. Her daughter, undoubtedly affected by her parents' tension, was acting out angrily. There was no one to lighten Marjorie's load. She felt her family didn't take her needs and difficulties seriously. "My baby son is the only one who doesn't give me any problems," she said. Their lack of attention and empathy, and her reluctance to demand help, meant that Marjorie never got the rest she desperately needed. It was an unfortunate confluence of terrible circumstances and human frailties.

"I feel worn out and it upsets me that I'm not being helped more. I have no leisure time. And this illness I have is practically terminal! I get very discouraged."

Marjorie described her depression. She couldn't stop thinking about her illness. "I misplace things, forget what I'm doing, forget what I'm supposed to do. I even forget what I'm talking about in the middle of a sentence. It's like the bottom has fallen out. The whole structure of my life is messed up. Everything is one big hassle."

She didn't see any way to shift the tide from her ceaseless caretaking to *receiving* the care she needed. Marjorie had felt trapped before her recurrence; now she saw no possibility of release. When everything became too much, she'd go into a room by herself and cry.

Marjorie stared at me point-blank and said, "I feel like the situation I'm in is hopeless. Just hopeless."

"Medically?" I asked.

"In every way," she replied.

Twelve months later, Marjorie died from the spread of her cancer.

Marjorie had had a strong spirit. Over the years, her spirit was dampened by acutely painful experiences. She never got along well with either of her parents, who fought constantly with each other and with her. "They never should have been married," she told me. As a child and as a teenager, Marjorie dealt with all this tension by being "super removed." She never complained, cried, or got angry. "I had a lot to say but I never opened my mouth."

Her suppression was her cover, her protection, and her way of keeping the tension level in her house to a minimum. But the lid came off when she was sixteen. No one remembered her birthday that year. At the end of the day, her mother scolded her: "This has been the worst year of my life because of you!" Marjorie couldn't take it anymore. In a suicidal rage, she smashed her father's car into a tree. Soon after, she was placed in a foster home. Her foster parents treated her well and she began to come out of her shell. Later, she gained enough distance to forgive her parents for their treatment of her—they had their own tragedies and limitations. Eventually she developed a much better relationship with her natural mother.

When she was twenty-two, and pregnant, Marjorie was diagnosed with a melanoma on her leg. The lesion was surgically removed and she was sent home. There was a great contrast between how she dealt with her original cancer and how she responded to its recurrence. The first time she was frightened, but she didn't get depressed or preoccupied. She had just gotten married to her first husband, was pregnant, and despite her painful past, she had high hopes for her future. After several years, she thought of herself as completely cured.

Then she went through a divorce and remarriage. Her new husband had his terrible accident. She lost a baby and became despondent. The stress of her job became insufferable. She had another child and felt deluged by responsibilities. One could speculate that, at this point in Marjorie's drama, her body suffered along with her mind, and her cancer defenses became weakened. Perhaps there were additional reasons for her recurrence, but one thing is clear: *eight years* after her supposedly curative surgery, the very same cancer was back. And it happened at the moment in her life when Marjorie felt more hopeless than ever before.

The cancer itself was one more intolerable stress. This time, she no longer had the inner resources to get her feet back on the ground. Perhaps the greatest tragedy was that Marjorie was beginning to change her pattern. "I've always been a person that doesn't say anything if something bugs me. I hold it in. Since I found out I have cancer, I've begun to change. If I'm treated unfairly or someone's upsetting me, I'll let them know. People don't know what to think. If it's someone I don't care about I'll tell them exactly how I feel."

Unfortunately, though, Marjorie was in a race against time. She was asserting her needs more in her job and with friends, but had a much harder time doing so where it counted most—in her family. Her drastic situation called for drastic measures. She may have needed intensive individual therapy and marital counseling. She may have needed at least a short-term break from her husband. His family could have been called in to assume caretaking responsibilities. These steps might not have solved everything, and Marjorie's cancer may have spread too far to be controlled by any means—*but there's no doubt that her quality of life was on the line.* Any one of these changes would at least have boosted her morale.

I can't emphasize enough that in situations such as Marjorie's, absolutely no one is to blame. Not her husband. Not her parents. Not her daughter. And most certainly, not Marjorie.

I thought about the differences between Marjorie and Gary, the patient who took the path of transformation and recovered from his illness. Both had endured painful traumas and unimaginable stress. You may be surprised to learn that I saw Gary as no more courageous or exceptional than Marjorie. I saw in Marjorie a reserve of good humor, deeply felt emotions that were not expressed, energy that had not been tapped, and a warm, vital spirit. The particularities of her adult life were like so many brick walls she'd have had to tear down to get her needs met. Gary was not encumbered by similar circumstances. While bad luck played a part for Marjorie, good luck might have made a difference. Had someone been there for her—a knowledgeable friend, a skilled therapist, a close relative—she might have been empowered to make some hard but self-preserving choices. Merely the *idea* that such choices are possible can make a difference.

In the final section of this book, I'll explain how you can procure the support you need as you take the path of transformation.

MAKING SENSE OF MIND-CANCER RESEARCH

In my reading of the mind-cancer literature, I found a number of clear, powerful trends, which I have described thus far. I also found certain seeming contradictions. The contradictions made sense to me once I developed the notion of Type C as a drama.

A tumor doesn't spring up overnight, and we don't cope with stress one way from the moment we're born to the moment we die. Cancer and coping are both *processes* that affect each other and play out over time. This helped me understand why different studies pointed to different mental factors in cancer, i.e., repression, depression, hopelessness, stress, trauma, etc. With regard to any particular study, I realized that one question made matters clear: *At what point in the Type C drama did the researchers assess the person's state of mind?*

According to the Type C script, researchers would not find depression or hopelessness in people decades before they contract cancer. Why? Because Type C's don't feel or acknowledge despair until the breaking point, which generally occurs soon before or soon after the cancer diagnosis. Researchers *would* find early evidence of Type C behavior—nonexpression, conformity, and self-sacrifice. As I showed in Chapter 6, the long-term studies conducted thus far generally follow this pattern. Type C behavior was detected years before the onset of cancer, and with one exception, depression was not.

My theory is supported by the findings of a 1989 study by the National Institutes of Health. Between 1971 and 1975, the Institutes sponsored a National Health and Nutrition Examination Survey, which collected data on more than sixty-four hundred healthy adults. The researchers relied on two short questionnaires to detect depression. Ten years later, they found no correlations between depression and later cancer. An editorial by Dr. Bernard H. Fox accompanied the published study, surveying the prospective studies of depression and cancer. He concluded that too little evidence exists to confirm any strong relationship between depression and later development of malignant disease.

Mainstream doctors and scientists tend to use such data to dismiss *any* connection between cancer and the mind. A misleading question is asked—Does depression cause cancer?—and a misleading answer is used to invalidate the mind-cancer relationship.

In his 1977 book, *You Can Fight For Your Life,* Dr. Lawrence LeShan related his discoveries from an intensive study of seventy cancer patients in psychotherapy. He described their "bleak hopelessness about ever achieving any meaning, zest, or validity in life." *But he made it clear that they hid their despair behind a "facade of benign goodness."* It took many therapy sessions before the despair emerged and could be dealt with directly. How could a pencil-and-paper test for depression pick this up?

Let's return to the Type C script again. As I've said, once the breaking point occurs, some patients change and fight, some remain the same, and others break down and give up. Therefore, well-designed studies of recently diagnosed patients have cataloged a variety of responses, including fighting spirit, Type C coping, and hopelessness. It's not until *after* the diagnosis that researchers will discover some patients in frank despair. Many researchers have taken this a step farther, and correlated hopelessness with rapid decline and mortality.

I understood the supposed contradictions among the major mind-cancer studies once I placed each study in the context of the lifelong Type C drama. In several published papers, I've shown how the findings of these studies fit neatly within the "dramatic" structure I've set forth here. All of which confirms an old bit of common sense: one can never make sense of the final act of a play if one hasn't grasped the developments of plot and character from the very beginning.

WRITING OUR OWN SCRIPTS

. . . each one of us develops throughout adulthood by stages. Between each stage are points of decision between progress

and regression where we are challenged to shed a protective
structure, and when we do we are left exposed and vulnerable,
capable of stretching in ways we hadn't known before.

—Gail Sheehy

When we are dependent children, our life scripts are essentially
handed to us. As we emerge through adolescence into adulthood,
we gain degrees of freedom that allow us to at first tinker with, then
edit, then finally rewrite our own scripts.

In *The Power of Myth,* the late Joseph Campbell, the world-
renowned authority on mythology, described this process as a journey:

We are in childhood in a condition of dependency under someone's protection and supervision. . . . You are in no way a
responsible, free agent, but an obedient dependent, expecting and receiving punishments and rewards. To evolve out of
this position of psychological immaturity to the courage of
self-responsibility and assurance requires a death and a resur-
rection. That's the basic motif of the universal hero's journey—leaving one condition and finding the source of life to
bring you forth into a richer or more mature condition.

I see the Type C person's confrontation with cancer as his
moment to change the course that's been laid down for him and
grasp control of his own story. But, as Campbell points out, this
requires a change of consciousness. Campbell was asked, "How is
consciousness transformed?" He answered, "Either by the trials
themselves or by illuminating revelations. Trials and revelations are
what it's all about."

For the Type C person, the stresses in his life, and finally his
illness, are trials in the sense Campbell means them. In order to
rewrite his story, the person must be open to illuminating revelations. I once read that the word *crisis* is written in Chinese with two
characters—one for *danger,* the other for *opportunity.* The cancer
patient who is open to revelations accepts both the danger and the
opportunity with which he is confronted.

The apex of the Type C drama is the diagnosis, and we know
a great deal about what happens to people during and after this
crisis. An unseen cellular process that's been unfolding for months

or years suddenly becomes known—the tumor is found—and the threat to the individual is assessed. The person becomes aware of his disease, aware that his body is fighting a battle for survival. His mind is now actively and consciously engaged in that fight. How he handles this awesome challenge will depend, in part, on early conditioning. But this challenge is so uniquely charged with meaning and emotion that surprising changes often occur in the weeks and months that follow.

The breaking point can jolt an individual into altering his style, often to the betterment of his recovery. A person could also conceivably *prevent* cancer by making changes *before* he reaches a breaking point of stress or disease. In this respect, I can compare our inner environment to our urban environment: we don't know how weak the structures of our buildings, highways, and bridges are until an earthquake hits. That's when we discover our invisible vulnerabilities, like hidden fissures or soft landfill. If we devoted our resources to detecting these problems early, we could fix them, preventing later destruction and loss of life. In the last section of this book, I'll discuss ways you can bolster your mind-body structure before it breaks down and becomes vulnerable to disease.

Type C is an early technique for survival that, later in life, cuts us off from ourselves. It reduces our resilience. At crucial points in the Type C drama, we have opportunities to rewrite our life script based on the rediscovery of lost parts of ourselves. Our new directions often arise from sparks of imagination and initiative left behind from childhood.

When we author our own story, we don't suddenly have the power to control every element. The path of transformation is not a royal road to fulfillment of all our fantasies. We must take that path knowing that no outcome is guaranteed—including recovery. But we can expect to overcome defeatism, open our hearts, discover parts of ourselves lost in the "bag," and make the best of our time. In my experience, this will certainly enhance our mind-body health and chance for wellness.

Whether we're sick or whether we're healthy, we can write our own script and bring about an unexpected, life-affirming conclusion. We can take the hero's journey.

PART III

MIND-BODY SCIENCE, MIND-BODY ETHICS

CHAPTER 9

Natural forces within us are the true healers of disease.

—Hippocrates

There is no such thing as a purely psychic illness or a purely physical one, but only a living event taking place in a living organism which is itself alive only by virtue of the fact that in it psyche and soma are united.

—Flanders Dunbar

In the beginning of my work, I matter-of-factly presumed that emotions were in the head or the brain. Now I would say they are really in the body as well. They are expressed in the body and are part of the body. I can no longer make a strong distinction between the brain and the body.

—Candace Pert

Type C and Mind-Body Science

Imagine the human organism as a magnificent, elaborately designed house with two wings, each of which contains many rooms. The central nervous system, including the brain, represents the most important room in the "mind" wing of the house. The endocrine, cardiovascular, digestive, and immune systems each represent a major room in the "body" wing. The mind and body wings are totally separate, with no connecting corridor to allow for the interchange of biological information.

Now you have a sense of how the mind and body have been understood by Western medical scientists for centuries. Today, all this is changing. Our perception of the human "house" has been permanently transformed. Scientific breakthroughs accumulated over the past two decades tell us that the mind and body wings are interconnected. They communicate, share information, and send messages through unrestricted passageways. What goes on in the mind profoundly influences what goes on in the body, and vice versa.

The old idea of a mind-body split, originally voiced by philosopher René Descartes in the seventeenth century, has ruled biomedical thinking for almost 350 years. In a doctrine known as Cartesian dualism, Descartes claimed that mind and body are totally dissociated. Though mind-body scientists now recognize that this separation is invalid, Cartesian dualism is still the basis for Western medicine. Our traditions of medical practice lag behind the recent discoveries in mind-body science. In coming years, these discoveries should change the face of medicine. What will emerge from the changing medical model is an approach that fully recognizes and harnesses the power of mind-body interactions.

When we talk of mind and body, what do we mean? Defining the mind has been an intellectual exercise of philosophers, psychologists, physicists, artists, and scientists for centuries. The scientific model tells us that the operations of the mind are rooted in the central nervous system and headed by the brain.

I recognize that the operations of the mind do not define *mind* in its totality. Mind is more than brain structures, cells, neurotransmitters, and neurons firing away. Some see mind as having no central location in the body; others see mind as part of a larger cosmic consciousness. I've relied upon the scientific model to illuminate the mind-body relationship, so for the sake of continuity, I will equate mind with the processes of the central nervous system. The brain is, at the very least, the physical seat of consciousness.

It's now clear that our mind/brain communicates with and modulates *all* the other bodily systems—most critically the cardiovascular, endocrine, and immune systems. The reverse is also true: our bodily systems communicate with the mind/brain. Yes, we tend to associate mind and body with different systems, but these systems are linked by all sorts of winding corridors. Messengers, in the form of certain mercurial molecules, travel freely from room to room, carrying information and instructions.

The mind-body house is a very busy place but, as in any house, the free flow of activity inside represents the functioning of the whole, the larger entity. In a real house, that entity is a family, a business, an organization. When we talk of the "family," for instance, we don't mean some mechanical equation: mother plus father plus son plus daughter. We mean mother and father and son and daughter, together, interacting—we refer to the whole unit. By the same token, when we talk of mind and body we must remember that the systems governing each are intertwined, interdependent, and, ultimately, defined by their interaction.

The messenger molecules that travel from room to room go by many names. The term used for the most ubiquitous of these molecules is *neuropeptides.* Candace Pert, Ph.D., a neuroscientist and leading expert in this area, wrote recently, "I can no longer make a strong distinction between the brain and the body. . . . Indeed, the more we know about neuropeptides, the harder it is to think in traditional terms of a mind and a body. It makes more sense to speak of a single, integrated entity, a 'bodymind.' "

Mind-body scientists have uncovered the existence of a dialogue between the brain and immune system, and this dialogue is the basis for my theory about the mechanisms linking Type C behavior and cancer. When a person chronically inhibits emotions, I believe that the brain sends biochemical signals that may restrain his anticancer defenses. The nervous system may also fail to transmit necessary "action" signals to his immune defender cells. In either event, the Type C person's defenses won't do their job efficiently. I'll return to this question, because research in the 1980s has yielded enticing clues about mind-body pathways in cancer. Scientists have even pinpointed brain chemicals that may be responsible for the Type C person's weakened immunity and susceptibility to cancer.

This chapter takes us headlong into the biological realm, so I'll be charting complicated terrain. Bear with me as I demonstrate, in the simplest terms, how mind states make their mark on molecules, cells, and tissues. Before I plunge ahead, let me ground you by describing recent breakthroughs in mind-body science. They provide the foundation for my subsequent focus on Type C behavior and the growth of cancer.

THE PNI REVOLUTION

Robert Ader, Ph.D., a psychologist at the University of Rochester conducted some of the most convincing research on mind-body connections. In 1979, he said, "There's been a huge transformation in the way we view the relationship between our mind and good health, our mind and disease. In many ways, it's nothing short of a revolution."

The mind-body revolution was wrought when scientists specializing in one field dared to cross boundaries into other medical fields. For instance, in the 1970s there were many previously unheard-of instances in which a psychiatrist and an immunologist collaborated on mind-body research. At the time, such a pairing was considered the scientific equivalent of the Odd Couple. But these were pioneers who made the imaginative and technological leaps necessary to discover intimate relationships among the brain, the hormone system, and the immune system. Today's high-tech biological research methods made the discovery of these linkages possible.

The biological evidence for mind-body connections is growing. It has been developed and gathered not only by psychiatrists and immunologists but also by neuroscientists, endocrinologists, cardiologists, psychologists, health-care workers, and behavioral scientists. In unusual settings and circumstances, these specialists have come together, shared data, and uncovered the heretofore secret passages between mind and body.

As a result, entire new fields of research have cropped up. The names they've been given reflect the strange sort of piggybacking that occurs when different disciplines are heaped together. George F. Solomon, M.D., first coined the term *psychoimmunology* in the 1960s. Later, Robert Ader came up with the tongue twister now commonly used for mind-body science: *psychoneuroimmunology,* also called PNI.

The breakthrough that helped put mind-body science on the map came in a series of studies Ader conducted in the early 1970s at the University of Rochester. He joined forces with Nicholas Cohen, M.D., an immunologist, to discover that rats could be trained to alter their immune functions in much the same way that Pavlov's dogs were conditioned. In Pavlov's experiments, dogs were repeatedly fed at the same time that a bell was sounded. Later, when no food was forthcoming, the bell sound alone stimulated the dogs to salivate. In a similar vein, Ader gave a group of rats a drug that suppressed their immune system at the same time they were fed saccharin-sweetened water. Thus, the rats learned to associate the sweet taste with immune suppression. Ader then stopped giving the drug and fed them only the sweet water. The rats' immune functions plummeted just as before. They had been effectively taught, through classical conditioning methods, to change their immune response.

Ader also used this technique in rats with lupus, an autoimmune disease in which out-of-control defender cells attack their own tissues. He trained them to inhibit their inappropriate immune response, and the result was astonishing: the rats' symptoms subsided, and they lived longer than an untrained control group.

Ader realized that the brain must be involved in immunity. How else could a rat learn to suppress its own immune system?

THE INNER SANCTUM OF IMMUNE CONTROL

How, Robert Ader wondered, was the brain telling the immune system what to do? What lines of communication existed between them?

Investigators before and since Ader's breakthrough have provided answers. One research group showed that the thymus—also known as the "master gland of immunity"—is richly endowed with fibers from the vagus nerve, a major nerve branch descending from the brain. The thymus, a walnut-sized gland located behind the breastbone, is like a training center for T-cells, the lead soldiers in our immune army. Another team found that a nerve network enveloped not only the thymus but also the spleen, lymph nodes, and bone marrow—the primary organs and collecting sites of the immune system. These studies proved that our defense network is essentially hard-wired to the brain.

In the mid-1960s, both Soviet and American research teams discovered the brain structure most responsible for immune regulation. The Soviet group produced changes in the immune system of rabbits by damaging a portion of their *hypothalamus*. This small cluster of tissue located inside the forebrain controls the glands that secrete stress hormones, regulate appetite and thirst, modulate body temperature, and play a key role in emotional activity. After the researchers destroyed parts of the hypothalamus, they observed a sudden drop in the rabbits' ability to mount an immune response to foreign invaders. When the American investigators destroyed parts of the hypothalamus in rats, their thymus malfunctioned and their T-cell defenses began to atrophy.

Based on these studies, I can liken the hypothalamus to the brain's headquarters for defense operations—a kind of inner sanctum of immune control. The fact that this same brain structure plays an important role in emotions provides us with a vital clue about the connection between emotions and immunity.

But the hypothalamus doesn't simply issue decrees to our immune army. Hugo Besedovsky, M.D., a Swiss researcher, measured the electrical activity in the hypothalamus of rats' brains before and after injecting them with powerful foreign substances (called *antigens*). Soon thereafter, he noted a 100 percent increase in electrical activity in the hypothalamus—at the same time the rats were gearing up a full-fledged immune response to the antigens. Clearly, the brain had received a message back from the immune system, saying, "The body is under attack." Then, acting as headquarters, the hypothalamus started buzzing with activity as it directed the necessary countermaneuvers.

The brain-immune interaction is a two-way street: messages are sent back and forth, and this dynamic relationship keeps the immune system finely tuned in its responses. Shortly, I'll describe the molecular "vehicles" that travel that street—the messengers that shuttle information between systems.

THE LIQUID ARMY

In his play *The Doctor's Dilemma,* George Bernard Shaw had one of his characters reveal the secret of physical healing. Sir Ralph Bloomfield Bonington said, "There is at bottom only one genuinely scientific treatment for all diseases and that is to stimulate the phagocytes."

Phagocytes are white blood cells that engulf and destroy foreign entities. It's an old term, not used much anymore because immunologists recognize how many different cells, with widely varying activities, fall under this umbrella. But Sir Bonington's point was made: no matter what the illness or what the medical treatment, it's ultimately up to our own immune systems to take care of the business of healing.

I've found that military metaphors, overused in so many contexts, fit the immune system perfectly. For this system is quite as breathtakingly complex as the defense department of a superpower nation. It has countless different divisions performing an endless variety of cooperative functions.

The greatest portion of this system has been called a "liquid army." It's an assortment of task-specific cells and substances that are constantly on the lookout for bacteria, viruses, microbes, and other foreign agents that threaten internal security. Each immune task force takes orders from a vast hierarchy, which includes other immune cells and substances, hormones, and nervous system products discharged by the brain. This hierarchy exists because the liquid army needs proper regulation to achieve success. It must respond to its target with specificity and just the right amount of firepower.

The body's immune response is therefore a fully coordinated effort. Command centers, clear signals to the "troops," and open-wire communications are needed to effectively eliminate the threat to the body. The precise degree to which the brain is involved still isn't fully known, but the fact that it is involved—centrally involved—is no longer in doubt. The immune system not only receives messages from the brain but also sends them back to the brain from the "field." Brain-immune communications ensure that our body's defensive maneuvers will be proportionate in strength and intensity.

Like a defense department, the immune system is labyrinthine in its complexity. It has two main branches, the cellular and humoral, with countless subdivisions. The number of different cell types alone boggle the mind. The cellular branch is led by T-cells, the "infantry" of the immune army. The T-cells are broken into major subdivisions, including T-helpers, which spur the troops into action; T-suppressors, which put the brakes on an invasion; and T-killers, which directly liquidate invading microbes, cells, and other substances. Heading the humoral branch are B-cells and the antibodies they manufacture to attack any one of a million different invaders. There are "natural killer" cells, preprogrammed to knock off cancer cells in a manner yet to be understood by immunologists. There is a smorgasbord of other white blood cells, including monocytes and their structural cousins, the macrophages, which are capable of releasing cancer-killing agents called by some "the body's own chemotherapy."

All of these cell types, and many more that I haven't named, perform multiple tasks. In their book, *In Self-Defense,* Steven Mizel, M.D., and Peter Jaret described the coordination that enables the immune system to function properly:

Virtually every cell of the immune system has the power to assist and enhance the activities of every other cell. In the intricate dynamics of a gathering immune response, one cell will activate another, which then activates a third, which may in turn enhance or assist the first. Working in concert, the cells of the immune system are capable of enormous violence.

How do immune cells activate each other? They hand out marching orders in the form of certain messenger molecules. These immune messengers go by different names (like "biological response modifier"), but the simplest is "biological." An immune cell literally squirts out a specific biological, which zeroes in on the proper recipient cell and delivers its biochemical message. These substances enable immune cells to inform, stimulate, inhibit, regulate, rouse, and trigger their comrades in arms. Were it not for these substances, the immune system would be like an army without the functions of command and control.

We've known about these immune messengers for decades. What we hadn't known about, until recently, are the neuropeptide molecules produced in the brain that also send messages to the immune system. What's also new is the discovery of the two-way, nonstop, effusive conversation between our brain and our defense system. Even more recent is our understanding of just how the brain and immune system "talk" to each other.

NEUROPEPTIDES AND THE MIND-BODY CONVERSATION

When Dr. Candace Pert was chief of the brain biochemistry section at the National Institute of Mental Health, she discovered that neuropeptides (*neuro* means they're made by nerve cells; *peptide* refers to their chemical structure) were the preeminent mind-body messengers. Along with Michael Huff, Ph.D., Pert showed that monocytes—those white blood cell defenders—are studded with molecules on their surface, called *receptors,* that are perfect fits for neuropeptides. Each receptor has a biochemical shape, exactly like the interior grooves of a door lock. It's designed precisely to receive a specific neuropeptide "key."

What does that tell us? That our defender cells receive messages sent by our brain and nervous system. Without those receptors, no communication would be possible. With them, the existence of a mind-body conversation is a sure bet.

How substantial is the mind-body conversation? So substantial, the evidence tells us, that calling it a dialogue is an understatement. It's probably more like a marriage. Candace Pert and Michael Huff have found that monocytes have not one or two different receptors for brain chemicals, *they have receptors for virtually every neuropeptide discovered to date,* which means that they can receive a wide variety of messages from the brain.

If monocytes were the only immune cells with these receptors, then the mind-body conversation might be nothing more than occasional chitchat. However, neuropeptide receptors have also been found on lymphocytes, macrophages, and natural killer cells. Not only are these primary cells of the immune system, they are all capable of killing cancer cells. In ways we have yet to fully understand, brain chemicals influence the growth pattern and the actions of our body's defenders, including the very cells we rely upon to protect us from cancer.

The success of an individual in a business, a group artistic endeavor, or a military exercise depends not only on her own skills but on those of her immediate supervisors, her higher-ups, and the vision of the men and women at the very top. By the same token, the success of our body's individual defenders depends on information from other cells in the immune hierarchy *and* from that great overseer, the brain.

MOODS, GUT FEELINGS, AND THE OPIATE SYSTEM

You may have heard about the discovery in the early 1970s of *endorphins,* chemicals produced in the brain that act on our systems like natural painkillers. Endorphins are one of several classes of *opiates:* neuropeptides that are the chemical cousins of morphine. (We usually think of opiates as a class of drugs. As it happens, we make our own opiates, in the brain.) Scientists, including Candace Pert, discovered that our brain cells have receptors for these opiates. Whether it's painkilling drugs we take or painkilling chemicals we make ourselves, both hook up to the exact same molecular

"lock" on brain and other nerve cells, thus altering our consciousness.

In experiments with people in a waking state, Wilder Penfield
and other neurologists showed that the limbic system (which includes the amygdala and hypothalamus) is the emotional center of
the brain. Candace Pert described their experiments: "The neurologists found that when they used electrodes to stimulate the cortex
over the amygdala, they could evoke a whole gamut of emotional
displays—powerful reactions of grief, of pain, of pleasure associated with profound memories. . . ." Pert and her collaborators
mapped the location of opiate receptors in the brain, and found
that the limbic system was "blazing with opiate receptors—forty-
fold higher than in other areas of the brain." This suggests the
crucial role of bodily made opiates in our moods and emotions.

Pert found other emotion-related peptides and peptide receptors in the limbic system and in other parts of the body as well. She
calls them "hot spots" of emotional reactivity.

"The entire lining of the intestine," she said in a recent talk,
"from the esophagus through the large intestine is lined with cells—
nerve cells and other kinds of cells—that contain neuropeptides and
neuropeptide receptors. It seems entirely possible to me that the
richness of the receptors may be why a lot of people feel their
emotions in their gut—why they have a 'gut feeling.' "

Which brings us back to the immune system. A host of immune-cell types have receptors for endorphins and other neuropeptides. These mood-altering brain chemicals can therefore "talk" to
the troops of our immune army. (I'll return to this point, an important clue to the Type C connection.) Therefore opiates, the chemical
conduits of our human emotions, play an intimate and intricate role
in regulating our defense system. And many of the defense forces
influenced by opiates are the ones responsible for cancer protection.

THE LANGUAGE OF BRAIN AND BODY

Candace Pert reports an even more astonishing development. Immune cells not only have receptors for various neuropeptides, they
also manufacture their own neuropeptides. Our defender cells, it
turns out, make some of the same chemicals that control mood in

the brain. In a recent interview, Pert referred to white blood cells as "bits of the brain floating around the body."

In addition, not only do immune cells make brain chemicals, brain cells appear to make immune chemicals, such as interleukin-1, a substance with anticancer activity. I've said that the brain and immune system communicate in order to orchestrate attacks against foreign invaders. Now we understand the true reciprocity of the brain-body dialogue. These discoveries have turned upside down the prevailing assumptions about the strict separation of biological systems. However, from a mind-body perspective such unexpected findings make perfect sense. Brain and body make and receive the same messenger molecules in order to communicate effectively. They "speak" the same language—the language of neuropeptides.

Neuropeptides are a universal language by which cells from different biological systems interact and alter each other's behavior. They are a medium of exchange, and what they share is information. That's why Francis O. Schmidt, an MIT neuroscientist, calls them "informational substances."

THE BODY'S OWN SURVEILLANCE SYSTEM

Now let's return to the question of cancer. Here, the mind-body research I've discussed is meaningful only if the immune system is indeed capable of combating the disease. To this day, some scientists dispute the "immune surveillance" theory, which claims that the immune system patrols the body and eliminates cancer cells before they form tumors. I've carefully reviewed the scientific evidence, and I believe it shows clearly that the immune system *is* able to prevent at least some forms of cancer. And there's no doubt that our defenses are able to halt the *spread* of existing tumors. Immune strength is not the only factor in stopping malignant spread, but it is a very important one.

To help you understand how immune surveillance works, I must explain how cancer gets started in the first place.

We begin with a single normal cell in the awesomely large community of our body's cells—we have about ten trillion of them. This normal cell becomes "transformed" into a cancer cell by a mechanism discovered only in the past decade. It all begins in the genes, the tiny units of DNA strung like beads on a string within the cell nucleus. Each cell has about fifty thousand genes, and each gene contains a blueprint for a vital cellular activity. On a large scale, these activities are the stuff of life. All our physical functions, our looks, our behavior, our personality traits are encoded within these infinitesimally small bits of DNA.

Beginning in the 1970s, molecular biologists discovered that certain "cancer genes" were the triggers that turned normal cells malignant.* These cancer genes began as normal genes that had a specific vital function within the cell. Most often, they served to regulate the cell's growth or energy metabolism. The turn toward malignancy started when this gene was improperly activated: probably it was switched on when it should have remained switched off. The "turned-on" gene causes the manufacture of proteins that make the cell change shape, proliferate madly, and inflict damage on neighboring cells. It's as if the switch on a factory assembly line became stuck, causing products to come barreling down at an unmanageable rate until they overwhelm workers, bottleneck, and smash into each other.

What causes the cancer gene to get switched on inappropriately? Scientists believe that carcinogens, viruses, and radiation are factors that disturb the machinery of the cell. However, they cannot always identify a specific agent that flips the genetic switch. For some cancers, the source remains a mystery. There are various explanations for these seemingly "spontaneous" cancer-causing accidents, including random genetic mutations, a disruptive rearrangement of genes, and the absence of a "suppressor" gene whose job it is to keep cancer genes in check.

We're all exposed to environmental pollutants, such as the chemicals in our air, water, and food. Many of us are exposed to cancer-causing viruses, and most of us are exposed to the ultraviolet rays of sunlight. But cancer researchers are certain that it takes several exposures to carcinogens for one of our cells to turn cancerous. These multiple assaults are required before the cancer gene "switch" will be flipped irreversibly: because there are many stages

*The fact that genes may be the fundamental mechanisms of cancer does not mean all cancers are inherited. In some instances, heredity plays a role, but not for most cancers.

to tumor growth, a single exposure hardly ever causes disease. Fortunately, we have many levels of regulation and defense before and after a cell turns cancerous. Our defense system stands poised to confront the threat at each and every stage of the cancer process.

We have immune sentries—white blood cells—that can surround, ingest, and neutralize carcinogens before they ever attack cells. If carcinogens do disturb our genetic material, our cells have DNA repair mechanisms—enzymes that literally "edit out" gene mutations by snipping them with a form of chemical scissors. Finally, if a cell does become malignant, we have soldier cells that may be able to detect and kill the interloper.

CANCER'S FINGERPRINTS

Our immune system is programmed to distinguish cells and substances that are "self"—that belong to the body—from those that are "nonself," or foreign. Once it recognizes something foreign— whether a bacteria, virus, or fungus—the alarm is sounded and soldier cells are rapidly recruited. We rely on our immune system's exquisite sensitivity in making such distinctions. Mind-body researcher Ted Melnechuk, Ph.D., once remarked that "The immune system is a sensory organ for molecular touch." It must be finely tuned, or we can start attacking our own cells, causing tissue-damaging diseases such as rheumatoid arthritis or lupus.

Cancer presents the peculiar problem of the double agent. The cancer cell started as one of us, a normal cell in the community. When it became cancerous, it switched sides from "one of us" to "one of them"—an invader. Fortunately, our immune cells are not only guards, policemen, and soldiers; they're detectives as well. They have to be. The outlaw cancer cell can, and often does, cloak its identity as a traitor to the community of cells.

Our immune detectives rely on molecular fingerprints to unmask these duplicitous cells. In many types of cancer, cell-surface molecules change when the normal cell turns malignant. These molecules once signaled "self"; now, they signal "nonself." They are the giveaway fingerprints that alert our immune detectives to the traitors within. These markers are known to immunologists as *cancer-specific antigens,* or *tumor-associated antigens.* According to the immune surveillance theory, T-cells and antibodies are the sleuths that recognize these fingerprints as belonging to a foreign agent. Once they do, they commence with a no-holds-barred counterattack.

But a great controversy still surrounds one aspect of this scenario—the part about fingerprints. For three decades scientists have debated whether these cancer-specific fingerprints actually exist. If not, the critics argue, then perhaps our immune systems can do little to protect us from cancer. To simplify an enormously complex and muddy scientific quarrel, the following is known:

Using the most most refined tools of biology, immunologists have isolated a handful of cancer-specific antigens on animal and human tumor cells, but only for certain types of cancer. These include melanoma and leukemia cells. For other types, the fingerprints found have been considered too "faint": they are neither sufficiently specific nor bold enough to be easily detected by the immune system. Furthermore, a few innocent normal cells may possess similar prints. Future investigations will unravel the mystery of whether specific markers exist on *all* malignant cells and we just haven't found them yet; or whether they exist only on some cells. The research in this area remains very promising, and someday, vaccines containing cancer antigens may be used to immunize people against the disease. Such vaccines are already in development for certain cancers, including melanoma and lung cancer.

SECRET WEAPONS

Today, there is new hope on the horizon regarding the immune system's power to fight cancer. The proof of this power may no longer rest solely on the existence of specific cancer markers. The reason? Recent research reveals that our defense system may not always need to "see" fingerprints. To be sure, our immune detectives—T-cells and antibodies—must recognize crystal-clear prints before going into action. They rely on absolute specificity.

But we also have *nonspecific* immune factors that *don't* require unmistakable markers. They are the secret weapons in our anticancer defense arsenal. Monocytes, macrophages, and natural killer cells are all capable of nonspecific action. They seem able to recognize cancer cells without detecting fingerprints, and head straight into battle with their appointed adversaries. Without marching orders from any other cell, these immune fighters literally grasp hold of malignant cells and pulverize them. What's more, these and other immune cells make biological substances capable of slowing down or even annihilating cancer cells. The interferons, interleukin-2, and tumor necrosis factor (TNF) are the most well known cancer-fighting chemicals produced by our own bodies.

Thanks to recombinant DNA techniques, scientists are now able to reproduce these agents outside the body and manufacture them in large quantities. The interferons, interleukin-2, and TNF have all been used, with some success, to treat cancer patients with established tumors. Stephen A. Rosenberg, M.D., of the National Cancer Institute has employed these substances clinically in a variety of creative ways. He's injected patients with immune cells activated by interleukin-2, and despite side effects, he's documented some remarkable cures. Rosenberg has just begun treating patients with advanced melanoma, using their own cancer-fighting lymphocytes. (These are the same types of cells I measured in melanoma patients to determine the strength of their defenses.) He's genetically altered these cells by inserting a gene that instructs them to produce TNF—a potent cancer-killing agent. Rosenberg hopes that these TNF-armed lymphocytes will home in on melanoma cells and eliminate them from the body.

Overall, the results of such studies have been mixed. But there's no doubt that some cancer patients have enjoyed complete remissions as a result of treatment with the body's own defensive chemicals. Cancer "immunotherapy" remains in the early stages of development, but it affords great hope for the future of cancer treatment. In the twenty-first century, potent "cocktails" comprised of the body's own products may supplant chemotherapy and radiation as the primary treatment for human cancer.

Lloyd J. Old, M.D., formerly of the Sloan-Kettering Institute and now head of the Ludwig Cancer Research Institute, is a codiscoverer of TNF, a substance with the uncanny ability to cause animal tumors to shrivel up, blacken, and die within hours of administration. Dr. Old is one of our leading cancer immunologists, and in a recent article he assessed the new medical therapies that put our own immune defenses to work against cancer:

If we are fortunate, the new treatments will consistently arouse the body's natural anticancer forces and produce the tumor regressions that have fueled the imagination of generations of cancer researchers. The forces exist; the task ahead is to find ways to unleash them.

All of this is testimony to the fact that our bodies house a powerful arsenal against cancer. The question should no longer be "Can our bodies effectively wipe out cancer?" but "Why *don't* our bodies effectively wipe out cancer?"

CANCER AND IMMUNE SUPPRESSION

One reason our defenses can fail has to do with the caginess of cancer cells. Malignant cells have been shown capable of slipping by our immune sentries to avoid destruction. How do they do it? They find a way to mask their molecular fingerprints. Some cancer cells actually shed the antigens that reveal their outlaw identity. They're like the cat burglar who commits his crime and quickly changes garb the moment he hits the street.

The other theory—the one I wish to focus on because it's most relevant to mind-body communication—is that tumors develop because our immune systems aren't doing their job. There's a malfunction somewhere in the defense network. For years, the data to support this has been spotty, but it's beginning to build. People with weakened immune systems are indeed more vulnerable to certain cancers.

We know that patients infected with HIV (the AIDS virus), whose immune systems are often damaged beyond repair, are highly vulnerable to cancers of the lymph glands and Kaposi's sarcoma, an aggressive skin cancer. Even more compelling evidence has come from studies of patients who have undergone organ transplants. For a period of time after transplantation, they receive drugs that suppress immunity so they won't reject the foreign tissue being implanted in their bodies. The unfortunate side effect is diminished immune strength and a rising risk of infections. Today it is clear that such immune-suppressed patients also have a greater chance of malignancy for years to come.

Compared with the general population, transplant patients have much higher rates of certain lymphomas, skin cancers, liver cancers, Kaposi's sarcoma, and cancers of the external genitalia. So says Irving Penn, M.D., professor of surgery at the University of Cincinnati, who helped found the Cincinnati Tumor Transplant

Registry two decades ago. It's the only registry of its kind, and Dr. Penn has accumulated data on more than forty-five hundred transplant patients with cancer.

"These cancers are clearly a result of being immunosuppressed," Dr. Penn said in a 1989 *New York Times* article. "If people have impaired immunity, they are predisposed to cancer."

Several medical teams have come up with a logical idea for treating transplant patients with cancer. They simply reduced the dose of immune-suppressing drugs, in the hope that the immune system would bounce back and destroy the cancer cells. In a majority of cases, that's exactly what happened. Thomas Starzl, M.D., a transplant surgeon who cofounded the registry with Dr. Penn, said that his patients' tumors "would shrink or disappear" when he dropped the dose of immune-suppressing drugs.

Ronald Herberman, M.D., director of the Pittsburgh Cancer Institute, has spearheaded research on transplant patients and cancer. He, too, has found that many lymphomas and most Kaposi's sarcomas literally "melt away" after patients cut back on their drugs. Michael Nalesnik, M.D., a pathologist on the University of Pittsburgh transplant team, commented, "The logical conclusion is that patients are rejecting tumors because of their normal immune response. And that normal people do this all the time without realizing it."

These findings suggest that "immune surveillance" must exist and function to prevent at least some types of cancer. Lewis Thomas, M.D., the renowned researcher and author of several books, including *The Lives of a Cell,* talked about the promise of cancer immunology in a recent talk:

> I am still convinced that the reason why about 75 percent of us will never develop cancer in a full lifetime is that 75 percent of us are equipped with an immunological apparatus sufficiently agile and sensitive for the first clone of neoplastic cells to be quickly recognized and gotten rid of. What needs clarification is the reason for the failure of immune reactivity in the approximately 25 to 30 percent of us who do develop cancer.

We don't know all the answers to Thomas's final question, but we do know that environmental agents, genetic inheritance, dietary habits, and psychological factors are among the elements that determine how strong, and how sensitive, our defenses will be.

THE THREAT OF METASTASES

While questions linger concerning the immune system's ability to prevent *all* types of cancer from developing, *there is little doubt that our defenses can stop existing tumors from spreading.* And that is cancer's greatest threat: it's capacity to spread, or *metastasize.*

Once a tumor has formed in the body, the greatest danger is that a single cell or cells will break away from the pack and enter the lymphatic system. From there, the cell can actually bore through lymphatic vessels and capillaries to enter the bloodstream, where it travels to distant sites. If the blood-borne cancer cell finds safe harbor in or near a vital organ, it can "set up shop" there and begin a new colony of malignant cells. This is the origin of a metastastic tumor. Invariably, these metastases, which spread from the original tumor, are the final triumph of cancer over the body. Once vital organs are affected, such as the lungs or the liver, the disease becomes vastly more difficult to treat.

A patient's original tumor is rarely the cause of death. "Metastases are what kills patients with cancer," said Lance A. Liotta, M.D., the chief of the pathology laboratory at the National Cancer Institute, in a 1989 article in *The New York Times.*

As it happens, we have a particular immune soldier that specializes in destroying wayward cancer cells—the kind that make their way into the bloodstream and create lethal metastases. It's the natural killer, or NK cell. Natural killers are unique in their ability to destroy blood-borne malignant cells without any help from other immune cells. In effect, they are capable of conducting a "quick strike" against cancer cells that have escaped recognition by the other soldiers of immunity.

NATURAL-KILLERS: LEADING THE RESISTANCE

NK cells provide us with the strongest evidence to date of the mind-immune connection in cancer. Leading the charge in NK research is Dr. Ronald B. Herberman, who discovered the existence of these cells in 1972. For over a decade, Herberman and Sandra Levy, Ph.D., former director of the Pittsburgh Cancer Institute's Biobehavioral Oncology Program, collaborated on a remarkable series of studies of psychological factors in the growth of breast cancer. Their work has been based on the assumption that NK cells really can stop the spread of cancer.

The ability of NK cells to vanquish cancer cells traveling in the bloodstream has been proved in many dramatic animal studies. Immunologists believe that animal immune systems—including those of mice—are sufficiently similar to a human's to infer that we, too, have natural killers that stop the spread of cancer.

John Hiserodt, M.D., former head of the Pittsburgh Cancer Institute Immunology Program, collaborated with Herberman and Levy in their mind-body research. In a recent interview, he described some astonishing animal studies of NK cell capabilities:

We have techniques to deplete the NK cells from a mouse, to totally wipe them out. Then, if you inject tumor cells, you wouldn't believe what happens to its lungs. They explode with tumors. So there's no doubt that NK cells are controlling the spread of tumor cells. There's also no doubt that if I put a tumor back into that animal, and then transferred back those killer cells, the tumor just shrinks and disappears. Whether NK cells can prevent a primary tumor from forming is uncertain. But once a tumor cell has escaped into the bloodstream, that is the point where NK cells are critically controlling things.

Later, Hiserodt stressed the crucial part these killer cells must play in the lives of cancer patients:

What do patients die of? They die of their metastases, not primary tumors. We can treat primary tumors, we can cut them out, we can melt them down with chemotherapy agents, but patients may still die of metastases. Therefore, ultimately, in terms of the cancer patient, the NK cells may be the most important thing that enables them to live.

PSYCHOLOGICAL FACTORS AND NATURAL KILLERS

A fascinating body of recent evidence concludes that psychological factors alter natural killer cell activity. Drs. Herberman and Levy provided some of the earliest and most compelling data.

They began their unusual and fruitful collaboration in the early 1980s at the National Cancer Institute. They continued to work together on mind-body research at the Pittsburgh Cancer Institute. (Dr. Levy also headed the Biobehavioral Oncology Program, a unique effort to provide psychological treatments for cancer patients and study mind-body relationships in cancer. In 1991, she left the institute to pursue training as an Episcopal priest, though she intends to remain a psychologist and scholar, and return to the field in some capacity. A replacement is now being sought who will take over all of her previous activities in mind-body-cancer research.) With Herberman's expertise in immunology and Levy's in behavioral psychology, the two found common ground in human studies of coping and cancer. They analyzed cancer patients' behavior and their NK cells using sophisticated lab tests measuring not only the number of killer cells, but also their activity—how effective they were in vanquishing target cells.

As I reported in Chapter 5, Levy found that breast cancer patients who appeared "adjusted" to their illness, fatigued, apathetic, and who lacked social support had more cancerous lymph nodes and weaker NK cells. Levy's profile recalled the passive, helpless style I'd observed among Type C patients.

Levy continued to track this group of breast cancer patients. Her data as of this writing is preliminary, but they add a new twist to the earlier findings. The passive patients not only sustained low levels of NK activity, they also tended to suffer earlier recurrences. Levy learned that patients with a Type C–like coping style may have increased vulnerability to the spread of cancer. Her successor at the Pittsburgh Cancer Institute will continue to follow up on this patient population.

How, exactly, could Type C behavior weaken immunity and leave people susceptible to cancer? The answer involves those chemical messengers, the neuropeptides, and possibly, a variety of molecules that make up the mind-body conversation. I'll return to this critical question later in this chapter.

Levy and Herberman addressed another crucial question: can

a cancer patient change her coping style and strengthen her natural killer defenses? Would this help prevent metastases and increase her chance of survival?

Levy and Herberman searched for answers to these questions. Along with Judith Rodin, Ph.D., a professor of psychology at Yale University, and Martin Seligman, Ph.D., a professor of psychology at the University of Pennsylvania, they conducted a pilot study of patients with melanoma and colon cancer to see if psychological treatments could boost the patients' natural immunity. Thirty patients were recruited. All received the standard medical treatment, but half were given an eight-week course in relaxation techniques and cognitive therapy. The relaxation helped the patients reduce stress and the cognitive treatments helped them cope with depression, regain control, and cultivate optimism.

In his book, *Learned Optimism,* Dr. Seligman described Sandra Levy's reaction when she got the first definitive results from their study:

"Holy Cow! You should have seen those numbers." I have never heard Sandy as excited as she was on the phone that November morning, two years later. 'The natural killer cell activity is up *very* sharply in the cancer patients who got cognitive therapy. Not at all in the controls. Holy Cow!' In short, cognitive therapy strongly enhanced immune activity—just as we hoped it would.

Not only did the therapy patients have stronger natural killers, they were less depressed and self-blaming. Rodin, Seligman, and their colleagues at the Pittsburgh Cancer Institute will track these patients to see whether therapy also increases their life span.

Levy, Herberman, and their collaborators have provided a sound scientific basis for a revolutionary concept: healthy coping can substantially bolster our *cellular* defense against the spread of cancer. I'll further explore the immune-boosting, cancer-protective role of psychological treatments in Chapter 12.

Herberman is now overseeing an enlarged research effort at the Pittsburgh Cancer Institute, which will include an entire team of immunologists along with Levy's successor. With the help of a large grant from the MacArthur Foundation, the group will expand its research on mind-immune relationships and the role of psychological factors in the development, growth, prevention, and treatment of cancer.

In a recent conversation, Dr. Herberman summed up his view of the role of the mind in cancer. "I wouldn't want to make the argument or even imply that psychological factors are paramount," he said. "But I think they represent one component of significant factors that regulate the functioning of the immune system." Herberman added that our natural defenses could perhaps be boosted with drugs, biologicals, psychological treatments, or a judicious combination of all three. "I don't see them as choices in conflict, because I'd like us to use as many different weapons as we can."

LONELINESS AND SELF-SACRIFICE

Our natural-killer defenses appear to be highly sensitive to subtle psychological influences. This is the conclusion of another mind-body research team specializing in NK cells. Janice Kiecolt-Glaser, Ph.D., a psychologist, and Ronald Glaser, M.D., an immunologist, collaborate on PNI investigations at Ohio State University. They studied first-year medical students and found that the stress of exams caused a drop in both the number and activity of natural killer cells. But here's the more telling discovery: the students who said they felt extremely lonely had the *least* active NK cells. Loneliness compounded the normal effects of stress and further weakened the students' defenses. The Glasers's finding was consistent with the conclusions of many other researchers who've shown that unless our needs for nurturance and social support are met, our immune systems and overall health can be threatened.

In a recent investigation, Kiecolt-Glaser and Glaser studied people who were caregivers for close relatives with Alzheimer's disease. When compared with a control group, the caregivers had suffered a marked loss of immune strength—especially among their T-cell defenses.

The caregivers found themselves in a grueling situation, having to endure difficult daily routines and the deterioration of a loved one. But they were not simply stressed; they were also forced by circumstances into a largely self-sacrificing role. These caregivers had to put their needs aside for the benefit of the patient. In some respects, they'd been thrust into a situation that mimics the one

Type C copers construct for themselves after years of conditioning. The Type C person puts her needs aside for the benefit of others— even in the face of painful losses or traumas. She, too, may experience a diminution of immune strength during times of great stress because she doesn't have the resources to take care of herself. In this sense, self-sacrifice and loneliness may be related. The Type C individual is often lonely because she is unable to get support or use the support system that's available to her. I believe that the Type C caregiver—or anyone put in that role—may retain her immune power by finding her own sources of nurturance. More on this in later chapters.

HELPLESSNESS AND THE OPIATE CONNECTION

I've said that the most dangerous mind states, in terms of their effect on our vital defenses, are chronic hopelessness and helplessness. In a number of experiments, researchers have found ingenious ways to re-create these mind states in rodents. The studies show that rats placed in situations where they are helpless to eliminate a source of stress suffer serious damage to their immune defenses.

One researcher has forged an intriguing new connection between helplessness and immune power. UCLA psychologist Yehuda Shavit, Ph.D., set up a study in which one group of mice received shocks to their tails but could turn off the shock by learning to press a lever. Another group received a shock at the same time as the first group, and had their shock turned off at the same time as their counterparts. But this second group had no control over ending the shock. In other words, they were helpless. Compared with the "in control" mice, the helpless mice had more sluggish NK cells and faster growth of implanted tumors. But Shavit also discovered that the helpless mice had higher levels of opiates, the painkilling chemicals made in the brain. In a series of elegant experiments, he found that the opiates were indeed *responsible* for the weakening of their immune cells and the rapidity of their tumor growth.

Shavit believes that the helpless animals go into a state of mind-body analgesia. Their brains react to stress that they cannot escape by releasing a gush of numbing biochemicals. The opiates, in turn, attach to immune-cell receptors and "instruct" them to put on the brakes. Hence, the sudden drop in NK-cell potency. The same mechanism may explain why people addicted to opiate drugs are particularly vulnerable to infections and all manner of diseases. (They are also exposed to many disease agents, including HIV, through needles.)

Shavit's mice who had control over their shocks did *not* have excess opiates. Nor did they have damaged immune systems. Scientists are now teasing out an intricate web of relationships between opiates and the immune system. On one hand, it seems that "normal" stress triggers the release of a quick burst of opiates that either has no effect or actually boosts immunity. (Exercisers who engage in moderately strenuous activity, like jogging, have been shown to benefit from a short-term rise in endorphin levels.) It's the body's innate preparation for an injury that may occur during our reaction to acute stress. On the other hand, prolonged or unavoidable stress may send our opiate systems into overdrive. Our brains then release a steady surge of narcotizing neuropeptides. This surplus of opiates is the possible culprit in the weakening of our defenses. Another explanation for this effect is that different classes of opiates are secreted during chronic, inescapable stress, types which down-regulate rather than up-regulate the activity of certain immune cells.

Perhaps this is why day-to-day stresses don't have a negative impact on our bodies. Many of us experience garden-variety stress in a positive light, as a challenge to be overcome. Studies suggest that "normal" stress can even *improve* health. But when a person confronts inescapable stress—or when he has a built-in tendency to react helplessly—he may let down, burn out, and give up. That's when he becomes illness-prone, like the helpless mice who could not control their fate.

TYPE C, OPIATES, AND HUMAN IMMUNITY

Now we have human studies showing that repressive (Type C) coping can compromise our immune defenses. While at the department of psychology of Yale Medical School, psychologist Gary Schwartz led a team of researchers studying 312 clinic-treated patients. Schwartz discovered that patients who were repressors had far fewer monocytes—key defender cells—than the rest of the sample. People who coped with stress in a "defensive high-anxious" manner had even lower counts.

You may recall my study with David Sweet, in which we found that defensive high-anxious patients had the thickest tumors. These were Type C individuals whose psychological defenses were coming apart at the seams. They felt anxiety but didn't have the experience, or the coping skills, to be able to express and resolve their anxiety. This left them prone to feelings of helplessness and hopelessness—the most dangerous mind states in terms of health.

Schwartz's findings mirror my earlier conclusions: Type C copers who blot out negative feelings (repressors) may sustain long-term damage to their immune functions. When their psychological defenses falter (as in the defensive high anxious), leading to unresolved anxiety or hopelessness, even more harm may come to their defense network.

Schwartz's repressors, and his defensive high-anxious individuals, had something in common biologically with the helpless rodents I told you about. After analyzing a series of blood and hormonal tests, Schwartz concluded that both groups had increased levels of opiates in their brains and bodies. The excess opiates, he said, were a result of repressive coping. And the excess opiates had helped cause the drop in their immune cells.

Schwartz's theory is one plausible and specific explanation for why Type C behavior makes people vulnerable to cancer. Certainly there are other mechanisms, other pathways between mind and body that underlie the cancer connection. In the next section, I will show how stress hormones, such as adrenaline, may be involved in weakening our cancer defenses. However, I've implicated two primary psychological factors in cancer: Type C behavior and underlying hopelessness/helplessness. Both seem to result in an overproduction of painkilling chemicals in our bodies. These opiates, in turn, may dampen our cancer defenses and therefore increase our risk for the growth of certain tumors.

THE MIND-BODY EFFECTS OF THE TYPE C TRAP

Here is a simplified version of what I see as an amazingly complex mind-body interaction. In our brains, emotional stress or pain is processed similarly to physical stress or pain. We respond immediately with the "fight or flight" instinct. For the Type C person, this instinct gets short-circuited. When he finds himself in an emotionally threatening situation—when he's made angry or scared—his past conditioning allows him no outlet.

Let's take the example of a Type C fellow who's regularly abused by his boss. During any given week, he is subjected to humiliating tirades. Were he to respond by yelling or even talking back, he's convinced he'd be fired instantly. On the other hand, if he simply walks away, he risks his boss's disfavor. For the nice guy, it's a classic double-bind circumstance. He has two alternative responses that would change the situation, and both have liabilities he can't bear. (This is also called an "avoidance-avoidance conflict.") All he feels he can do is stand there and take it with a smile.

Like our animal brethren, we humans respond to threat with the fight or flight response. Our bodies are pitched at a state of readiness for either action or retreat. *Our Type C fellow can't respond to the threat with fight or flight.* But the threat isn't diminished—the boss keeps abusing him—and his inner tension builds. When he keeps up this behavior for months and years, his body responds to the unrelieved stress with a steady stream of opiates. He'll be fatigued, lack spark and energy, and remain passive in the face of life's vicissitudes—much like Sandra Levy's NK-depressed cancer patients. He makes his way in the world like an automobile with the emergency brake on. He may feel tired or distressed, but he won't realize that his body's immune army is being depleted.

Repressors react to stress with comparatively more physical tension. Experiments have shown that they have increased heart rate, breathing rate, and skin resistance in response to stress. This supports the "discharge" theory of emotion: if anxiety and anger aren't expressed, the person is constantly agitated just below the surface.

When an animal or human experiences the fight or flight response, his body is primed to act. His mind-body will go through the cycle that begins with assessing danger and quickly moves to bodily readiness, physical action, emotional discharge, and finally, back to a resting state. If he neither fights nor flees, he's stuck at the stage just prior to action, where stress hormones—such as adrenaline—are surging through his body, along with the opiates I told you about. These hormones, which include corticosteroids, have also been shown to deplete our immune systems. (T-cells and other immune defenders have receptors for many stress hormones and are influenced by them.) So repressors not only suffer from opiate overload, they may also have higher levels of the stress hormones that suppress immunity. The overall result, as I've discussed, is damage to our T-cell forces, our cancer-killing macrophages, and our ever-vigilant NK cells.

Indeed, the entire mind-body communications network I have described—starting with the emotional centers in the brain, mediated by neuropeptide messengers such as the opiates, and stress hormones like adrenaline, and ending with changes in the actions of our immune-cell defenders—appears to be involved in the relationship between Type C behavior and the growth of cancer.

If we're constantly stuck in a no-man's land between fight and flight, we never diffuse the mind-body tension experienced during stress. This chronic tension, a product of feelings unresolved and actions never taken, gradually erodes our best defense against disease.

TYPE C AND OTHER DISEASES

Type C's are prone to other diseases as well. He or she may be vulnerable to infections and autoimmune disorders, which result from immunological imbalance. Studies have linked the repressor personality to asthma, arthritis, and high blood pressure. In the 1960s, George F. Solomon, M.D., while working at Stanford University, studied the personality of patients with rheumatoid arthritis, that painful disease causing inflamed joints. Solomon and his colleague, Rudolf Moos, Ph.D., described the arthritis patients as generally "quiet; introverted; reliable; conscientious; restricted in their expression of emotion, particularly anger; conforming; self-sacrificing, tending to allow themselves to be imposed upon; sensitive to criticism; distant; overactive and busy; stubborn; rigid; and controlling." The first eight characteristics have been explicitly described as part of the Type C constellation.

Type C may even play a role in HIV infection and AIDS. AIDS patients endure a rapid deterioration of their immune system. Dr. Solomon and I hypothesized that psychological factors might influence the progression of the disease. With the help of several colleagues, we conducted long-term studies of patients with

AIDS and HIV-related symptoms. We discovered several connections between psychological coping and immune strength in these
patients. For example, among eighteen AIDS patients (including a
number of long-survivors of the disease), we found that patients
who were less anxious and fatigued, who were able to withdraw and
nurture themselves, and who were able to say no to requests for
favors they did not want to do, had more or better-functioning
immune cells of various types.

The AIDS patients who had more favorable immune profiles
appeared to be less stressed, more assertive, and more able to take
care of their own needs. They were able to resist the temptation to
be the nice guy in the face of their illness. In pilot research, Solomon
and I interviewed a small group of long-survivors. Our informal
findings showed what our formal research later helped to confirm—the survivors had meaning in their lives, they were problem-
solvers, they had a sense of control over their lives and fate, they
expressed their needs and feelings, and they took charge of their
medical care.

All these factors imply that AIDS patients with a better prognosis, including long-survivors, are *not* Type C—they are active,
expressive, and assertive. The inverse may also hold true: AIDS
patients with Type C characteristics may be at risk for faster disease
progression. I must add that the number of patients we studied was
small and our findings are preliminary. More research is needed to
confirm and expand upon our research.

Dr. Solomon believes that Type C–like behaviors can lead to
a variety of diseases of immune dysfunction. Why, then, would
some Type C copers get cancer, and others, say, arthritis? For the
answer, we must return to the dynamic model of medicine, which
tells us that many variables contribute to a person's illness. Undoubtedly, heredity will dictate "predispositions"—constitutional
weaknesses for one disease or another. (Rheumatoid arthritis, for
example, has a genetic component.) Environmental pollutants,
viruses, and dietary factors can tip the balance toward a specific
disease entity. Nonetheless, I believe that Type C behavior takes a
particular toll on those divisions of the immune army responsible
for cancer protection.

THE MYSTERY AT LIVERMORE LABORATORIES

In 1979, there was a strange cancer scare at the Lawrence Livermore Laboratories in California, a research facility for the production of strategic nuclear arms. A high incidence of malignant melanoma was uncovered at the facility. Health officials, fearing the presence of some unknown source of radiation or other environmental hazard, conducted a full-scale investigation. They never found a definite cause, but their efforts included extremely careful screening of every employee for undetected melanomas. To everyone's surprise, they uncovered a sizable number of people with very early stage melanomas. Most of these patients were easily cured with surgical removal of the primary tumor.

This occurred just as I began my research on melanoma patients from the UCSF Melanoma Clinic. I decided to conduct a separate pilot study with the people from Livermore, all of whom had either precancerous lesions or extremely small, thin tumors. I interviewed many such patients and studied the videotapes carefully. I saw no psychological pattern like the one I'd discovered among the scores of melanoma patients from the clinic. The patients from Livermore were decidedly *not* Type C.

I soon came upon a likely and telling explanation for this phenomenon: these early tumors would never have been detected without the extensive screening by health officials. Does that mean all of these people would have gone on to develop thicker, life-threatening melanomas? No, I thought. The original group of melanoma patients that caused the scare may have been just a fluke. But the early stage patients found later were discovered only because they were examined with a fine-toothed comb. I believe that, in most cases, their own immune defenses would have kept their tumors in check or even eliminated them.

Likewise, if everyone in your hometown were checked head to toe for early melanomas, I wouldn't be surprised if larger-than-expected numbers turned up. The point is this: we all have an innate ability to control some tumors, especially if they are small and localized.

How were the Livermore patients different from my UCSF melanoma patients? I believe that the non–Type C patients from Livermore had their immune defenses intact, while the Type C patients at UCSF had suppressed immunity. That's why the Livermore group had limited tumor growth and the clinic-based patients had more aggressive and dangerous tumors.

The Livermore episode provided me with early clues to immune suppression among Type C individuals. Later, I turned up data that validated my theory. That was the study, described in Chapter 5, in which I found that emotional expressors had slower-growing tumors and a stronger immune response, and nonexpressors had faster-growing tumors and a weaker defense.

There may be other mechanisms our mind-body uses to prevent the growth of tumors. Each and every cell has a DNA repair apparatus that can circumvent cancer, and one recent study, led by Dr. Janice Kiecolf-Glaser, found that emotional distress can harm this built-in protection. Hormonal imbalances, influenced by the mind, may cause some malignancies, including breast cancer. Perhaps emotions play an important role in maintaining proper hormone balance and warding off tumors. But the best evidence we now have indicates that cancer and the mind are linked through the immune system.

Can Type C patients reverse the harmful physical effects of their behavior? Can behavior change actually boost recovery, and if so, what changes really work? The research to date teaches us that expressing emotions can awaken mind and body and fortify the natural power we all have to resist cancer. But expressing emotions is no simple prescription, and it's not the sole factor in transforming Type C behavior. In the final chapters of this book, I'll show how cancer patients, and people wishing to prevent the disease, can change their pattern to enhance wellness.

CHAPTER 10

Disease can be a real opportunity, and it can be an opportunity without your having to lay a guilt trip on yourself. In other words, disease is not caused by a lesson you are giving yourself but, if you choose, you can turn disease into something to learn from, or something to motivate you toward more balance or harmony in your life.

—Ken Wilber

An appropriate sense of guilt makes people try to be better. But an excessive sense of guilt, a tendency to blame ourselves for things which are clearly not our fault, robs us of self-esteem and perhaps of our capacity to grow and act.

—Harold S. Kushner

I must confess that I find the notion of 'positive' emotions a disturbing concept and perhaps even a dangerous one. At best, it implies that there is a way to live, a certain set of attitudes that may guarantee survival. At worst, the concept of positive emotions can degenerate into self-tyranny and may lead the individual into some kind of mind control. Many people now seem to fear harboring "negative" emotions or "wrong" thoughts in the same way people used to fear having evil thoughts.

—Rachel Naomi Remen, M.D.

I am content to follow to its source
Every event in action or in thought;
Measure the lot; forgive myself the lot!
When such as I cast out remorse
So great a swellness flows into the breast
We must laugh and we must sing,
We are blest by everything,
Everything we look upon is blest.

—W. B. Yeats

Blaming the Victim and Other Traps

Knowledge of the human mind has both the potential to help people grow and the potential to cause suffering. The same holds true for most areas of knowledge. Nuclear physics can be used to produce energy or make atom bombs. Medical knowledge can be used for unethical experiments or lifesaving clinical applications. Knowledge of history can be used by despots to rule or by liberators to spawn democracy. In my field, mind-body treatments can be used responsibly to help people achieve wholeness and health, or they can be abused, causing people the undue suffering of self-blame.

When the mind-body connection is understood correctly, and applied with care, therapists and patients alike know—on a gut level—that no one is to blame for their illness or its progression.

I've told you about the role of Type C behavior in cancer, and in upcoming chapters I'm going to show how changing Type C behavior can aid in the prevention and treatment of cancer. I call this program *Type C transformation,* and it is one form of mind-body medicine. Other mind-body practitioners emphasize relaxation, guided imagery, visualization, and dream analysis. These are all methods for mobilizing our own natural healing abilities to help in the fight against cancer.

When misapplied and misunderstood, mind-body approaches

can lead patients to believe that they caused their own cancers. This theme of self-inflicted illness has several variations. Some patients think they brought cancer on themselves by living "wrong." Others feel they are being punished for a lifetime of "bad" behavior. Patients have also been known to blame a relapse on their "failure" to use their minds effectively to combat the disease.

These beliefs are mental traps, often set unintentionally by mind-body "healers" or other trusted individuals who unwittingly give vulnerable patients distorted ideas about mind and body. In my clinical work with cancer patients, I've helped them to avoid the trap of self-blame. As I've said throughout this book, even though Type C behavior may contribute to cancer development, the pattern itself carries no implication of blame. The Type C person's coping difficulties came about *unintentionally* as a by-product of early conditioning. Patients should be encouraged to identify their behavior pattern while, at the same time, to learn the art of self-compassion as an antidote to blame. They need to recognize that their behavior originated as a survival technique when they were dependent children with no other choice. How could they possibly be at fault?

A few basic realizations can help patients overcome self-blame:

Type C behavior is not intentional and it is not shameful.
Type C behavior is not a sign of psychological or spiritual impoverishment.
Type C behavior has been your best attempt to handle pain and stress.
Type C behavior is only one of many factors in cancer risk and recovery.
Cancer is not your fault.
Cancer is no sign of weakness, failure, or personal inadequacy.
Cancer is not a result of your basic "personality."
Your fight for recovery is no test of character.

While these are simple statements of fact, accepting them is not always so easy. That's why patients need to find sources of self-love that enable them to embrace these basic truths. This allows them to diffuse self-blame in every area of their lives, including the blame they heap on themselves for their behavior patterns, problematic relationships, addictions, unhappiness, *and for their illness.* All of this self-blame is harmful, it is toxic, and it is common in Type C individuals—that is, to people who have trouble expressing emotions and standing up for themselves.

Certain cultural myths fuel the self-blame that occurs among cancer patients. When I work with Type C patients, I help them get rid of blame by dismantling these myths. They include the "mind-over-matter" myth, the "self-inflicted illness" myth, and the "macho cancer-fighter" myth. Later in this chapter, I'll describe these myths, explain why they are groundless, and why Type C people are so susceptible to them. By tackling the problem of self-blame, these patients do more than eliminate guilt for their illness. For the first time, they develop real self-compassion.

Many conservative doctors and scientists have decried all of mind-body science, citing the specter of self-blame. In my view, their overreaction represents a tragic turn backward. It's like saying, "This knowledge can be dangerous in the wrong hands, so let's pretend it doesn't exist." Rather than push aside this knowledge, we should learn to apply it with intelligence and care so that people with serious illness can cultivate hope and empowerment instead of unnecessary guilt.

In my view, hope and empowerment are what mind-body medicine is all about. I'm afraid that doctors who dismiss the entire field are unknowingly robbing patients of a sense of control over their fate. This loss would be as hurtful to them as self-blame. Telling a patient that his mental state is irrelevant is another form of victimization. The message is, "You're deceiving yourself if you turn within for any source of emotional or spiritual energy that could be said to bolster your physical recovery." This leads to passive faith, in which patients can only pray that the god of medicine or God above will look well upon them. In my research, I've found that patients do best when they say, "I'm going to participate in my recovery and do everything in my power to see that the drug (or radiation or surgery) works."

I know that cancer patients can recognize and change Type C behavior without self-blame. Moreover, when patients identify their own pattern, they often feel relief. "That's me!" they say when reading or hearing a description of Type C. "You've hit the nail on the head—that's how I've always been." They feel less alone and more understood, as do people with other addictive patterns when they step forward at a twelve-step meeting and share their experience with a group. They give their pattern a name that acknowl-edges their problem, unites them with others who know the same pain, and provides them with pathways to transformation. When they see connections between their behavior and their ill-health, they open to the possibility of life changes that not only improve their quality of life but also their quality of health.

Most of my colleagues, and many of my patients, care deeply about this issue. We are concerned that some within our ranks have unintentionally contributed to self-blame. But we reject efforts to disparage all mind-body medicine on the pretext of concern about self-blame. We don't want the baby thrown out with the bathwater. We know there is a way to tap the healing potential of the mind that not only avoids blame but redresses the problem of self-blame at the deepest levels.

In the following pages you will hear the eloquent voices of those who've spoken out on the problem of blame. They are voices struggling to come to terms with difficult questions, searching for the most realistic, compassionate, and useful way to apply mind-body medicine. These voices belong to doctors, therapists, and cancer patients themselves.

SPEAKING OUT ON BLAME

The crux of the blame problem can be summed up in one question: how do we embrace our own power to heal illness without taking on the burden of self-blame?

One of the cancer patients I've had in therapy gave a passion-ate answer. Ron, a forty-year-old man with melanoma, was in the process of changing his Type C pattern. He had faith that the transformation he was undergoing would bolster his recovery on all levels—emotional, spiritual, and physical. He was exceptionally open and articulate. In one of our sessions, I asked him whether he blamed himself for his cancer and whether he would blame himself if he suffered a recurrence. Here is how he responded:

> I want to explore my behavior. I know it affects me on all sorts of levels. That includes my health. I'm trying to take responsibility for the ways in which my behavior has kept me unhappy and unfulfilled. Otherwise, how could I change it?

How can anyone change unless they take responsibility? I know that people worry about blame. I don't blame myself for anything. I'm trying to take a hard look at where I've been, where I am, and where I'm going. None of this means that I'm punishing myself for past mistakes. I've learned how pointless that is. It's not fair and it's not true. In fact, the harder I look at this, the more I see that I'm *not* to blame for the years I've spent denying myself.

Later in our talk, Ron referred directly to his cancer:

I guess some people think it's OK to say that your behavior can make you miserable, but it's not OK to say that your behavior can make you sick. Why do we have to draw the line at the body? I suppose I'll never know for sure, but yeah, I think my past behavior had something to do with my illness. I don't think that means I got cancer because I'm messed up or because I made mistakes or because I wanted to get cancer. I never wanted to be unhappy, to deny my feelings, to let people take advantage of me. And I certainly never wanted to get sick! I was stuck, and now I realize how deep-seated it was and how hard it is to change. What I am trying to do is face reality and care for myself at the same time.

Soon after her mastectomy, Naomi, age thirty-two, went into treatment with a therapist and a group whose purpose was to help her change Type C behavior. When I met her, she recounted her journey, which began long before she contracted cancer. Yet Naomi's diagnosis "was like an earthquake" that caused her to do some serious soul-searching.

After joining group and individual psychotherapy, Naomi was able to chart her path toward illness. She realized that she'd been under extraordinary stress for the year and a half prior to her diagnosis. Naomi had been working a full-time, pressure-filled job with abused and neglected children, *and* she'd entered a teachers' college full-time. Her enrollment in school depended on her full-time job status, and improving her job prospects depended on staying in school. She felt she had to do both.

At the same time, Naomi's brother was in prison and she and her family were collaborating with lawyers on an appeal. "Every time I didn't absolutely kill myself to do that work," she said, "I felt like the worst person in the world, because my brother is rotting in jail and here I am too tired to type another letter." She summed up the whole period as "just more than I could bear."

Despite all of this, Naomi never told me that stress caused her cancer. She believed that letting the needs of others take precedence over her own, and the resulting emotional exhaustion, contributed to her illness. She also told me that she constantly suppressed a mammoth rage and mounting frustration, punishing herself rather than finding constructive outlets. This tendency was exemplified in her relationship with her mother, who had helped to mold Naomi into the nice-girl pattern.

"After the operation, my mother came to see me, and I really couldn't stand her being there," Naomi told me. "But I felt that I'd rather die than say to her 'get out of here.' That was the motive of my life. I'd rather die than say 'this is the way I want to live and to hell with all their needs.' Dutifulness is a very strong part of my problem."

Naomi wondered if her cancer *had* been some form of punishment. Somehow she had failed to live up to others' expectations, and her own, and this was the result. When she went farther in therapy she realized that she'd been punishing *herself,* and she saw this as a cause of her physical breakdown. Her illness, and the insights that followed, led her to nurture herself more, to abdicate such heavy responsibility for others. She stopped turning her rage against herself. Finally, she felt free to live her own life.

"I thought, now I'm sick and I can be nasty if I need to. I don't have to take care of everybody else. Yes, [the illness] gave me the legitimation to take care of myself. Sometime after starting therapy, I began to feel really happy for the first time in my life. All of a sudden I saw a choice, and I enjoyed living in a way I never had before."

When I met her, Naomi had thoroughly beaten cancer. She didn't blame herself for getting cancer, and told me that she wouldn't blame herself if the disease recurred. She did believe, however, that her behavior pattern played a role in her cancer, and that her life changes strengthened her recovery.

Cancer does not occur in order to teach anyone a lesson. It may, however, be a sign that something is wrong with the body's immune defenses. Behavior affects these defenses and, hence, our body's protective and regenerative capacities. Naomi took on more than she could handle and punished herself in countless ways. For her, cancer became an opportunity to quit punishing herself and lift that burden from soul and body.

WE DON'T CREATE OUR OWN REALITY

I recently read an inspiring story of one cancer patient's struggle to take charge of her recovery while rejecting self-blame. Treya Killam Wilber discovered that she had cancer ten days after her marriage to Ken Wilber, an author of many books on transpersonal psychology. Treya was soon deluged with help and support from the couple's many friends who were part of the holistic-health movement. Friends were there to give advice, offer a shoulder to cry on, and help in any way they could. Some, with the best of intentions, offered insights that were not so helpful. These were friends who looked askance at her decision to go ahead with chemotherapy, and instead lobbied for their own favorite alternative treatment.

At times, Treya expressed great rage, sorrow, and fear about her ordeal and her future prospects. Some friends counseled her to have a more positive outlook. But she didn't want to be told what to feel; she simply wanted someone to be there for her.

A few friends even asked, "Why did you choose to give yourself cancer?"

That question, and others like it, caused Treya considerable anguish. Because she believed that we have a good deal of control over our lives and health, she wondered whether she was, in some dark way, to blame for her illness.

Treya explored these issues in depth. She struggled to develop self-understanding and insight. She sought the most nurturing kind of social support. She undertook a medical program involving a combination of grueling cancer treatments (surgery, chemotherapy, and radiation) and alternative nutritional and psychological therapies. Part of Treya's exploration stemmed from her attempt simply to understand which therapies and supports helped and which didn't. She tried to reconcile her own personal philosophy—that we have responsibility for our health and some power to determine our well-being—with her friends' New Age belief that we "create our own reality." It was hard. Accepting her friends' doctrine meant that she'd somehow brought on her illness and two subsequent recurrences. But, she wondered, if she rejected their view, did that mean her state of mind had nothing to do with her cancer or her recovery? If so, was she personally powerless over her illness?

For Treya, both extremes—total control versus no control—seemed unacceptable. She hit upon these insights:

> Probably everyone who becomes ill, especially when they are young (I was thirty-seven), will struggle with some form of the question "Why did this happen? How was I responsible?" This can be a helpful issue to raise, especially when we deny responsibility for our lives or feel like victims of fate. But I have found it to be helpful only when done without judgement. . . .
>
> I'm certain that I played a role in my becoming ill, a role that was mostly unconscious and unintentional, and I know that I play a large role, this one very conscious and very intentional, in getting well and staying well.

Treya touched upon the heart of the issue of blame when she used the terms "unconscious" and "unintentional." For Type C behavior, or any other mind-body state that weakens our defense system, is unconscious and unintentional. At an early age the Type C person makes a choice to stifle her needs and feelings, but that choice is not conscious. As she gets older, she has even less awareness of her behavior and its significance, unless or until a growth process, or a series of adverse events, disrupts the pattern and brings it to her attention. Even when she does become aware of her pattern, she rarely realizes that it can compromise her health.

Treya also found the flaw in the logic behind "you create your own reality." She realized that we simply *can't* create our own reality because there are too many impinging factors over which we have no control. In terms of cancer risk, some factors are external, well outside our sphere of influence. Can we wish away environmental carcinogens? Do we somehow bring radon or pesticides or electromagnetic fields into our lives? Of course not. Believing that we do is a monumental form of narcissism, an attempt to pretend that we're more than human. Even smoking, an addictive habit most of us know causes cancer, is driven by forces over which we have only partial control.

What about our immune systems and the mind-body factors that influence our health? Don't we have control over them? Treya had come to realize we don't have total control even over these internal factors. As I've said, the Type C pattern is not a path that anyone consciously chooses, and changing it can be difficult. We don't have complete mastery over our feelings and behavior. The idea that we do is a denial of the imperfect, limited, often irrational side of our human nature.

On the other hand, Treya accepted that we have a degree of power to change the internal factors. Those of us hit with catastrophic illness are often put in touch with parts of ourselves that have lain dormant for years. Commonly, we see our coping style clearly for the first time and start looking for better ways. Through introspection or therapy, we can throw a strong beam of light on our unconscious needs and feelings, all to help navigate ourselves through the darkness. The reward may be some illumination in terms of self-awareness and growth. We may or may not have bettered our physical health, but we have taken responsibility for an aspect of our well-being. Here's how Treya put it:

> I try to focus on what I can do now. . . . I am also very aware of the many other factors that are largely beyond my conscious or unconscious control. We are all, thankfully, part of a much larger whole. I like being aware of this, even though it means I have less control. We are all too interconnected, both with each other and with our environment—life is too wonderfully complex—for a simple statement like "you create your own reality" to be simply true. A belief that I control or create my own reality actually attempts to rip me out of the rich, complex, mysterious, and supportive context of my life. It attempts, in the name of control, to deny the web of relationships that nurtures me and each of us daily.

Two years after writing this, Treya died. In a moving piece in *New Age Journal,* Ken Wilber talked about her death, her life, and her contributions to the lives of others, especially to other cancer patients in the Cancer Support Community in San Francisco, which she helped found. He spoke of the spiritual awakenings they shared together and the richness of her last years. The aching sense of loss he conveys is profound, but no more so than the joy they both felt right up to her final moments.

The cancer patient who changes, who fights, who seeks spiritual enlightenment, is often motivated by the belief that his efforts will bolster his physical recovery. That's a perfectly valid reason, and in many cases he may achieve just that. But no matter what the physical results, *the transformation has intrinsic value that can't be measured by the amount of time his life is extended.* Gilda Radner, the *Saturday Night Live* comedienne, also taught us that lesson in her book *It's Always Something.* Gilda told of her struggles with ovarian cancer and her participation in the Wellness Community, a support group for cancer patients in the Los Angeles area. Gilda believed that her will to live, and her humor, were the foundations of her fight against cancer. The fact that she eventually succumbed did not lessen the poignancy, truth, and power of her story.

MOVING BEYOND BLAME

Roger Dafter, Ph.D., is a Jungian-oriented clinical psychologist who works with cancer patients. He recently published an article on the problem of blame in mind-body healing. Dafter reported several extraordinary case histories of self-blaming patients whom he helped in therapy. One of them, named Leah, had cancer of the spinal cord and brain stem. She was described by Dafter as someone who "recognized that she had been passive throughout her life; she could not name even one instance where she had expressed anger. She felt that she was 'boring' and that people only tolerated her presence because she was associated with her husband, without whom she felt invisible." Dafter did not appear to be familiar with my work, but his description of Leah was a precise rendering of the Type C pattern.

Type C people are particularly prone to self-blame, and Leah was no exception. "While lying by herself at night between operations," wrote Dafter, "she heard a faint, nagging voice within her say that she was responsible for her cancer and that she had no right to live." Leah told Dr. Dafter that she had been beset by "bad feelings" before her illness but had been able to push them away. Since being diagnosed, however, they had come to the surface—she cried uncontrollably and couldn't sleep due to terrifying nightmares. She feared that her "bad feelings" had caused her cancer, and now, they would cause it to recur.

Leah's self-blame had arisen naturally, not because she'd picked up wrongheaded messages from books, friends, or self-proclaimed "healers." It grew out of her profound sense of shame about herself, her needs, and her feelings. One can only imagine what happens when someone like Leah is also exposed to distorted ideas about mind-body, i.e., "You create your own reality." She has no healthy defense against them. "Of course," she will surmise, "I am to blame."

Here is how Dr. Dafter helped Leah:

> I assured Leah that "bad feelings" in people's lives are always amplified by catastrophic illness. She could not expect to feel overjoyed, since she had the difficult task of enduring great physical *dis-ease* and integrating life changes imposed by her illness. She would be crazy to feel happy about the suffering she was experiencing from cancer. I shared with her that there was no conclusive evidence that "bad feelings" caused cancer. On the other hand, if she worked with these "bad feelings," she could probably feel better about her life and present suffering, and this was a worthy goal in itself. I assured her that all of us have the opportunity to attain peace in the soul, and when this is the emphasis, there are only winners; there are no scapegoats in mind-body healing work, despite the life or death outcome.

I couldn't agree more with Dr. Dafter's approach. "Bad" feelings don't cause illness; working through them can promote healing. In Chapter 13, I'll describe how Dafter worked with Leah to change her behavior, explore untapped regions of her psyche, and develop a fighting spirit. His efforts helped her to slough off self-blame and, incidentally, to recover fully from her lethal cancer. I believe that changing Type C behavior accomplishes both goals of eliminating self-blame *and* improving one's chance for wellness.

Mind-body healing, approached with balance and perspective, yields empowerment, not blame. The proper perspective is vital, though, because it prevents empowerment from becoming a false sense of omnipotence. The fantasy that we possess limitless power in our struggle with disease can lead to feelings of failure if we somehow "lose the battle." The healthy alternative is a belief in our own healing abilities balanced by a realistic sense of our all-too-human limits. I tell patients that a healing middle ground exists between the dangerous extremes of helplessness and omnipotence. One way to develop that proper perspective is to leave behind the myth of mind over matter.

THE MIND-OVER-MATTER MYTH

In June 1985, the powerful *New England Journal of Medicine* published the results of a study of the role of the mind in cancer conducted by Barrie Cassileth, Ph.D., a sociologist at the University of Pennsylvania Cancer Center. Cassileth tracked 359 patients, most with very advanced cancers, after studying their psychological responses to cancer. After three years, the study showed no relationship between her measures of patients' mental states and cancer survival. The *Journal* published an editorial in the same issue that criticized mind-body medicine as baseless and blame-inducing.

The study and editorial caused a donnybrook in the press, with articles in *Time* magazine and elsewhere. It was an odd episode, considering the study that caused the firestorm. Cassileth and her team addressed very few psychological factors in their research. There were no measures of anger, anxiety, or expression of emotions, factors I believe to be of great importance in cancer. They did not look at Type C behavior or any construct like it. They did examine "general life satisfaction," social ties, adjustment to illness, job satisfaction, and hopelessness/helplessness. More significant, the only measures they used were portions of questionnaires—a few brief questions to cover each factor. There were no complete standard tests, no one-on-one interviews, no videotaped sessions. A slew of letters to the *New England Journal of Medicine,* many from respected mind-body scientists, described the methods used in the Cassileth study as inadequate.

But there was an even more profound problem with the Cassileth study. The majority of the subjects had metastatic cancer—advanced disease that had spread to other parts of the body. For most of these patients, no form of medical therapy could be expected to overcome their disease, and the same holds true for attitudes, mind states, or mind-body treatments. Mind-body therapies rely on bolstering the immune system's ability to recognize and destroy cancer cells in the body. Once distant metastases are present, the immune system is generally incapable of the herculean task of turning the tide against the spread of cancer. Any therapy aimed at strengthening our natural defenses—whether it is medical, nutritional, or mind-body—has the best chance of helping during the early or middle stages of cancer progression. Every responsible mind-body practitioner knows this. That doesn't mean it's wrong for patients with advanced cancer to harbor hope—miracles do happen, and some patients do go on to defy the statistics. But there's a difference between hope and reasonable expectations.

Dr. Cassileth herself recognized this limitation. Despite this, and the other problems with her research, the deputy editor of the *New England Journal of Medicine,* Marcia Angell, wrote an editorial that used the study as a launchpad to begin a broad attack on mind-body research and practice. She stated that "the medical literature contains very few scientific studies of the relation, if there is one, between mental state and disease." In one stroke of her pen, she brushed aside decades of published findings in psychosomatic and behavioral medicine, along with recent breakthroughs in psychoneuroimmunology.

Angell went even farther, though. Her editorial included this passage: "It is time to acknowledge that our belief in disease as a direct reflection of mental states is largely folklore. Furthermore, the corollary view of sickness and death as a personal failure is a particularly unfortunate form of blaming the victim."

Dr. Angell misstates the way responsible mind-body scientists today view the problem. We don't see disease as "a direct reflection of mental states." Rather, we view mental state as one contributing factor in an interactive mix of many factors. Angell is actually referring to the old mind-over-matter myth, which most mind-body scientists abandoned long ago. She's right in one respect—some people and certain practitioners have swallowed this myth. They've watered down mind-body science and reduced it to homilies like "You gave yourself that illness and you can cure it," "All you need to recover is the proper attitude," etc. Angell unfairly attributed these dangerous simplifications to *all* of us who are working to explore the complex truth of mind-body interactions.

The mind-over-matter myth tells us that mind controls body, that by properly focusing our mental energies we can alter every bodily function, prevent any illness, vanquish all disease. Treya

Wilber's friends, the ones who said. "You create your own reality," had succumbed to a New Age version of mind over matter. People who accept this myth, whether it's the old or the New Age version, will doubtless feel guilty when they get sick. If they suffer setbacks during their illness, they wonder, Why can't I lick this thing? And they decide it's because they don't have the right attitude. Or emotional state. Or meditation practice. Or guided visualization. Or spiritual awakening. The New Age movement has made contributions to human potential, but this type of thinking is not one of them.

The new, dynamic model of medicine is leading us to equally dynamic therapies—new approaches that "package" different forms of treatment to address the multiple factors in disease prevention and recovery. Dynamic mind-body medicine—whether you label it "biopsychosocial," "systems," or "complementary" medicine—involves the whole person in a comprehensive plan for recovery. We stress the need for medical therapies (surgery, chemotherapy, radiation, immunotherapy) alongside other physical (diet, exercise) and mental approaches (i.e., psychotherapy, behavior change, relaxation, imagery, and spiritual development) in judicious combinations that speak to the needs of the individual.

Whenever I speak on the subject of mind-body—to individuals, groups, or at scientific meetings—I say that we *don't* simply control our bodies via the mind, and we *do* need multifaceted approaches to get well and stay healthy. There is both logic and beauty to this idea—perhaps even some justice. For complete control would be too great a burden; it would be a form of spiritual test, with a "survival of the fittest" mentality being foisted on those afflicted with dire illness.

A more modest belief—that we don't control but rather *influence* our biological reality—cuts closer to the truth and liberates us from the burden of total responsibility for the outcome of an illness. I like to think of our bodies as being governed by a pluralistic democracy of many forces rather than a dictatorship of the mind. Our capacity to influence rather than command bodily functions means that mind-body approaches are no guarantee of recovery in any illness. Therefore, although we need hope, our day-to-day focus in healing should be less on the goal of physical recovery and more on the process of self-discovery and change.

We have a choice: we can use our knowledge of mind-body communication to punish ourselves with regret over the "shoulds"—lists of everything we should have done differently. Or, preferably, we can use it to understand what patterns of living are healthful, what risk factors are controllable, and what we can do about them. We accomplish this by accepting our innocence, our weakness, our denials, and our oversights as part of our human imperfection.

THE MYTH OF SELF-INFLICTED ILLNESS

In my contact with melanoma patients, I found a small number who wondered whether they had, in some way, caused the disease in themselves. These were patients who literally believed they had given themselves cancer, or gotten cancer as a direct form of punishment for some terrible moral or behavioral sin.

It's interesting to me that the idea of self-inflicted illness is more apparent in cancer than other diseases. Despite the fact that many people are aware of the Type A connection with heart disease, it's far less common for heart patients to feel guilty about their condition. And there's far less concern in the media and medical establishment over heart patients blaming themselves, even though the role of the mind in heart disease has been studied and discussed for decades. Diseases such as asthma, peptic ulcers, irritable bowel syndrome, and rheumatoid arthritis all have been linked with an emotional component, but no one worries that patients will blame themselves for these conditions.

I think there are two reasons for this disparity. One is cultural—the stigma long associated with malignant disease. It harkens back to the days when the word *cancer* was never to be uttered. In her book *Illness as Metaphor,* Susan Sontag identified the harmful literary and political metaphors we apply to cancer. They imply that cancer is "the epitome of evil," and that cancer patients, as host to this "evil" force, must suffer from a profound spiritual or character weakness. Sontag argues that these metaphors are a form of projection: we map our fears onto cancer and cancer patients. We stigmatize patients because they embody a condition we associate with "the enemy." And the "enemy," really, is death. Our denial of death then becomes a denial of the humanity of people with dire illness.

Sontag attacks the fallacies about cancer with the full force of her intelligence. *Illness as Metaphor* has relegated these moralistic and punitive myths to the cultural dustbin. I agree with Sontag that all of us—patients, doctors, therapists, loved ones—must discard the notion that cancer is a sign of personal failure or spiritual impoverishment. I disagree only with the passages in her book in which she disavows the mind-body connection, for fear of the blame she says it implies. In my view, Sontag's critique is valid only when applied to distorted versions of mind-body; it's not valid when applied to dynamic mind-body approaches, which, as I've explained, carry no implication of blame.

There's another reason why blame is a greater concern among cancer patients. I suspect it is related to the prevalence of Type C behavior in the cancer patient population. The Type C person already feels shame about herself, her needs, her body. The person who can't express anger in defense of herself often turns anger against herself. She tends to blame herself for any personal short-coming or unhappy event, no matter whether she had control over the circumstances.

We live in what Sontag calls a "blame" culture. In such an atmosphere, everyone is looking for scapegoats. We see that there is the problem of self-blame among some cancer patients. Right away, we think, *Who can we blame for this blame?* The mind-body adherents who have distorted ideas? The medical establishment, which victimizes some patients? The patients themselves? In my view, none are to blame but all are responsible in different ways. In my field, even among those who are careful, compassionate, ethical, and scientific, we have yet to define our position with enough clarity to help patients transcend blame.

That said, I think it's important to recognize that some patients do participate in their own victimization. That *doesn't* make them to blame for their self-blaming! It *does* mean that we must encourage them to develop self-compassion. When they do, they become less susceptible to the wrong people, books, ideas, hucksters, and healers. It's their psychological seedbed of low self-esteem that makes them vulnerable to the voices of blame. I can compare this with the notion that people don't commit violent acts simply because they watch too many violent movies. The violent tendency was there to begin with, only to be triggered by media images. For many people with cancer, the blaming tendency was there, only to be triggered by external voices of blame.

Those with cancer need to find the strength to reject the voices of blame and accept voices of self-love and empowerment. Those who care for someone with cancer can help him or her to find that strength through love and nonjudgmental support.

That's why self-blaming cancer patients benefit the most—not the least—from psychological change or therapy. The Type C person can begin a process of dismantling her entire inner system committed to self-negation. John Bradshaw calls this "shame-based" behavior. With support from professionals and/or friends and family, the person with shame-based behavior can understand the origins of her pattern, free herself from blame, and take some responsibility for her health and well-being. This time, she won't take responsibility out of guilt; she'll do it as an act of self-care.

THE MACHO CANCER-FIGHTER MYTH

The New Age movement is not the only cultural trend responsible for the legacy of blaming the victim. The macho ethic, exemplified by a spate of films starring such actors as Sylvester Stallone, Clint Eastwood, and Arnold Schwarzenegger, also contributes to the problem, albeit in strange ways.

How is this possible? Dr. Barrie Cassileth, the medical sociologist whose controversial study I mentioned earlier, claims that the problem starts when cancer is viewed as an evil enemy. According to Cassileth, we are culturally conditioned to respond to "the theme of the power of the individual to beat insurmountable odds; to single-handedly conquer the enemy. It is the theme of immensely popular movies."

People with cancer may be seduced by such images, or are drawn to them while in a state of despair. The Stallone/Eastwood/Schwarzenegger mythology of beating an enemy through sheer force of will, through teeth-gnashing determination, has its appeal. But the downside is a false belief in one's own absolute power, and the terrible letdown patients feel when they discover that they can't live up to it.

Fighting spirit can help patients recover, but the macho ethic is not synonymous with genuine fighting spirit. Confident fighters have enough self-esteem so they don't have to build themselves up with images of inviolability. They accept their weaknesses; they don't judge themselves or others only in terms of strength, power, and success. True fighters have the will to live but are smart enough to know that willpower is not the only force that matters. Self-awareness, compassion, and the courage to admit needs are healthy values that stand in stark contrast to the macho ethic.

The dark side of the macho ethic, as expressed by Cassileth, is the possibility that those who "fought equally hard and with equal grace and who lost the battle" will be blamed for their "failure."

While "courage" and "heroism" are not useless terms, they have a pernicious underside when applied to cancer patients who are asked to develop these qualities and are implicitly told that their failure to do so may result in relapse. I don't believe in issuing a whole new set of behavioral laws for people to live by based on my idea of heroism. The most courageous acts come under the heading "being one's self," not "being a hero." Being one's self is fostered in an environment in which doctors, family, and friends encourage autonomy. No patient should ever feel he has to keep a "stiff upper lip," "take it like a man," or "behave with utmost dignity" all the time.

We can look back at someone's success in fighting cancer and describe those grand efforts as heroic. But many patients who have succumbed to cancer are no less heroic or courageous than those who have been fortunate enough to survive.

WHY TYPE C BEHAVIOR IS BLAME-FREE

I've been asked, "How can you say we're not responsible for our *behavior*?" On some level we are responsible, but we are not to blame, especially when the pattern developed in our early years as a modus operandi for psychological survival. Here's how Lawrence LeShan addressed the issue when I spoke with him:

> We are long since past the stage where we should believe that because there are emotional factors pressing on us, it's our fault. When a patient asks if it's true that I'm causing cancer in myself, or my attitudes are causing cancer, the answer I give is absolutely no. I am only saying that we all fall into emotional traps when we are young—when our brains are technically unfinished—and we are wounded by life in certain

ways and don't know how to handle it. Our bodies react to the stress, and our abilities to maintain health are weakened.

LeShan's statement mirrors what I tell my cancer patients. How do I know they are blameless? I insist that at least one—if not many—of the following statements applies to *every* Type C cancer patient:

- In the past, you were not aware of your Type C behavior.
- You were aware of your Type C pattern but did not recognize it as a psychological impediment.
- You were aware of your Type C pattern but you did not know it could affect your health.
- You were aware of your Type C pattern but you did not know you could change it.
- You were aware of your Type C pattern and its effects, but you were not able to change. Your inability to change was due either to lack of self-understanding; lack of social support; social pressures at work or in your family; or your own human limitations—not character flaws.

These statements of fact enable my patients to understand how Type C behavior is unconscious and unintentional. They also learn that their attempts to take control of their health and behavior *now* does not mean they are at fault for what happened *before*.

Sadly, Type C's often grow up with so much shame that they can't even look at their behavior without believing that it's all their fault. As Karen Horney has written, they say to themselves, "Although I was helplessly exposed to this atmosphere, I should have come out of it like a lily out of a swamp."

Horney added that, "It is a sign of progress when the same patient at a later period reverses his position and rather gives himself credit for not having been crushed by the early circumstances."

Once embarked on a process of change, most Type C patients forgive themselves for past mistakes, patterns, feelings, or relationships over which they feel shame. They recognize how deeply ingrained was their pattern, how ignorant they were of its ill effects, and how truly difficult it is to change. They develop, to borrow LeShan's phrase, "a fierce and tender concern for every part of themselves," especially for the child within who stifled needs and feelings in order to maintain harmony in his family.

IS GUILT ALWAYS UNHEALTHY?

While self-blame cuts off the potential for change, guilt can sometimes be a necessary stage in a dynamic process—the inner search for responsibility and a measure of control. Anyone who undertakes that search is liable to experience some short-lived feelings of guilt.

When I met her, Marie was in her late forties, two years past a difficult divorce from her husband of nineteen years, and recently diagnosed with breast cancer. Stunned by the news, she wondered whether there was any link between her unresolved feelings about her divorce and her illness. She decided to do some research on emotions and cancer.

From the very start, Marie believed that she played an important part in her recovery. "I don't think anything is ever a hundred percent," she said. "There are circumstances outside of my control. But I am responsible for what I can be in control of." She also believed that emotional factors contributed to her illness. For several years before her diagnosis, she had been under severe stress. While working six days a week ("burning the candle at both ends," she said), she was still wrestling with the tumultuous feelings caused by the end of her long marriage.

"I knew at the time that I came down with cancer, I was still holding on to resentment," Marie commented. "Even though I had worked through some of the emotions about my divorce, I still had not closed the door on it. I decided that this was an area I had to deal with."

After her mastectomy, Marie went to a local church group for people who were separated, divorced, or widowed. She also went back to her therapist and joined a support group for cancer patients. The group encouraged members to express emotions, explore past and present conflicts, and use relaxation and imagery techniques—all in addition to their medical treatment. Marie was undergoing chemotherapy, as her breast cancer had spread to her lymph nodes.

Marie's guilt feelings followed soon after her diagnosis. She wondered whether she "did it to herself" by allowing herself to be so stressed. She felt she "should have known better." Her previous experience in Alcoholics Anonymous signaled to her that she was falling into a trap, that guilt was preventing her from making progress. Then, in her group, she got the kind of nonjudgmental support that enabled her to see clearly that cancer was not her fault.

> I needed to talk about it. I just needed to bounce it off others, to get it out in the open. When these kinds of thoughts and feelings come, it's better for me if I share it with somebody, rather than just let it stay within me and kind of twist around there . . . but [the guilt] didn't just dissipate overnight. I have found that what you know intellectually has to sift through until it meets your gut. That's why it took a while for me to realize that *I wasn't guilty of it.* To let go of that. I finally accepted that it was nothing intentional, but now that I'm aware of it, I can do something about it.

Marie viewed the way she had handled stress—by cutting off feelings—as a product of her past: "This is the way I was brought up, but that doesn't mean I can't change now. A lot of the patterns I grew up with seemed natural, but I realize now they're not healthy."

Marie's story shows how guilt can be a relatively common, brief stage that a cancer patient passes through soon after diagnosis. If the person isn't susceptible to intense self-blame, and is not exposed to misguided ideas about mind-body, the guilt will be transient.

Such guilt is a side effect of self-exploration, especially among people struggling to take charge of their health. While searching for an antidote to helplessness, they may subject themselves to painful self-questioning: "What have I done to contribute to this illness?" Their pendulum swings to the extreme end of a sense of responsibility. With the proper support or professional counseling, such as Marie received, the pendulum will move back toward the healthy middle ground between omnipotence and helplessness.

Marie's self-exploration flourished in therapy and in her group. She resolved her resentment toward her ex-husband, and she used visualization as a way to reconnect with her emotions. "Something that I don't think I was ever able to do at this level was to pay attention to my own gut feelings," she said. She realized that she'd stifled herself in her marriage. Soon thereafter, Marie met a man who supported her desire to go back to social-work school—something her ex-husband had never done. She finished the work of the past and got on with her present and future. Within a year, she was engaged to the new man in her life. She was reenergized by social-work school and dreams about her new career. Marie was one of the patients who told me that cancer "was one of the best things that ever happened to me."

We need to distinguish between normal guilt, based on self-questioning and conscience, and unhealthy guilt, based on a deep sense of shame and worthlessness. People suffering from unhealthy guilt need especially sensitive psychological support in order to cope healthily with their illness. How can you tell the difference? Ask yourself, Do I feel guilty about my illness because I blame myself for *everything*? Is it because I feel worthless and this is my just desserts? Is it because I feel shame about my body? Is it because I believe I've sinned in some horrible way? If these are among the reasons, you can rest assured that your self-blame is based on deep inner conflicts and has no basis in reality. You can begin a process of transformation that will reverse the self-denial and repression upon which your shame is based. If your guilt is like Marie's—part of a process of searching for clues, causes, and potential cures—then you'll soon dissolve or work through these feelings.

THE "POSITIVE ATTITUDE" TRAP

In our culture, the mind-body connection has been diluted and distorted in subtle ways. One simple phrase, uttered constantly by doctors and family members to their patients and loved ones, sums up the problem: "You've got to have a positive attitude."

Originally, this maxim had meaning. In its overuse, however, it has taken on very questionable shadings. In fact, "positive attitude" is often interpreted to mean the exact opposite of what, in my view, is a healthy way of coping with cancer.

In his 1979 best-selling book, *Anatomy of an Illness,* the late Norman Cousins helped start the positive-attitude trend. He told of his struggle to overcome ankylosing spondylitis, a degenerative disease of the connective tissue of the spine. Cousins decided to take charge of his medical care. Armed with his own research, the support of an unusually open-minded physician, and a belief in the regenerative powers of the body when allied with the mind, Cousins embarked on his plan. His key strategies were to take large doses of vitamin C and to make a systematic effort to summon up positive emotions. In a by-now-famous anecdote, Cousins had a projector installed in his hospital room so that he could watch Marx Brothers movies and laugh his way toward health.

Cousins fully recovered within a matter of months. He developed a concept of mind-body interactions that captured the imagination of doctors, patients, academicians, and just about everyone interested in health. But his ideas were subsequently simplified by readers and critics, and boiled down to the adage, "You've got to have a positive attitude." A close reading of *Anatomy of an Illness* and Cousins's subsequent books, articles, and statements shows that he did not intend to purvey a magical Dr. Feelgood approach. Yet the watered-down concept made it easier for people to integrate and apply something they feel instinctively—that the mind-body connection really matters.

Rarely does the purveyor of positive attitude have anything less than the best of motives. But the catchphrase has a serious downside. It communicates, "Be up, be optimistic, feel good, have energy—and you will get well." What effect does this dictate have on a recently diagnosed patient? Cancer patients, especially in the initial weeks and months, are often scared or numb or depressed or angry. Emotional and sometimes physical pain is part of the experience. During this period, urging a patient to stay positive is tantamount to telling him to keep a mask over his pain. It's a bit like inviting Bobby McFerrin to sing his famous song "Don't Worry, Be Happy," at the site of a natural disaster.

That said, the confusion is somewhat understandable. We all want those we love who are sick to feel hopeful and to avoid suffering. Unfortunately, the flight from suffering sometimes prolongs and even exacerbates despair. Although patients should do all they can to remain comfortable and pain-free, it's best for them to acknowledge their existing discomfort, fear, and sadness when possible. These sensations and emotions can't be wished away, and they are important signals indicating what the person needs. We mustn't unwittingly ask our loved ones to hide their true feelings.

I've also found that there is profound confusion about hope

and negative emotions. Some people misread anger and particularly sadness in patients as signs of total despair. Our tendency is to
rush in to prevent their sadness as if it necessarily meant they felt
hopeless. It doesn't, as I pointed out in Chapter 7, when I explained
how to distinguish sadness and temporary hopelessness from
chronic hopelessness. Often, we intervene anxiously because their
sadness makes *us* uncomfortable. We should allow our loved ones
to feel sad if that's what they feel. We can encourage them to be
hopeful without throwing a blanket on their sadness.

Unfortunately, physicians, oncologists, and surgeons are often
the first to toss off the positive-attitude dictum. The awesome power
they hold in the eyes of the cancer patient can sometimes lend their
advice the force of a command. But doctors are rarely trained
psychologically, and given our current system of health care, rarely
have the time to deal with their patients one-on-one. So the positive-attitude maxim becomes a substitute for sustained psychological follow-up. Well-meaning physicians may thus add to the burden
of patients who feel they must swiftly produce the "right" attitude
in order to get well—just at a time when they may need to grieve.

For Type C patients, this actually amounts to a *reinforcement*
of their behavior pattern. The positive-attitude message can be
taken as another rationale to hold back negative feelings. And the
Type C person is particularly prone to putting up a good front for
the sake of his family. If the positive-attitude dictum creates only a
forced optimism, a swallowing of sadness or anger, a mask over
pain, then it can make the patient worse, not better. We must
remember that Type C individuals are already browbeaten internally by the "shoulds"—having been told from childhood how they
should feel, act, and behave in all circumstances. (I am reminded
here of Horney's phrase "the tyranny of the shoulds.")

For family and friends of cancer patients: the best thing you
can do for your loved one is to allow her the freedom to be herself,
whether she is sad, angry, joyous, enraptured, empty, confused,
irritated, frightened, or just plain depressed. When she has that
kind of support, the natural process of grieving will resolve itself.
Then, under the best of circumstances, she can galvanize her energy
and optimism for the struggle ahead.

"It was not helpful when people warned me that worrying
about a recurrence might make it happen, or when they pressed me
to think positively," reported Treya Wilber. "I needed to plunge

into the depths of my fear, to face the truth squarely; only then could a genuinely positive attitude emerge."

The positive-attitude idea, when taken too far, is an extension of "magical thinking," a throwback to childhood fantasies. During certain stages of infancy, the person believes that if she wishes something, no matter how otherworldly, it will happen. For an adult facing dire illness, magical thinking can emerge in the belief that living "right" can somehow undo the wrongs of disease and death. I'm thinking of cancer patients who believe that changing their diets, their attitudes, or their personalities should absolutely and quickly eliminate their tumors. I'm also thinking of family members and other helpers who encourage patients to indulge in magical thinking.

Given our fears of suffering and death, and our need for hope, such lapses are understandable. The tragedy occurs when these hopes become demands upon the ill to live up to our fantasies. Some New Age thinkers—those who believe cancer is caused or overcome *only* by psychospiritual factors—have this "let's pretend death doesn't exist" perspective. They believe that visualization, meditation, prayer, or faith healing, if practiced "purely," will surely vanquish disease and hold back death. Here the macho ethic is dressed up in New Age clothing.

Visualizing a healthy immune system destroying weak cancer cells can be a useful procedure as an adjunct to conventional cancer therapy. Studies have shown that it can ameliorate the painful symptoms of cancer, but claims for its capacity to reverse the disease itself remain inconclusive. However, imagery techniques have helped many patients develop a sense of control, inner harmony, and relaxation. They have demonstrable positive effects on some immune functions. One day, it may be shown with certainty that visualization helps people recover. But it is far from a panacea.

While there are many responsible teachers of visualization, some practitioners make overblown promises. Ken Wilber believes this approach also harkens back to magical thinking. According to Wilber, a leading interpreter of Eastern and Western metaphysics, such practitioners think that ". . . in all cases you should be able to cure the disease by thinking it away, by visualizing it away, poof! And that poof!, I tell you, is pure magical thinking. . . . There is no support for this type of thinking in the world's great mystical traditions." Spiritual factors can play a part in recovery and should not be downplayed. But so do psychological, social, and biological factors.

Those of us who are members of the cancer patients' support system need to listen more to our loved ones rather than trying to impose on them our idea of what they should be feeling. By the same token, those of us who are patients can benefit by overthrowing the "tyranny of the shoulds" in our own minds and hearts.

PART IV

TYPE C
TRANSFORMATION—
FOR RECOVERY

CHAPTER 11

Every "victim" is a survivor who doesn't know it yet.

—Rachel Naomi Remen, M.D.

You must be vulnerable to be sensitive to reality. And to me being vulnerable is just a way of saying that one has nothing more to lose.

—Bob Dylan

It became apparent that those whose bodies healed, as well as those who completed their life before they died, had the same process in common: a receptivity, a commitment to work directly with their illness. Each seemed to enter, in their own way, and as fully as possible, the feelings, fears, and hopes, the plans and doubts, the love and forgiveness that arises in the course of healing.

—Stephen Levine

Type C Transformation— For Recovery

I was sitting by Ralph's bedside in his hospital room, talking with him about the chemotherapy treatments he was receiving for his leukemia. Ralph spoke softly, as always, and I had to lean forward to hear him. A nurse popped in abruptly and blurted out, "Could I give you a shot now?" Nurses, I understand, have schedules to meet, but Ralph and I were in the middle of one of the therapy sessions we had agreed to have together in the hospital.

"Oh, sure. Fine," replied Ralph.

"What?" I said to him, with some gentle emphasis.

Ralph thought for a moment. Then he looked up at the nurse, and said, "Um, what I meant to say was . . . we're talking right now. Would you mind coming back later?"

"All right," the nurse said, unperturbed. She whisked out of the room. Ralph smiled, and I felt we had made some progress.

That seemingly minor incident took place after I had had several sessions with Ralph. Before, he'd never have questioned the nurse's prerogative for any reason, no matter how minor. Ralph was an extreme Type C coper who not only didn't express his needs, he barely recognized them. Ralph had a severe, debilitating form of leukemia, and the doctors did not hold out much hope for his recovery. Yet here was a man who didn't seem to know when he was tired. Once, he sat up in the chair in his hospital room well into the night sorting out medical bills, until he finally collapsed into bed, exhausted from the strain of pushing himself.

Ralph was one of a number of cancer patients with whom I developed an experimental method for changing the Type C pattern. I call this therapeutic program "Type C transformation." It is a form of mind-body medicine, an approach that, alongside regular medical treatment, is designed to improve the patient's quality of life and optimize his chance for full recovery. I've found that changing Type C behavior is beneficial both for recovering cancer patients and for healthy people who wish to prevent cancer and other illnesses. In this chapter, and the next two, "Small Victories: From Diagnosis to Recovery," and "Stories of Hope, Change, and Survival," I will describe Type C transformation for recovering cancer patients.

From the beginning, Ralph exhibited some form of Type C behavior almost every minute. As an integral part of his treatment, I directed his attention to his automatic thoughts and behaviors, constantly asking him what he really wanted or felt, and supported his slowly blossoming awareness of his basic needs. It became a painstaking process of redirecting almost everything he was doing in his life.

The simplest interactions, like making an appointment, had to be restructured.

"What time would you like me to come back?" I asked.

"What time is convenient for you?" he replied.

"No. What time would *you* like me to come back?"

"I don't know."

"I have a slot between two and three next Monday that's free."

Ralph hesitated, looking sheepish.

"There is something wrong with that hour, isn't there? Why don't you tell me what it is?"

"Well, I was planning to see someone else then."

"Oh, fine," I said softly. "Why didn't you say that?"

I made sure the latter reply was said without judgment. It was meant not to berate but to call Ralph's attention to one modest truth: he had every right to tell me that was a bad time for him and to ask for a more convenient one. I was prodding him to constantly question his guilt about his own needs and to replace that guilt with simple, directly stated requests. That way, Ralph could change his Type C behavior and learn that others—in this case, myself—could still accept him. I wasn't asking Ralph to become a different person, to switch overnight from "nice guy" to "tough guy." I was teaching him that he could assert and satisfy his basic needs without destroying the fabric of his social relationships.

Ralph and I devoted several sessions to talking about his relationships with those who visited him in the hospital. Initially, he said everything was fine—he was grateful for all the visits. After he began to open up, Ralph admitted that sometimes his visitors absolutely exhausted him. I told him to try an experiment. Over the course of a week, I asked Ralph to tune in to himself and recognize when he felt exhausted. With whom did he feel especially tired? How long did it take before he became fatigued? What was going on at the time? Was he doing most of the talking or was the visitor? What subjects were being discussed? Did any visitors make him feel good? I was prompting Ralph to become his own mind-body diagnostician, his own best doctor.

When I met with him a week later, Ralph shared with me some revealing insights. He became exhausted only with certain people. We talked about each individual at length, and it turned out that visitors who were not close friends or family tired him out almost immediately. He was less comfortable with them and felt more obliged to be cheerful for their benefit. I asked Ralph to imitate his behavior with them. He launched into a hail-fellow-well-met routine that, I'm sure, had exhausted him even when he was 100 percent well!

On the positive side, Ralph also became cognizant of who made him feel good, who energized him. I encouraged him to see more of these friends and family members.

"What do I do about the ones who tire me out?" he asked.

"You have several choices," I explained. "You can kindly explain to them that you are not in the mood for too many visitors right now, but you appreciate their support. You'll see them when you feel better. Or, you can see them but curtail your hail-fellow-well-met behavior. Don't feel obliged to entertain them—let them entertain you. And know that you can politely ask them to leave if you become worn out."

Ralph was not comfortable with telling these friends not to visit. He still cared intensely what they thought about him. He preferred to let them come and to practice his new plan for self-protection. Ralph would concentrate on preserving his energy in their presence. It was hard at first, but he began to make strides at preventing visitor-induced burnout.

For the first time in his life, Ralph was beginning to think about his own physical and emotional needs. In a sense, he used his cancer as an excuse to express his desires. We tend to think of people who "use" their illness as being manipulators, self-indulgent types who milk any infirmity for all it's worth in favors and attention. For Type C patients, just the opposite is true. Remember, these are individuals at the other extreme, who have spent most of their lives denying their wants. If they use cancer as an "excuse" to start expressing them, we and they should consider it a blessing.

Ralph's good-guy behavior was so deeply rooted that he not only held himself to stringent standards in front of others, he did so even when alone. I learned that he'd sat up all night paying bills when I came to see him the following day. He was so tired he could barely speak. I asked him to explain what happened. "I had to pay these bills," he said. "And so I didn't get to sleep until late." While that seemed simple enough, I knew that I had stumbled upon an example of his behavior worthy of further examination.

I asked Ralph to recount the whole evening to me in great detail:

LT: Were the bills late?
Ralph: No.
LT: Did you have to pay them all that evening?
Ralph: Not really, I guess.
LT: How long were you in the chair?
Ralph: Two hours, from twelve to two in the morning.
LT: How did you feel during that time?
Ralph: Not bad.
LT: Are you *sure*?
Ralph [after hesitating]: I actually remember feeling more and more fatigued and achy.
LT: Did you stop only after finishing?
Ralph: Yes.
LT: How did you feel then?
Ralph: Really tired.
LT: What did you do?
Ralph: I collapsed on the bed.
LT: What were your sensations when you hit the bed?

Ralph: Incredible relief.

LT: Can you compare it to anything?

Ralph: Lying down after running a twenty-six mile marathon.

LT: At any point did it occur to you that you could stop and finish tomorrow, or later in the week?

Ralph: Yes, briefly. Maybe for a split second or two, but then I'd push that thought out of my mind.

LT: Why?

Ralph: Once I start something, I can't stop myself. I'm on automatic pilot.

I saw it as my task to help Ralph shut off his automatic pilot and go back to "manual." How so? When someone is operating an airplane (or any other vehicle) on automatic pilot, he is an observer of a process over which he has little control. He doesn't have to pay strict attention to his own perceptions, i.e., Am I on course? Do I have enough fuel? For Ralph to revert to manual, he had to start paying strict attention to his own perceptions of his emotional and physical needs. For example, he could have grasped the one-second realization that he could pay his bills later, stopped himself, and gotten back into bed—hours earlier than when he collapsed from exhaustion.

Therefore, in my work with Ralph, I focused on those one-second realizations. That's why I made him report his every thought and move from the previous evening. We all have the capacity to tune in to our self-perceptions and go back on manual—but first we must rediscover those fleeting moments of awareness of our real needs. They seem so obvious, and their message so simple, but for those of us trained to ignore them, they are elusive and slippery. I told Ralph that he didn't need me to tell him what to do; he had that self-preserving voice within him. He only had to know that the voice was there, find its frequency, and pay attention to its dictates. Ralph was struck by my insistence that his one-second realizations were the key to his transformation, and he referred to them again in our later sessions. It was a benchmark for him. He had discovered his inner guide.

One day I went in to see Ralph for one of our scheduled appointments. He looked haggard and ill at ease.

"I'm really feeling tired now because of the treatments. Could you come back tomorrow?" he said.

It was a mild-mannered statement, but I was floored. He never would have said that before. I don't believe he would have even consciously entertained the thought.

As we worked together, the changes appeared to solidify and cut deeper. Ralph had a daughter in college from whom he had been estranged. They hadn't spoken to each other since his illness. Little bit by little bit, Ralph talked to me about the conflict between him and his daughter. I helped him to realize that he would gain emotionally, not lose, by confiding in me. I soon became his combination sounding board and testing ground. In our later sessions, Ralph admitted the hurt he had felt but suppressed for several years. Finally, he called his daughter and began a process of reconciliation. Ralph had journeyed from complete denial to expression to direct action.

Ralph's Type C pattern was changing shape. He was learning to cope in a more self-nurturing way. He was becoming more assertive with his friends, family, and medical personnel. At the same time, his health began to improve. Before I began therapy with him, Ralph's platelet count, one sign of the vigor of his immune system, was dropping precipitously. His prognosis was poor. Weeks after we started sessions, his blood counts began to improve almost daily. He regained much of his old energy, and the palor left his face.

One day I came in to see Ralph, and he told me the good news: he was well enough to go home. He lived a long distance from the hospital.

"How are you going to get home?" I asked.

"Well, nobody in my family is available then. I guess I could take the bus."

I just looked at him blankly, something I had done countless times before. He got the message and smiled.

"You have a car, don't you?" he said.

"That's right."

"Maybe you could give me a ride?"

I drove Ralph home from the hospital, and a very gratifying drive it was.

Unfortunately, Ralph lived too far away to become a regular private patient of mine. I encouraged him to continue his program of change on his own and to seek another therapist if he could.

According to my last report, one year after he finished treatment, Ralph was still alive and thriving.

What accounted for Ralph's improvement? I credit his doctors, his chemotherapy, and mostly, Ralph himself, for the fortitude and courage it took for him to change. Although it is impossible to prove, I believe that a combination of his medical therapy and Type C transformation worked together to enhance his recovery.

My method for Type C transformation has not yet been formally tested in clinical trials. I have, however, developed and fine-tuned this program in my work with cancer patients like Ralph. In the majority of them, I observed a clinically significant turnabout in their Type C behavior. Many patients also got better physically and surpassed their doctors' expectations for recovery.

Type C transformation is designed to change your pattern on the level of thoughts, feelings, and behavior. In creating this approach, I've combined established methods of behavior therapy and psychotherapy, along with techniques I devised specifically to modify the mindset that underlies Type C behavior. My program differs from "regular" psychotherapy in its special emphasis on emotional expression and assertiveness, and in its features that are custom-tailored for cancer patients. While addiction recovery programs often seek to change certain Type C–like behaviors, they don't address the problems of medical patients and they're not designed to stimulate physiological healing.

Most mind-body therapies for cancer revolve around group support or meditation or visualization. I accept the validity of these approaches, though my treatment is distinct in its direct and primary focus on changing the Type C pattern.

I am certain that Type C transformation will reduce the pain and suffering that attend your illness, increase your sense of personal authority, and help you to attain psychological wholeness. The question remains: What scientific evidence exists that Type C transformation, or related mind-body approaches, can contribute to *physical* recovery? Recently, a number of studies have demonstrated the positive biological effects of mind-body therapies. The best known of these studies involved a form of group therapy that, in my view, effectively changed the patients' Type C behavior.

SCIENTIFIC EVIDENCE FOR THE LIFE-EXTENDING EFFECTS OF MIND-BODY THERAPY

Twelve years ago, David Spiegel, M.D., associate professor of psychiatry and behavioral sciences at Stanford University School of Medicine, began an investigation of group therapy for cancer patients. A rigorous and respected researcher, Dr. Spiegel approached his study with modest expectations. His goal? Simply to find out if group therapy designed specifically for cancer patients could minimize their suffering. He was not a mind-body advocate, holistic practitioner, or New Age acolyte. He did *not* believe that group therapy would extend the life span of cancer patients. He wanted to see only if it helped them to cope better.

"We did not focus on wishing away the cancer, but on living as fully as you can," Dr. Spiegel told *The New York Times.* "It was psychotherapy, with the main issue being how to redefine yourself in the face of imminent mortality."

Spiegel recruited for his study eighty-six women with advanced, metastatic breast cancer, all of whom received similar medical treatment. But one portion was randomly assigned to the group therapy program, and the rest received only the routine medical care. After ten years, the researchers found that the women in therapy lived almost twice as long as those who did not participate in therapy. The treatment group had survived an average of thirty-seven months from the outset of the study, while the nontreatment group lived for a mean of nineteen months.

Metastatic breast cancer carries a very grave prognosis, and only three women were still alive after ten years. But all three had been in the therapy group.

"We were shocked when we saw the magnitude of the effect," said Dr. Spiegel. "We expected no biological effect from the psychological one."

Dr. Spiegel's shock spurred a change in his attitude. He now believes that social and emotional factors may indeed play a *biological* role in recovery. His study was published in the *Lancet,* the most prestigious British medical journal. The *Lancet* placed an editorial on psychological cancer treatments in the same issue, which concluded with high praise for Spiegel's study. His scientific methods were said to be "beyond criticism," and the editors commended his "intellectually honest approach." Soon, other mainstream medical experts weighed in with their support for the study's validity.

Both the editorial and Spiegel said that it remains to be seen what aspect of his group therapy accounted for its influence on survival. I believe that we need to understand how the group therapy had its impact. Here is a description of the groups, much of it in Spiegel's own words, from a recent report in *The New York Times:*

> The weekly support groups met for an hour and a half. During the group sessions, the women were encouraged to express their feelings about the illness and how it affected their lives. They compared notes on radiation treatments and chemotherapy and the side effects. All of them were also taught a self-hypnosis technique to help them control pain. The women also encouraged one another to be more assertive with their doctors.
>
> "One woman told how her oncologist would sit there coolly typing his notes of her progress, and would ask her to leave when she started crying about having to take chemotherapy, which she dreaded," Dr. Spiegel said. "She'd spend the next three days upset about how he treated her."
>
> The woman learned to be assertive with her oncologist. "She told him, 'On any given day, I'll decide if I'm ready for chemotherapy, and I'll cry at first because it upsets me. But then I'll stop,' " Dr. Spiegel said. "Her oncologist was more understanding after that."
>
> A strong bond of support for each other formed among the women in the group. Many felt that the other women had a special understanding of their predicament that someone else without cancer, no matter how well meaning, simply could not have.
>
> They would visit each other during hospitalizations, and they held their own memorials for members who died during the year the group met.
>
> "The groups spent a good deal of time grieving for members who died," Dr. Spiegel said. "It reassured them that they would be grieved when they died."

Facing and mastering fears about dying was another focus.

While some of those problems had to do with such medical issues as side effects of treatment, others had to do with questions of life priorities.

"The challenge was to make the best use of whatever time remained for them," Dr. Spiegel said. "For some, that meant saying no to social obligations they didn't really care about. For others it meant repairing relationships that were valuable to them. One left her husband and spent her time with her children. Another wrote two books of poetry."

The groups were led by a psychiatrist or social worker, along with a therapist who had breast cancer in remission. Notably, the therapists never told the patients that the purpose of the groups was to extend life; they were only supposed to enhance life. "One role of the group," wrote Spiegel in his *Lancet* paper, "might have been to provide a place to belong and to express feelings."

In 1983, Spiegel published a report on these groups (just a few years after they commenced—long before he had any idea what his survival results would be) containing an analysis of group expression of emotion and the content of group discussions. He found that the most time was spent expressing negative emotions, though a great deal of time was also spent on positive and neutral emotions. Spiegel concluded that there was "balance" in terms of emotional expression; though group members expressed a great deal of negative affect, there was *not* a pervasive atmosphere of despair. There *was* a "confrontation with dying [that] became an occasion for mastery and problem-solving rather than demoralization."

I have spoken with Dr. Spiegel and read his reports. I doubt it would be possible to pick apart the groups to find one key ingredient that accounted for their life-extending effects. That would be like trying to isolate the one healing ingredient of chicken soup. But I can distinguish certain core elements in his groups—and I'm sure you can as well, from reading the above descriptions. They provided each patient with social support, with encouragement and skills enabling them to express their feelings, and with empowerment—a sense that they had a right to participate fully in every aspect of their care. These elements undoubtedly blended together and became, for each participant, a whole human experience.

Broadly speaking, these same elements—social support, emotional expression, and empowerment—are the pillars of my program for Type C transformation.

CAN MIND-BODY THERAPY STRENGTHEN YOUR CANCER DEFENSES?

I believe that any therapy or process that helps patients change Type C behavior will strengthen their recovery process. Groups are one way, but in the event that a patient lacks access to a group, there are other ways to achieve similar ends. There is no single road to health. However, social support, emotional expression, and empowerment are guiding principles that, in my view, will enhance any patient's recovery.

Several other recent studies point to the immune-enhancing and potentially life-extending benefits of mind-body therapy for cancer patients. They include:

- Dr. Sandra Levy and her colleagues at the Pittsburgh Cancer Institute have preliminary evidence that psychological interventions that might increase cancer patients' optimism, reduce feelings of hopelessness, and teach them to relax can strengthen their NK (natural killer) cell defenses (as fully reported in Chapter 9).
- Dr. Fawzy I. Fawzy and his colleagues at the UCLA School of Medicine studied melanoma patients who were given group treatment to improve their coping skills and counteract helplessness. These patients became significantly less depressed and had higher counts of natural killer cells, when compared with a control group of patients who did not participate in the groups. These effects strengthened over the course of one year after the study began.
- Dr. Steven Greer and his colleagues at the Royal Marsden Hospital in London have designed a targeted therapy that demonstrably reduces feelings of hopelessness and boosts cancer patients' fighting spirit. He awaits long-term results to determine if his therapy lengthens survival time.

Drs. Levy and Fawzy have shown that our anticancer defenses are materially strengthened by mind-body therapies that increase patients' participation in their recovery—what I call *empowerment*. Until they follow their subjects for many more years, we can't say whether these patients' immune enhancement will translate into life extension. But we do know from Dr. Spiegel's work that life extension is possible with psychological treatments.

Michael Lerner, Ph.D., head of the Commonweal program for cancer patients in Bolinas, California, suggests that Dr. Spiegel's results may partially vindicate the findings of earlier scientists who used less rigorous methods. Dr. O. Carl Simonton and Stephanie Simonton-Atchley studied the effects of their mind-body therapy, which included group support, stress management, and visualization, on 159 "incurable" cancer patients. Two years later, sixty-three were alive; 22 percent had "no evidence of disease," and 19 percent had tumors that were shrinking. Lawrence LeShan has said that almost half of the "terminal" patients in his early clinical studies outlived their doctors' predictions. Although their research methods lacked precision, the Simontons and LeShan may none-theless have been on to something—the same intangible "thing" that Spiegel found in a more scientifically rigorous study.

The effects of psychosocial and group support may be even more powerful than most researchers have imagined. A recent, surprising study by Dr. Jean L. Richardson and her associates at USC Medical School assessed the effects of an educational program designed to increase cancer patients' compliance with their medical regimen. Patients in the educational program got several hours of special instructions on medication and self-care; they also got considerably more time and attention from health-care providers. Remarkably, these patients, all of whom had cancers of the blood system, survived significantly longer than a control group who received the same medical care but did not participate in the educational program.

Patients in the program did take an antinausea medicine more regularly, and tended to keep their doctors' appointments more often, but the influence of the educational programs on survival appeared to be completely independent of medical compliance. In other words, some other factor was at work. In their conclusions, the authors, who never expected these results, speculated that the additional care and concern of health care personnel may have reduced the patients' anxieties and enhanced their sense of control. If Dr. Richardson's study could be repeated, we would have additional evidence to support a startling conclusion: more human consideration from and contact with health care providers not only makes patients feel better, it may help them live longer.

The work of the future lies in discovering which therapeutic methods offer cancer patients the best hope for psychological and physical recovery. Now let's explore the essential features of Type C transformation.

THE BASICS OF TYPE C TRANSFORMATION

Type C transformation is best achieved with the help of a professional therapist who can guide you through a gradual, profound process of change. You can also change your pattern through group support, by connecting with others who share the same stresses, pains, and revelations. But I realize that not everyone has access to individual or group therapy. That's why I'm presenting a program that you can initiate with or without therapy.

This program has nine specific goals, tailored to meet the needs and capacities of people recently diagnosed with cancer:

1. To develop awareness of your needs
2. To discover your inner guide
3. To reframe your ideas about your feelings
4. To learn the skills of emotional expression with doctors, nurses, friends, and family members
5. To take charge of your medical care
6. To get the social support you need
7. To secure your legitimate rights
8. To work through hopelessness
9. To cultivate fighting spirit

In the case of Ralph, you've seen a patient who got in touch with his needs, found his inner guide, elicited more quality social support, and began to learn the skills of expression and communication with nurses and family. As a result, he not only *felt* better, he *got* better—quickly and unexpectedly. As we move through the program, I will tell you about other patients who took charge of their care, worked through hopelessness, and developed fighting spirit.

Remember, though, that Type C transformation does not guarantee recovery. *Nor is it a substitute for conventional medical treatment.* I recommend only that cancer patients use therapy or behavior changes in *conjunction* with the proper care of a cancer specialist. First and foremost, your purpose in changing Type C behavior should be for its psychological benefits. The program will help you to live your life more fully and meaningfully and to open your heart to others. If you also beat the odds, you can count that as a marvelous by-product of your commitment.

Then, in Part V, "Type C Transformation—For Prevention," I'll show how those of you who are physically healthy can change your Type C pattern to achieve psychological wholeness and disease prevention.

What, you may ask, is the difference between Type C transformation for cancer patients and for healthy people? When you're told you have cancer, you're struck abruptly with a massive load of stress, during which time you have to make vital medical decisions and ride waves of emotional upheaval. You're unlikely to make sudden, radical alterations in your long-held patterns of coping. However, certain aspects of your Type C behavior come into play instantly, and you have much to gain by changing them as you fight your disease. You can learn to relate to your family and friends so that your needs for privacy, communication, and support are met and respected. As a Type C person whose habit has been to do only what you're told to do, you'll have to alter your nice-guy pattern in order to become an assertive participant in your medical program. These modifications are within your grasp and have a substantial positive effect on mind and body.

My focus in changing Type C for *prevention* of illness is to help you express and manage anger in a constructive way, to stand up for yourself in your work and relationships, and to find the source of your creativity. I've developed a program you can apply in daily life to restructure Type C behavior over the course of months or years.

For those of you with cancer, once you've gotten through the tough times of medical treatment and you're beginning to heal physically and psychologically, you can embark on the same long-term changes I recommend for healthy individuals. Long-term Type C transformation will help you as a recovering patient to consolidate the healthy changes you've already made. These modifications may also help prevent a recurrence of your illness.

For any one of us, the mere idea of such changes is threatening. In following this program, you may be surprised to discover that after the first few difficult steps, the rest is a surprisingly natural, organic process, as when snakes shed their skins. My hope is for you to gradually glide out of old protective defenses and slip into new ways of coping that bring self-esteem and pleasure into your daily life—even as you confront the hardships of illness. A passage from the *I Ching* says it best:

> After a time of decay comes the turning point. The powerful light that has been banished returns. There is movement, but it is not brought about by force. . . . The movement is natural, arising spontaneously. For this reason, transformation of the old becomes easy. The old is discarded and the new is introduced. Both measures accord with time; therefore no harm results.

WELCOME YOUR HEALTHY SELF INTO THE WORLD

One way we repress emotions and restrict self-awareness is by mis-perceiving inner signals. In so doing, we also develop ideas that justify our misperceptions. Ralph, the leukemia patient, thought he *had* to stay up all night in the hospital to pay his bills. He ignored his exhaustion and rationalized that he had to go on "automatic pilot" to get the job done. Ralph was a good guy who not only paid his bills on time, he paid them early. Even his debilitating illness couldn't throw him off track; on the contrary, it made him feel *more* compelled to get his bills paid early.

This is the catch-22 and the danger of Type C coping in cancer patients. Underneath his facade, Ralph was experiencing tremen-dous anxiety. And he coped with his fear of worsening illness and death by doing what he had always done, but *even more so.* I call this the "five times" rule. People deal with severe stress by doing what they always do with five times the frequency and intensity. This holds true for many people who are hit with life-threatening illness, or job loss, or retirement, or divorce, or loss of a loved one.

If they were controlling before, they become five times more controlling. If they were appeasing before, they become five times more appeasing. You can fill in the rest.

Ralph was coping by becoming five times more conscientious, reserved, nonexpressive, "nice." The catch-22 is this: his old way made him feel temporarily more safe and secure, but it also prevented him from getting his very real needs met. Hence, Ralph continued to ignore his inner signals even more completely than before, and put himself in circumstances that exhausted his mind and body: paying bills in the hospital, spending time with people toward whom he felt responsible; keeping up a false front for others, etc. Dismantling his old ways was therefore a great challenge, because the need for change came at a time when it seemed to him the most formidable task he could undertake.

That's why changing Type C behavior often requires the intervention of a caring therapist or group who can help you get over the first big hurdle. That hurdle is the realization that *you can get in touch with your needs and assert them without losing love and support.* It's a simple lesson, but it's the critical step in changing the Type C pattern. I've called the cancer diagnosis a breaking point, a moment when you can follow a path of resignation, or entrenchment, or transformation. When you discover, through a relationship or through self-discovery, that you can change without losing your support—indeed, while gaining more genuine and nourishing support—you are on the path toward transformation.

Ralph's old style had worked for him, in a limited way. He had gotten respect and kudos from friends and coworkers for being such a friendly fellow, always cooperative, ever reliable. But Ralph had so severely lost touch with his needs that, when I met him, he lacked the strength to fight for recovery. He had that strength in him, but it was drowning underneath waves of fear. My goal—and this is crucial in Type C transformation—was not to point out to Ralph what was *wrong* with him, but to help him find what was *right* with him. While I did help Ralph recognize his misperceptions about his needs and feelings, I made sure he knew these were mental traps, not signs of a deficient personality. I enabled Ralph to find his inner guide, and when he discovered that guide, he felt renewed self-confidence and surges of energy. I wasn't saying "change your damaged self," I was saying "discover your healthy self and welcome him out into the world."

YOUR INNER GUIDE TO TYPE C CHANGE

In my work with Ralph, I continually asked questions like: When do *you* want me to come back? Who would *you* like to come visit? Do *you* want our visit interrupted by the nurse?

My insistent queries had one purpose: to help Ralph find his inner guide, the voice in his head and heart that told him exactly what he needed and felt. You can do this for yourself by asking yourself the same questions. Let's say you have just undergone surgery and are awaiting chemotherapy treatments. Let every experience be an opportunity to tune in to your body and emotions. Ask:

> *Am I too tired for company?*
> *Can test schedules be altered to meet my needs?*
> *Am I satisfied with my doctor's explanations, or does he leave me*
>   *feeling confused and anxious?*
> *What part of me hurts, and what can I do to alleviate the pain?*
> *Would I prefer a different meal than the one served?*
> *Which friends lift my spirits?*
> *Who can I confide in?*

Ask yourself these questions, and your answers will be launch-pads for appropriate new behaviors—healthier ways of coping. As in: *I can ask the nurse to perform the test later. I can request more information from my doctor. I can ask for more pain medication. I can demand a different meal. I can call up the friends who lift my spirits and say, "I'd love to see you again if you can make it."*

Type C transformation is a two-stage process: first comes awareness, then action. Both are difficult to come by for Type C's because normally, your awareness of needs and feelings is blocked and you shy away from assertive actions you deem to be "inappropriate." *Once you find your inner guide, however, the impetus to take action is much stronger.* You realize: I'm hungry, therefore I must eat. I'm in pain, therefore I must find out why and deal with the cause. I'm angry, therefore I must redress the unfair situation.

My concept of an inner guide differs from some others put forth by mind-body practitioners. Finding this guide is not a mystical search, and the guide itself is not a bearer of transcendent messages. While meditation practices may help bring out your inner guide, they aren't absolutely necessary. Your inner guide for Type C transformation does not search for heavenly illuminations; it searches only for your unconscious needs and emotions.

- Your guide is an internal voice that constantly asks, "How do *I* feel right now?"
- Your guide is always on the lookout for your best interests, through all your illness-related tribulations.
- Your guide can play the mild-mannered skeptic whenever it hears evidence of self-betrayal. When you say to yourself things like "I shouldn't burden my guests with any more requests," or "I shouldn't bother the nurse for another blanket," or "I shouldn't ask the doctor too many questions," your guide can instantly perk up: *Wait a minute, I'm very sick right now. Don't I have a right?*
- Your guide is a voice with many different tones: loving, outraged, reasonable, vigilant, at times yielding. But it is always staunchly on the side of your innermost self.

Another image that works for some is that of inner guide as a ringside fight trainer. He's someone who's always in your corner, who has got a deep and abiding vested interest in your health and well-being. You step into the ring to face your opponent and, during breathers between rounds, he is there to massage your neck, whisper words of encouragement, and give you pointers about the other guy you couldn't possibly see in the heat of battle. He can tell you what parts of your body you're leaving unprotected, what punches you could be throwing. I don't mean that your doctors, nurses, friends, or family are opponents—just that you are a fighter in a tough battle who needs the best advice and protection you can get. The stronger your inner guide, the more secure you feel; the more secure you feel, the easier it is to form a healing partnership with doctors and a gratifying relationship with the people in your support system.

MACHINES TO MONITOR FEELINGS?

In working with patients who are severely out of touch with their emotions, it often takes many sessions before they successfully increase their feeling awareness. Some have a very difficult time contacting their inner guide. In one of those ironies of our techno-logical age, it sometimes takes a machine to help a patient recognize lost parts of her humanity.

Edith, a middle-aged woman from Utah, had a severe case of malignant melanoma. She exhibited extreme Type C behavior—she said she never expressed anger. In my therapy sessions with Edith, I sensed the anger beneath the surface when she talked about her relationship with her husband, but she remained unconscious of any negative emotions. I decided to try an experiment.

Biofeedback is a mind-body technique that uses instruments hooked up to register bodily processes. There are machines that monitor brain-wave activity, pulse, heart rate, skin-surface electri-cal activity, and muscular tension. All these functions change when a person experiences anxiety, anger, pleasure, or tension. People can use biofeedback machines to tap their inborn capacity to achieve a state of deep relaxation. I used biofeedback for a slightly different purpose: to show patients how they blocked their emo-tions.

I brought Edith into the biofeedback room at UCSF, which was replete with a dizzying array of electrical equipment. I had her hooked up to a machine that measures muscular tension. An assist-ant videotaped her reactions as I asked Edith a series of questions. I kept watch on the dial measuring levels of tension. First I asked some benign questions, like How did you get to the office today? and What do you think of this rainy weather? both to get her relaxed and to determine baseline levels of tension. I showed her the minimal movement of the dial when she answered these questions.

Then I said, "Would you tell me the last time you were really angry?"

She sat quietly, thinking. "I don't really remember anything," she finally said.

"Is there anything at all?" I asked.

"Well, I guess it bothered me a little bit when my husband refused to do the dishes last week."

"Did you get mad at him?"

"No."

"What happened?"

"I didn't say anything. I don't think it's a good idea to get into fights," she replied.

"Do you think it's unfair that he didn't do the dishes?"

"Well, I wished he had. I don't know if it's unfair. I wouldn't go that far. He works so hard all day long. I feel bad for him when he comes home so bushed."

"But you said you were angry," I reminded her.

"Not so much," she said. "Now that I think about it, I really wasn't mad."

"Can you think of any time in the past when you were really mad?"

After a long pause, Edith said, "No. I just can't."

Each time she answered, I took down the biofeedback readings. (I preferred that she not see the dial, as she might become self-conscious while answering my questions.) Afterward, I showed her the results. As soon as I asked her the first question about anger, her tension level shot up dramatically. It stayed high throughout our dialogue. It elevated even more when she mentioned the fact that her husband didn't do the dishes, and got still higher when she backtracked and said she wasn't angry.

I explained that the rise in her biofeedback reading probably indicated that she was angry with her husband, and that her denial made her inner tension even greater. We went over the videotape of her answers and matched the readings to her responses. I emphasized how her voice and facial expressions remained the same—showing little emotion—while her muscular tension rose. I treated it as pure mind-body education; we were learning how Edith responded to negative emotions. I did not, in any way, scare or cajole her into feeling that her behavior was "bad." My tone was this: together, we can discover how you handle your feelings, and learn new approaches that are good for your state of mind and health. She responded with interest and enthusiasm.

I returned to the issue of Edith's husband and the dishes. We delved more deeply, and she realized that she was still recovering from surgery and desperately wanted more help from her husband. Her focus on his exhaustion served only to take the focus off her own needs. This also kept her anger at bay. But she saw that her denial *made the silent anger grow and fester,* because she never said to him, "Listen, I need more help."

Using biofeedback, I was able to impress upon Edith the fact that her behavior pattern had physiological consequences. The lesson learned was simple: it's healthy to recognize and explore feelings like fear and anger. Your body registers them whether or not you consciously feel them. What's more, when you keep them buried—and never take constructive action to remedy them—the physical effects don't decrease, they increase. This tension can take a toll on your body, including your cardiovascular and immune systems. No one instance of repression will make you sick, but a long-term pattern may compromise your health.

I told Edith that her Type C reactions were like any other unhealthy habits. You can only do your best to change these stubborn behaviors. It's better to change out of a positive desire for health rather than out of some terrible guilt. Behavior modification tactics that exploit fear and shame are less effective and less humane than those emphasizing positive health benefits, whether the habit is smoking, drinking, or Type C behavior. However, an occasional shock of recognition can help, as when a person splashes a bit of cold water on her face to wake herself from a deep sleep. The biofeedback session made a strong impression on Edith, and in later therapy sessions she began to acknowledge fear and anger. She was developing emotional flexibility. Her newfound awareness was a tool, I explained, to sharpen her state of mind-body health. I used biofeedback this way with a number of patients, with similar good results.

Many of us share Edith's tendency: we deny our needs, suppress our anger when those needs aren't met, and rationalize our own or other people's neglect. One moment, our anger peeks out from its hiding place; the next moment, we make excuses like Edith's: "He works so hard, why *should* he help more?" We can get away with that mentally but our bodies won't let us forget. Still, our minds continue to play tricks by nudging us to ignore or grossly misinterpret the physical symptoms of our distress. We get a headache; we take an aspirin. We feel run down; we drink more coffee and continue our ceaseless pace of work and self-sacrifice. Our chests and necks hurt from chronically holding back emotions, so we drink alcohol or take painkillers to calm the tension. Instead of falling back on these addictive substitutes, we should be learning the art of tuning into ourselves.

How can we best monitor our feelings? Obviously, we can't rely on machines. But our inner guide can function in the same manner as the biofeedback machine. We all have within us the equivalent of sensitive dials that read out our stress levels, bodily needs, and emotional states. Our job is to locate those "dials" and pay attention to the readings. Many of us, however, can't begin to get readouts on our most troubling emotions. Our inner guide has been silenced for years. In order to contact and honor our sadness, anger, and fear, we'll need to change deep-seated ideas that have served to stunt our emotional growth.

REFRAMING YOUR IDEAS ABOUT YOUR FEELINGS

In my studies of cancer patients, I discovered what I believed was the linchpin of Type C behavior: *people have wrong ideas about their feelings, ideas that serve to keep feelings unconscious and unexpressed.* Later, in my clinical work, I found that if I could change these wrong ideas, patients would begin to liberate emotions that they'd long ago stuffed in their "bag" of lost parts of themselves. That bag had been sealed with rationalizations and beliefs based on misguided cultural clichés.

Cognitive psychotherapists use the term *reframing* for the shift in thinking that brings about a shift in feelings and behavior. Commonly, cognitive therapists show their patients how their false ideas are the cause of depression or anxiety. For example, Mr. X is depressed after his wife leaves him. He believes he will never meet another woman who will love him. His therapist shows Mr. X how this belief is the source of his depression. He'll challenge Mr. X's notion and help him substitute a healthier one: "Others have lost spouses and met new mates. So can I." By confronting, questioning, and then replacing negative thoughts with more rational and positive ones, the patient becomes less depressed and anxious.

These methods can be useful for certain cancer patients. However, for Type C patients, *I used reframing not to reduce depression or anxiety, but rather to increase feeling awareness.* This set off a chain of events that, in a rather different way, helped patients to become less depressed, more optimistic, and more in control of their medical care and their lives.

Reframing your ideas about your feelings involves a subtle shift that makes a world of difference. You may have seen double-image pictures, which look like one thing one moment and seconds later appear as utterly different. There's one that seems to be either a chalice or two heads in profile; another looks like an old witch who, in the blinking of an eye, becomes a beautiful woman. I'm suggesting that you find a new perspective on old feelings and sensations. Put simply, this shift is from perceiving "negative" emotions negatively to perceiving them as part of your full humanity. If you're open to the possibility, the old witch can be seen as a beautiful woman. Once this takes root in your mind and heart, your inner guide to feeling will make its appearance. You'll begin responding to inner dictates, not outer dictates from doctors, family members, or peers.

The final three sections in this chapter will help you reframe your ideas about your emotions. This shift will enable you to more readily contact and honor your real feelings.

Negative Emotions Aren't Negative

Nowadays, the word *negative,* when attached to the word *emotion,* carries a bevy of misleading connotations, like "bad for you," "bad for your immune system," and "bad for society." Our culture has passed along these meanings, and unfortunately, many holistic and New Age followers have magnified this error. I've had patients tell me that they felt guilty about crying, because their depression might weaken their cancer defenses. Guilty about *crying?*

Remember that primary emotions like anger, fear, and sadness do not have any harmful effect on our bodies. They alter our physiology, but so does every natural biological function. It's only when we habitually block feelings that they become the "toxic" states associated with weakened immunity: anger becomes resentment or chronic depression; fear turns into panic; sadness yields to hopelessness. Even though depression, panic, and hopelessness can be harmful, they, too, carry important information. We can no more wipe out these conditions than we can discard our primary emotions. None of us should succumb to what sociologist Philip Slater calls The Toilet Assumption—the principle that we should flush down any mind state (on a personal level) or social problem (on a mass scale) that upsets our false sense of contentment. Toxic states tell us that we've ignored primary emotions, which have backlogged to the point of bursting. They also tell us that something is wrong in our world—something that disturbs us but which we have not dealt with adequately. The way to reduce depression, panic, and hopelessness is neither to deny nor indulge them, but rather to work through and transcend them. The next time, you may be better able to recognize their predecessors and to avoid experiencing those toxic states at all.

Stop labeling your emotions as "negative." Begin to identify sensations you associate with the emotions of anger, fear, or sadness. *Heed them not as signs of weakness or indications of a failure to maintain a positive attitude, but welcome them as important messages.* Though unpleasant, you are far better off receiving these messages than you are shooting the messenger. They provide you with invaluable information about who you are, what you need, and what actions you must take in the best interests of your mindbody. Viewed this way, emotions empower you to change the conditions that give rise to your discomfort—and ultimately, to *reduce* your distress.

I once had a therapy patient, Jimmy, a young man with melanoma whose depression wouldn't go away. He told me how hard he had tried to lift himself out of this depression by working, watching TV, and otherwise distracting himself. Obviously, this wasn't working. I had the image of Jimmy attempting to pull himself out of quicksand. Married, with two young sons, he was terrified he might lose his bout with cancer. Yet, in the two months since his diagnosis, he hadn't once cried. When I explained that he didn't need to run from depression, he began to accept his sorrow. He was able to cry about his fear of losing his life, and the effect this might have on his wife and sons. He began talking to his wife about his worries. Soon his depression lifted, because he'd experienced the sadness and fear. No longer denied and repressed, the feelings lost their subterranean grip on him.

SIGNPOSTS ON THE BRIDGE BETWEEN MIND AND BODY

While our thoughts enable us to make decisions about how to act, our emotions motivate us to act. When we're angry, we're *moved* to correct an unfair or threatening situation. When we're sad, we're *moved* to find comfort and contact. When we're afraid, we're *moved* to deal with or escape the source of danger. Emotions are therefore a bridge between mind and body, stimulus and action. When we chronically deny, split off, or repress emotions, we're destroying this bridge. Many years of repression create cracks and fissures in the bridge until it is essentially dysfunctional.

One of the healthiest moves cancer patients can make is to patch up the mind-body bridge. You can rebuild that bridge and use it to get back to your sensate body. How so? Begin by paying attention to your inner signposts.

Imagine you're on a country road late at night. A thick fog hangs over the road and visibility is poor. You can't see a thing, so you flick on your brights. Suddenly, the brilliant beams of your headlights illuminate the phosphorescent surface of a stop sign—just a few yards before you reach an intersection. You have a millisecond to react. For those of us who need to rediscover lost emotions, illumination of our inner signposts is just that fleeting. But they *are* there and you *can* see them.

Consider this hypothetical example, drawn directly from my experience with several Type C patients. You've just had surgery and, despite your medications, you still have pain—enough to keep you from getting a good night's sleep. Your doctor visits you in your hospital room, and asks if everything is all right. You tell him you still have discomfort. You're waiting for him to offer more pain medication, but he doesn't. For one split second, the thought flashes, *I need relief from this pain and I better ask him for help.* Just as quickly, the thought recedes, because you override it with *He knows best,* and *He might get annoyed if I ask him outright.* You let it go, and remain stoic in your pain. Your inner signpost was obscured by thoughts that only served to maintain your shame-based Type C style. Indeed, you're so habituated to this way of thinking that you endure your pain in the belief that nothing more could be done for you. Your needs are in *his* hands, not *yours,* so if he didn't offer more medicine, he must have had some very good reason.

If you'd been on the lookout for your inner signposts, you'd have quickly identified *I need relief from this pain and I better ask him for help* as it flashed in front of your mind's eye. It would have been accompanied by an anxious buzz, but instead of ignoring the buzz you'd have recognized its meaning: *Deal with this now, or I will lose an opportunity to take care of my pain.* Having read and heeded the sign, you'd have blurted out your question: "This pain is quite bad and I wonder if more medication would help?" He'd have probably concurred, but even if he hadn't, you'd have opened a dialogue that enabled you to tell the whole story. You'd have been able to say what you hadn't before—that your pain was interfering with sleep. He would have had more information to go on and more reason to grant your request.

Those of you who are Type C copers have the same signposts as everyone else. The only difference is, you can't read them, you ignore them, or you talk yourself out of the meaning of the message. Once you pay attention to the signs, you'll automatically make the right turn—you'll take proper action. Here are examples of inner signposts, and how you might respond once you've discovered them:

> "I'm exhausted by so many guests." / *I have to rest, so I'll ask them to leave.*
> "My friend isn't listening." / *I'm going to ask him to let me talk more.*
> "I'm scared that the aftereffects of surgery will restrict my physical activities." / *I'll ask my doctor, and if there will be problems, I'll find out how I can best overcome or adapt to them.*
> "The nurse's massage made me feel ten times better." / *I'll tell her that, and ask her for another one tomorrow, even if it might put her out.*
> "My father hasn't visited me much in the hospital." / *I'll tell him I miss seeing him and how much I look forward to his visits.*

I'm not suggesting that you wallow in sadness or neediness, and I don't mean you should cherish anxiety and anger. For those of you with Type C tendencies, it's hard enough to even recognize these feelings. Once you can, the goal is not to dwell on them but to accurately discern the information they carry. These messages motivate you to change your behavior in ways that ultimately bring gratification, joy, and fulfillment—even as you confront serious illness. Seen this way, negative emotions are not an indulgence but rather a spark for positive changes that give your life dynamism.

ELIMINATE MENTAL ROADBLOCKS TO
FEELING AWARENESS

I recently met a man with lung cancer who, when he discovered my line of work, asked me a spate of questions. He was confused when I talked to him about negative emotions. "I thought you had to replace negative emotions with positive emotions in order to get well," he said. I explained that I didn't counsel patients to wallow in negative emotions, but rather to experience them, take appropriate actions, and move on. Once they've done so, they are free to feel the range of emotions, including positive ones. This was a revelation to the man, who confided that he had trouble staying positive and optimistic since his diagnosis.

The man had been bitten by the societal bugaboo against negative emotions. We all have a vast array of ideas that prevent us from feeling our feelings. Most are cultural baggage transferred to us in our families. They are clichés that creep insidiously into our lives, like the positive-attitude trap. Cancer patients especially should be on the lookout for these clichés, to challenge and debunk them as forcefully as possible. Ultimately, they only serve to keep us alienated from ourselves. Here is a short list of these ideas; they are all misguided.

1) I must exhibit courage at all times.
2) Depression, anxiety, and anger will make me sicker.
3) I must never question my doctor's actions or prescriptions.
4) I can't allow myself any negative thoughts.
5) I must conquer my fears.
6) I have to be strong for my family.
7) I shouldn't burden my friends with my pain.
8) I am going to be the perfect patient.
9) Everyone's been so good to me—how dare I complain?
10) I must get well quickly; people are depending on me.
11) If I express my pain and sadness, people will think I'm a sentimental jerk.

Watch out for these beliefs, because each one of them reinforces repression. You can contest and replace all of these dangerous ideas with the following affirmation:

I am very sick. My mind and body need as much rest and relaxation as possible. In order to get well, I must pay attention to my needs above all else. This may seem self-centered, but I know that I'm a very giving person—I have been my whole life—and now I need to be indulged a bit. I have to take care of myself so that I have the best chance for recovery. If I try to be courageous at all times and strong for other people, I'll be falling back into my old pattern. I realize now that it's depleting to play that role. I'm optimistic about getting well but I can't simply rid myself of all negative thoughts. I'm going to give myself permission to be sad, grumpy, and scared. I find it a great relief to allow these feelings to come out with other people—it was a strain to hide them all the time. I want to be a "good patient" but I can no longer live up to the label "perfect patient." I'm going to take as much time as I need to get well. These are gifts I'm giving myself, and they make me feel good about myself and my recovery.

When you can make this affirmation your own, you are rejecting the repressive myths that keep you from your inner guide. Read it over and over until you feel you've internalized the meanings. Once you have, you'll find yourself contacting needs and emotions you didn't know you had. This is the beginning of your Type C transformation.

The way to achieve real optimism during your bout with illness is to ride the highs and lows of experience, to accept everything about yourself, which includes your pain, sadness, and anger. To live this way is not to sacrifice dignity. You can express the total spectrum of emotions without lapsing into self-indulgence, histrionics, or sentimentality. I'm not suggesting that you live out some disease-of-the-week TV movie, in which patients, doctors, and family members cry on cue as the plot thickens. Only you know what "appropriate expression of emotions" means for you. Trust your instincts and don't be manipulated in either direction, whether toward repression or forced expression. When illness gives you permission to surrender some of the roles, obligations, and false fronts of the past, you will find yourself thrust suddenly into the moment. That's where you want to be.

CHAPTER 12

Out of such abysses, from such severe sickness one
returns newborn, having shed one's skin, more ticklish
and malicious, with a more delicate taste for joy, with a
more tender tongue for all good things, with merrier
senses, with a second dangerous innocence in joy, more
childhood and yet a hundred times subtler than one has
ever seen before.

—*Friedrich Nietzsche*

Becoming a pathfinder requires small acts of courage . . .
doing the sometimes tedious, sometimes terrifying work
of making a normal life passage and fully completing it.
Or by refusing to go under in the onslaught of a life
accident and emerging victorious, finding in the process a
catalyst to growth.

—*Gail Sheehy*

I've got to admit it's getting better
A little better all the time.

—*John Lennon and Paul McCartney*

Small Victories: From
Diagnosis to Recovery

I've described the experience of cancer as a crossroads in your life, when you are confronted with both danger and opportunity. Once you're diagnosed, certain pivotal questions arise. Often, you don't focus on them consciously, but they are there. How will you decide on your medical program and relate to the doctors in whom you have entrusted your care? How will you handle the fear and sadness that will course through your mind and body in the days ahead? How can you open your heart and find your way toward a fighting spirit? What changes must you make to turn this experience from what (at first) may seem like a prison sentence into an opportunity for healing and a better life?

The answers lie in small changes carried out in every phase of your life, including your medical program—changes that accumulate over time until they become a genuine transformation of your Type C style. In broad terms, these changes enable you to move from inhibition to expression, isolation to connectedness, and passivity to empowerment.

I can't overemphasize how minimal these alterations in your behavior may seem to you or to others in your support system. You can avoid the dreadful mistake of judging yourself harshly as you endeavor to change, by remembering that each change, no matter how minor, is a small victory to be celebrated and a spur to the next small victory.

Other recovery programs for cancer patients extol the virtues of peace, relaxation, and love as promoters of healing. I have no argument with them, but it's far easier to prescribe peace, relaxation, and love than it is to help people reach these states. I once attended a group for cancer patients where the leader talked for two hours about inner peace but never dealt with the distress that was blocking his patients from finding it. The tough question for a cancer patient is, How, in the midst of this trauma, can I find peace? The Type C transformation program offers new approaches that involve working through distress—not avoiding it—as a means of achieving tranquility and wholeness.

The process of change stimulates opposing emotions that are inextricably bound to each other: sadness and joy, fear and pleasure, anger and love. Put simply, one can experience both negative and positive emotions and learn the skills of emotional expression, which allow one to "move through" different feelings and then "move on"—not get stuck in one emotion or another. In this chapter, I will take you through various postcancer phases and explain the specific skills you'll need during each phase.

STEPS IN THE HEALING SEQUENCE

Karen was a melanoma patient who always had difficulty asserting her needs. In the months after her diagnosis, she found herself lucky to have many friends visiting her at home, but not so lucky when she found herself too tired to entertain and too anxious to absent herself, for fear of hurting people's feelings. Changes sparked by her psychotherapy enabled her to assert her need by announcing, "Excuse me, I have to go into the other room to meditate." Although Karen was a meditator, she didn't really need to leave the room to achieve higher consciousness. Most of the time, she just wanted to lie down. But Karen didn't feel comfortable saying "I want to lie down," fearing that this reason wasn't good enough and might cause some of her guests to bristle. Eventually, she would be able to tell them the truth without guilt, but at that time, her meditation excuse was the easiest way to get her need met and retain her sense of social support. Before Karen's diagnosis, even *that* simple strategy would have been impossible—she'd have thought it rude and selfish on her part. Small steps, small victories.

James W. Pennebaker, Ph.D., a professor of psychology at Southern Methodist University in Dallas, has spent the better part of his career studying the psychological and physical benefits of processing emotions and confiding in others. In Chapter 14, I'll discuss Dr. Pennebaker's research on the immunologic and health consequences of expressing emotion. In his 1990 book, *Opening Up: The Healing Power of Confiding in Others,* Pennebaker confides the origin of his life's work. He explains that he married his wife right out of college and, three years later, they found themselves questioning the foundation of their marriage. This sent him reeling into the first depression he'd ever experienced. He didn't know where to turn or how to cope. He began drinking and smoking more, and isolated himself from others. One day, out of desperation, he turned to his typewriter and began pounding out all his feelings about his marriage, parents, career, sexuality, and death. After doing this every day for a week, he felt fatigued but also much freer. For the first time in years, Pennebaker explained, he was in touch with the meaning and purpose of his life. This led him to realize his deep love for his wife, and enabled the two of them to resurrect their marriage.

Pennebaker's victory started with one small step—admitting his feelings to *himself* through writing. This induced a chain reaction that relieved his alienation, brought him out of depression, and led him to resolve his marital conflicts. This is what I call a healing sequence: first came awareness of emotions, then actions based on those feelings, which led to resolution. For cancer patients, the same small moves—such as writing down one's feelings—can also lift depression, enhance meaning, and spark actions that contribute to recovery.

Stephen Levine works with people with serious and terminal illnesses. In his book *Healing Into Life and Death,* Levine describes the manner in which he helps patients open their hearts. They move through and transcend what he calls "heavy" emotions like fear and rage by accepting them without guilt. In his own way, Levine embraces what I call the "small steps" approach:

At first, of course, it will be difficult if not impossible to open to such immensities as rage or terror. They are too big. But one can build the capacity to open to such primal holdings by working with the little angers and the everyday fears. Thus we will be able to see them sooner, before they become full-blown rage or terror. But if we started to work with the 5-pound weights and then the 10-pounders, with willingness and resoluteness we would eventually build our strength to its maximum capacity. Just as it is not skillful to try to press that 300-pound weight without long preparation, so it would not be appropriate to dive into a state as dense as rage, thinking, "I should be able to make this stuff float!" Good luck! And welcome to the world of the limping and the herniated.

We will not be able to overcome the 300-pound hobgoblins on first approach. In fact, if we are thinking in terms of overcoming anger or fear, we will just feel overcome each time they arise. But meeting them wholeheartedly, we come to know them like the backs of our hands or, more accurately, the backs of our minds.

The way to Type C transformation, and to recovery, involves "working with the little angers and everyday fears." Let yourself know what they are. Your newfound consciousness will then motivate you to take constructive actions to address the needs underlying these feelings: the need for respect, privacy, a sense of safety, bodily integrity, creative expression, communication and contact with your loved ones, the giving and receiving of affection.

Before I take you through the stages that occur after a cancer diagnosis, and the changes possible in each stage, I want to emphasize the healing approach you can adopt throughout: that of *taking charge.*

TAKING CHARGE OF YOUR MEDICAL CARE

One of my therapy patients, Lorraine, had breast cancer that had metastasized to her bones. Lorraine's doctors held out no hope for her recovery. She was confined to her bed, in a great deal of discomfort, but was primarily concerned about her husband, son, and daughter. All her hopes and fears were focused on their well-being. "What can I do to help them through this?" she asked me. Despite her deteriorating condition, she refused to be seen without makeup and perfectly coiffed hair. Lorraine was not about to remove her mask of composure and self-sufficiency.

I realized that Lorraine's pattern was deeply entrenched. I also knew that she might not have long to live. It seemed that there was no point in my attempting to help her reverse decades of self-denial and repression. I wasn't even sure she could make the small, incremental changes that would revitalize her emotional life. I wondered, How can I help her?

I had heard about a clinical trial of an experimental chemotherapy drug for patients with metastatic breast cancer. I told Lorraine, and she was interested. After consulting the doctor heading the trial, she was told that she didn't meet the study's protocol and could not receive this new form of chemotherapy.

Lorraine was ready to give up. I knew, however, that the drug had already been approved for use by the FDA. While it was mainly being used in experimental trials, its use was not restricted to such tests. I thought that the doctor might administer the drug to her outside the clinical trial for which she had been rejected.

Lorraine had trouble understanding that she could simply ask the doctor for the drug. "The experiment was to help him," I explained. "The drug is meant to help you." I encouraged her to call the doctor and discuss it with him. She feared his response. "He'll think I'm being pushy," she said. I gently reminded her what was at stake.

A week later I was at my home giving a party for scientists from the Soviet Union. It was a big noisy affair that had taken days to prepare. The phone rang in the midst of this mayhem. It was Lorraine. "Listen, this is not a good time to talk," I explained. "It's important, I have to tell you something," she replied. Suddenly I realized that Lorraine was asserting herself with me in an extraordinary way. "Can you wait two hours?" She called me back as soon as the party was over. Her voice was filled with pride as she recounted her conversation with the doctor. She asked him outright for the drug, and when he balked, she insisted in no uncertain terms. Finally, he acknowledged that the drug might help her and agreed to begin treatments right away. For many, this action would be considered a minor victory. For Lorraine, it was a big victory, a playoff win in her fight for recovery.

In contrast to her usual Type C behavior, Lorraine had taken charge of her medical care. She responded well to the drug, and as of this writing, she's alive—living longer than her doctor expected. Whether she lives two more years or twenty, her health and self-esteem have certainly benefited from her moment of courage. In Lorraine's case, changing Type C behavior had positive effects on *two* levels: it had a life-affirming influence on her mental and physical state, and it resulted in a significant improvement in her medical care.

Norman Cousins, in *Anatomy of an Illness* and other books, has championed the cause of patients' taking charge. In the following sections, I'll describe specific skills for self-assertion with doctors and medical personnel. Use these skills to take responsibility for every phase of your medical program. Develop the "healing partnership" with your doctor described by surgeon Bernie Siegel, M.D., in his book, *Love, Medicine, and Miracles.*

Remember that ultimately it's you who makes the final choices in your cancer treatment. But you can make choices only if you take responsibility for understanding the risks and benefits of every procedure. You do this by asking questions and insisting, in every way you know how, on crystal-clear answers.

THE BASIC QUESTIONS

As a start, here is a list of basic questions you should ask your doctor. It was prepared by Neil A. Fiore, Ph.D., author of the superb book *The Road Back to Health: Coping with the Emotional Side of Cancer.*

1. Doctor, what disease do I have?
2. If it's cancer, what kind of cancer?
3. If it's cancer, has it spread?
4. What treatment plan do you recommend?
5. What are the alternatives?
6. What are the risks in waiting or doing nothing?
7. What are the side effects, the risks, and the benefits of this treatment?
8. Why surgery? or Why surgery first? or Why chemotherapy or radiation?
9. What will these tests determine? What are the risks of taking these tests?

10. What is the purpose of this medication? What are the side effects and warnings?
11. Doctor, who do you recommend for a second opinion?
12. What can I do to aid the treatment and improve my health?

YOUR OWN PLAN FOR RECOVERY

In addition to asking questions and asserting yourself with your doctors, taking charge of your medical care involves:

- Deciding what doctors and specialists should be on your case.
- Getting second opinions to make sure your treatment plan is the best available and suits you as an individual.
- Doing your own research on your type and stage of cancer, and the treatments commonly employed, so that you are knowledgeable when you discuss your case and make decisions with your doctor(s).
- Exploring alternative health approaches to use alongside your conventional treatment. Such alternatives include nutritional programs, psychotherapy, and mind-body therapies.
- Determining your overall health needs and meeting them. In the process, you may embark on a cancer-prevention diet, meditate for relaxation, exercise for physical and emotional well-being, etc.

You don't have to pursue all these approaches in order to become a "take charge" cancer patient. But each level of involvement represents a commitment to health and recovery. The only criterion is that you follow your *own* plan, one based on your individual needs and carried out as you see fit. Otherwise, you are doing someone else's bidding—a throwback to your Type C pattern of helplessness or dependency.

In our study of a small group of long-term survivors of AIDS, Dr. George Solomon and I found that they were assertive, and they shared the trait of choosing health measures appropriate to them as individuals. Patients who exercised regularly—but only when they felt up to it—had more active natural killer cells. How much they exercised didn't matter. Many of them used guided imagery, but not because someone had told them to. And they used visualizations that suited them, not ones they read about in books or were instructed to use.

When your decisions flow from inner directives, then whatever approach you take—meditation, diet, or visualization—will give you a sense of control over your own destiny. That sense of control may be as important as the treatment itself.

When Ilana, a middle-aged commercial artist, was diagnosed with melanoma, her doctors prescribed a cancer vaccine and administered it weekly. "That's all we can do for you," the head of her team remarked. "Now let's hope it works."

Despite the fact that Ilana was getting high-tech medical care at a prestigious cancer institute, she felt vaguely unhappy about her prospects. The melanoma on her leg had spread to the lymph nodes in her groin, and she knew that her outlook for five-year survival was considered gloomy. It wasn't until she attended a mind-body workshop for cancer patients that she learned how much *she* could do to facilitate her own recovery. Overnight, Ilana felt more in control and she embarked on a multifaceted program, including a macrobiotic diet, a meditation practice with guided imagery, yoga exercises, and group therapy with other cancer patients. I'm sure that each of these facets contributed to her well-being. However, in my interview with Ilana it became clear that *the mere fact of her taking charge* in all these areas had the greatest positive effect on her energy and outlook.

In group therapy, Ilana learned to take charge of her care, and the participants supported changes in her Type C style. But the process of change was not smooth and easy. Soon after her diagnosis, Ilana went to a well-known holistic health center for recommendations on diet and other alternative treatments. She was nervous to begin with, and the clinic's director did little to make her feel at home. She was put off by his condescending manner, and upset when he told her to spend an additional four hundred dollars on another service in order to obtain a printout of available alternative therapies. What then, she wondered, was she doing *there*? The center had been advertised as a place where she could get expert advice on a spectrum of alternatives. Even worse, the clinic director wasn't very reassuring about the benefits she could gain from *his* clinic.

The next thing she knew, Ilana was shuttled downstairs for a long series of medical tests. She'd been told not to eat that day, so by late afternoon she was starving, exhausted, and only halfway through her workup. The emotional and physical strain was too much, and Ilana announced to the medical personnel that she couldn't continue and would return in a few days to finish the tests. (Ilana told me that she probably would have stayed there and exhausted herself, had she not learned lessons about assertiveness in her group therapy.)

When she returned to complete her tests, Ilana told the clinic's receptionist that she wanted a word with the clinic director. The receptionist tried to brush her off with the usual, "He's busy." But Ilana was persistent. "I'm going to be here all day and I'm sure he'll have a few minutes to see me." She got her wish, but as she walked toward his office she began to feel like the cowardly lion approaching the ghastly oversized head of the not-so-kindly Wizard of Oz. As it turned out, her image was not far off. She entered and explained in a quavering voice that she was upset by their earlier meeting and had not understood why he recommended another service before telling her the benefits of his service. The director rose from his chair and proceeded to berate her, leaving her in tears. He stormed out of his office, went downstairs to upbraid the receptionist for letting Ilana in, and left the building! Now, five years later, Ilana laughed over the memory of this incident. She found it hilarious that the director had prefaced his tirade by saying, "Well, I understand that it's necessary for cancer patients to express their feelings, but . . ."

Days later, Ilana recalled, she received a phone call. It was the clinic director. "He offered what for him was close to an apology." She felt better and realized that, although the scene had been unpleasant, *she'd done the right thing on her own behalf.* She'd never have had the gumption to express her feelings before cancer and before therapy. Ilana recalled the confrontation as a watershed— the beginning of a vital change in her behavior pattern.

Ilana's Type C behavior pattern gradually metamorphosed. She also received the benefits of excellent medical care along with a healthier diet and a more physically fit body. Eight years after her initial diagnosis, and six years after a recurrence in her lymph nodes, Ilana is alive and in excellent health.

Ilana confronted and overcame the obstacles in her way by

taking charge not only of her medical care, but of her psychological well-being. As I take you through the stages from diagnosis to recovery, I will demonstrate how you can apply this "take charge" approach.

REACTING TO YOUR DIAGNOSIS

When your doctor tells you that you have cancer, the shock can be overwhelming. People have widely varying responses, depending on their unique coping characteristics and the severity of the cancer. Sometimes, the doctor can tell you right away what your chances are for a full recovery. Other times, more tests are needed before a clear prognosis can be determined. Either way, you are dealing with the fact of cancer and the frightening associations that word carries.

You may feel numb. Your greatest desire may be to put all of this out of your mind immediately. Or you may be terrified. You might cry for hours, or you might not cry at all. You might become instantly depressed and stay that way for days.

Don't question the validity of any of these responses. They are all *normal.* Follow the dictates of your mind and body. If you need to be alone, be alone. If you need to cry, cry. If you crave contact and support, ask yourself, *Who would make me feel better?* Ask that person to visit you. If you wish to avoid thinking about cancer, do so. Don't feel obligated to confront the reality of cancer immediately. If you're depressed, don't listen to any voice—internal or external—that says *Depression is bad for you.* That simply adds a layer of guilt to your depression. If all you want to do is watch Marx Brothers movies, give yourself permission. Even if it's Jerry Lewis flicks you crave, go right ahead. My point is, don't be embarrassed by whatever measures you wish to take to get through this difficult period. Your top priority is identifying and meeting your needs.

This is a period of enormous adjustment. You need time to get used to the information that is bombarding you. The numbness of shock serves a purpose: it enables you to bear up under the stress, to prepare yourself for difficult emotions and circumstances. Similarly, denial as a coping mechanism is like the formation of a scab. A wound has been delivered to your psyche, and it needs time to heal. In the first days and weeks after your diagnosis, you may wish to stay insulated from facts and feelings about your cancer. This, too, is normal. In time, you can make a healthy adjustment toward acceptance, both of your illness and the accompanying emotions. If you tune in to your underlying emotional state, you will know when to start grappling with reality. Eventually, you'll be able to follow Norman Cousins's advice: "Don't deny the diagnosis, just defy the verdict."

Ask yourself, Do I need to share my feelings with someone? Is there anyone I trust—my spouse, parent, or friend—who I know will listen and understand? Don't choose the person (or people) you feel you *ought* to trust. Choose the ones your intuition points you toward. You might not feel completely comfortable with your spouse, perhaps because you're worried that you'll add to his or her distress. Eventually, it's best to work through obstacles to open communication with your partner, but for the moment, a person removed from your family may offer support without any extra burden. For many, your spouse is just the person—perhaps the only one—you can trust in such moments of anguish. Whomever it is, don't feel guilty about seeking the support of someone you trust to hear and accept your feelings, whatever they are.

One patient, Freda, wasn't ready to open up to her husband. Later on, she discovered why. She had spent years trying to please him and had forsaken her own need for support as she took on the role of his caretaker. Underneath, she didn't trust him to be there for her and didn't know how to express her needs. During her process of transformation, Freda confided mainly in one of her female friends. In time, however, Freda's behavior change took root in all areas of her life. She started asking for her husband's support in small matters and he responded, until the trust reentered their marriage and she felt comfortable talking to him about anything, including her struggles with cancer.

Try not to judge your emotional or social predilections. Don't feel guilty if you're not ready to open up. *My point is not to foist another set of expectations upon yourself—i.e., "you better express your feelings or else."* You'll be able to share your emotions about having cancer when you're ready. The process of change always takes time, so don't put pressure on yourself to "get all those feelings out." I only suggest that you carefully ask yourself: what are my real desires? If communicating your anxiety to others is one of them, then honor that need as best you can. When it comes to acknowledging and sharing your pain during this time, taking small steps is the most natural and healing way to proceed.

IN THE HOSPITAL

After your diagnosis, you will have a series of consultations with your doctor about your treatment plan. Most of the time other specialists—surgeons, oncologists, radiotherapists, and pathologists—will be called in to devise a complete medical program for your recovery. Surgery is often combined with chemotherapy or radiation treatments. You are usually required to stay in the hospital for an extended period. The treatment plans for cancer patients are extraordinarily varied and depend on hundreds of variables, including the type and stage of a particular cancer. But it's important to remember that 50 percent of all patients are cured of their disease. Certain types and stages of cancer are *completely curable,* and the new technologies of cancer therapy continue to improve.

You will confront many situations in the hospital that will call on your skills of communication and expression. Whether you're dealing with nurses, doctors, family, or visitors, these skills can help ease the loneliness, fear, or discomfort of your hospital stay.

Relating to Nurses

Nurses play a pivotal role in your recovery and hospital experience. You may get more medical feedback and emotional support from them than you will from physicians. You'll certainly get more day-to-day help with your physical hardships. On the other hand, a difficult nurse can be an obstacle to your psychological and physical wellness.

Being able to assert your needs with nurses is one of the early testing grounds for changing Type C behavior. For example, a nurse will enter your room, on schedule, to deliver certain drugs. You may wish to know the purpose of your medication. Understanding your medical procedures is both a right and a furtherance of your "take charge" approach. Feel free to politely ask, "What is that drug?" Then, "What's it for?" If your nurse refuses to answer directly, you can say, "Listen, I want to feel like I'm part of this treatment. It will ease my mind to know the purpose of my medication. Can't you tell me?"

This kind of communication is effective. The latter statement is honest; it reveals your vulnerability and states your need explicitly, but it doesn't alienate the nurse. I teach my patients communication skills that enable them to express their desires without offending other people. For Type C individuals, this is especially important. The motivation to change increases as you learn that *appropriate expression works*—rarely does it result in rejection or humiliation. The term *appropriate* means there are ways to communicate needs and feelings while maintaining respect for others. You don't have to throw a tantrum, cause turmoil, or bring down someone else's wrath on your head in the process.

You can apply this method in many contingencies: you might need to ask your nurse for physical help in getting around the hospital; to request a meal change; to ask about the side effects of treatment; or to request a change of bedding, dressing, or a back rub. Remember to state your need directly, stand your ground, and treat her with the same respect you want in return. A caring, professional nurse (and most are) will respond with warmth and consideration.

RELATING TO DOCTORS

Relating to doctors can be your greatest challenge. We've all been taught to perceive them as godlike figures, and many of us have a preexisting (Type C) tendency to comply with authorities. Add to that your sense of vulnerability as a person recently diagnosed with cancer, and you have a prescription for timidity. One way to become assertive with your doctor is to alter your belief that he holds your life in his hands. *You* hold your life in your hands, and at best your doctor is an ally who supports your own healing abilities.

Make sure you have the right doctor from the start. You shouldn't have to struggle with him to be heard and understood. Consider a change if he's not answering your questions, not treating you with respect, or making you feel worse by dint of his attitude. How can you find the courage to fire your doctor when you've always tried to please people in authority, from your school teacher to your boss? By focusing on your rights as a cancer patient and a human being, and by paying strict attention to your feelings, which tell you when and if those rights have been violated.

We all have the right to harbor hope for recovery, no matter how "unfavorable" our prognosis. One patient with advanced breast cancer, Collette, found a surgeon whom everyone told her was "tops" in his field. (That most overworked descriptive term for cancer specialists cuts two ways: it makes you feel secure about their technical proficiency, but it can also intimidate you into submission.) Collette had strong faith in her recovery, and she wanted doctors who believed in her. When this "top-notch" surgeon came to visit her in her hospital room, she was dismayed. "He walked in and I could see on his face that he thought I was going to die. I just couldn't have that in my room."

Collette was in touch with the anxiety she felt upon noticing the look on the surgeon's face. His words were not much more encouraging. That was all she needed to propel her to action. It didn't matter that he was "tops" in the field.

Collette discovered that this vaunted surgeon had an associate who was equally skilled but who reinforced her own positive outlook. She insisted that he take over her case. Then she proceeded to assemble an entire team of doctors—including a physician and oncologist as well as the surgeon—who were both experienced and compassionate. This took time and effort, as she consulted many specialists before making decisions on the final team. But it was time well spent.

"I rejected certain people if I didn't like their bedside manner," she said. "If I was a number in their rounds, they were out. I needed doctors who came in and treated me like Collette, not bed 37B. And I was lucky in putting together a team that did."

Collette is alive and free of disease after four years—despite the fact that one specialist had "given" her less than a year. That doctor, of course, never made it past Collette's first round of auditions.

COMMUNICATION SKILLS WITH YOUR DOCTOR

In order to be an integral part of your own medical care, you'll need to hone your skills of expression and communication with your doctors. No one else can provide you with as much information about your diagnosis, prognosis, and treatment options. Asking them questions, such as those listed on pages 278–79, and getting answers is one means by which you ensure that you are a true partner in your medical program.

While you may go through periods in which you'd rather know less than more, I suggest that you become a knowledge-seeker. Taking charge is a learned function, and one you can develop. Invariably, your doctor will provide you with only a certain amount of information. I don't know how many times I have left a doctor's office only to realize that, in the rush of events, I'd forgotten to ask him a critical question.

Write down the missing information you need. You may need to know how long the side effects of chemotherapy will last. Or how long it will take to determine whether the treatment is working. Or whether the surgery "got all the cancer out." Or whether your sex life will be affected by your surgery. Rehearse these questions before your next meeting. When you're sharp, you'll discover unanswered questions while he's still with you, and you can ask proper follow-up questions immediately. Here is a sample dialogue, derived loosely from actual patients' experiences. You can follow this example to learn communication skills with your doctor.

Patient: How many chemotherapy treatments will I receive?
Doctor: Twice a week for six weeks.
Patient: Will there be any side effects?
Doctor: It shouldn't be too bad. Don't worry about it.
Patient: Can you be more specific?
Doctor: There could be some hair loss.
Patient: What are the chances of that?
Doctor: Listen, I know you're concerned, but it's not a good idea to dwell on the downside of this.
Patient: I understand. But actually, it makes me feel more positive and less scared when I have a handle on what's going to happen to me. That's just the way I am.
Doctor: OK. Well, there's a fifty-fifty chance you'll lose a lot of hair. But it almost always grows back to normal within a few months. OK?
Patient: Thanks. That helps.

Doctor: Well, I have to go see another patient now.

Patient: Doctor, I know you're a busy man, but could I take another minute of your time?

Doctor: [Looks at his watch.] All right.

Patient: I've heard that there's really bad nausea from these treatments. Is that true?

Doctor: Yes.

Patient: How bad?

Doctor: I wouldn't focus on that.

Patient: Like I said, I'm better off when I'm prepared.

Doctor: It can be pretty bad. You may vomit a lot.

Patient: Is there anything I can do to prevent that?

Doctor: Actually, there's a new program in this hospital that uses behavioral techniques to reduce nausea and vomiting.

Patient: Can I participate?

Doctor: Sure. I'll send someone from the behavioral medicine unit.

Patient: That's great.

Doctor: I'll be on my way.

Patient: It really helps when I can talk to you about my treatment. I feel like we're in this thing together.

Doctor: We are.

Most physicians are more forthcoming than this one. But you may, at one time or another, confront doctors who withhold information or support. The above dialogue shows how you can handle his or her inaccessibility. Our sample patient did one thing consistently: *he stood his ground.* The doctor tried to give as little information and time as he possibly could, but the patient kept him from walking out the door without answering specific requests for information. These were prefaced by positive statements that appealed to his humanity and his desire for a constructive relationship with his patient.

When you handle interactions this way, you're unlikely to alienate your doctor. If he has integrity, he'll respect your steadfastness and clarity. Don't assume that he'll be annoyed by your persistence. However, if he is, talk to him openly about your concerns. Tell him you want his support, that you wish to see him as a partner in your treatment.

In your relations with your doctor, bear in mind that the issue at stake is your health. You may not realize it, but every time you take charge of your medical care, you are helping to ward off hopelessness. Acts of self-assertion can be as powerful as anti-depressants.

There are a few simple guidelines you can follow for communicating with doctors. They can also be applied to many other similar relationships:

- State clearly and directly what it is you want and need from your doctor. Begin your requests with "I want —" or "I need —."
- Avoid criticizing your doctor. Like other human beings, he is more likely to respond to feelings than judgments.
- If your doctor has been unresponsive or insulting, don't accuse him of insensitivity. Instead, tell him how what he's done has made you *feel*. For example, "I was angry when you said that I ask too many questions," or "I was scared when you cited all those statistics," or "I was hurt when you cut me off during our consultation." Statements of feeling are far more likely to be *heard* and *understood* than accusations, like "you obviously don't care about my needs or my input."
- Listen carefully to your doctor and acknowledge his statements and feelings as well. You will be far more likely to establish a partnership with him if the relationship is a two-way street.

THE RIGORS OF CANCER TREATMENT

The three mainstays of conventional cancer treatment are surgery, radiation, and chemotherapy. Each carries certain risks and side effects. Many books are available that describe the different cancer therapies and help you prepare for, and cope with, the potential pain, side effects, and long-term consequences of each.* Consult these books—and your doctor—for detailed information about what you can expect. Here, my purpose is to encourage you to take

*See *The American Cancer Society Cancer Book,* Arthur I. Holleb, M.D., ed.; and *Choices: Realistic Alternatives in Cancer Treatment,* by Marion Morra and Eve Potts.

actions that reduce your fear and distress and increase your sense of control and participation.

Cancer therapy, by its nature, can cause you to experience a loss of control. As you face surgery, and the side effects associated with chemotherapy and radiation, you may come to feel that these medical interventions are being done *to* you, not *for* or *with* you. The dehumanization that often occurs in hospitals can make you feel like an object, not a person. By contrast, every action you take to be the *subject*—the principal actor in this medical drama—can have untold beneficial effects on your psyche and the healing potential of your immune system. You can:

- Make sure your doctor has explained your surgery fully and respects your need for involvement, emotional preparation, and support from him and other medical personnel.
- Visualize positive outcomes of your surgery.
- Express your fears about surgery to your loved ones. Have them stay with you as long as you need up until surgery. Imagine the faces you most wish to see when you regain consciousness—whose presence would comfort you most?— and ask them to be there.
- Identify specific fears about your chemotherapy or radiation and address them. For example, if you fear hair loss, ask to speak to other recovered cancer patients (many hospitals have volunteers) for tips on coping. You'll find that their hair has grown back—visible proof that you will get there, too. Most of all, they are living testimony that cancer can be overcome.
- Ask your doctor about available pain treatments. This can help you prepare for the pain you fear is ahead or deal with pain you are actually experiencing. Find out if there is a pain clinic at your hospital. There are new and better drugs being used all the time. There are also new and effective nondrug treatments for pain, including hypnosis, relaxation, and other behavioral techniques.
- Find out if group therapy or individual counseling is available at your hospital. Don't think that you must have psychiatric symptoms to benefit from support or counseling. Most patients benefit from expressing their feelings in a group setting.

■ Consider meditation and guided visualization to help you cope with the side effects and pain of cancer treatment. These methods have been proven effective, and they add significantly to your sense of control.

One breast cancer patient I interviewed, Ellen, underwent a mastectomy and was terribly afraid of the chemotherapy treatments she would have to endure. She entered a support group in which she learned visualizations that enabled her to see her chemotherapy drugs entering her body and performing heroic tasks on her behalf. This helpful technique dramatically altered the mental vantage point from which she approached her treatments. "I was very fortunate, because—to my surprise—I was never sick from my chemotherapy. Yes, I lost hair, and I got fatigued. But I wasn't nauseated, scared, or incapacitated. I didn't miss a day of work. I wouldn't have been able to do that without the skills I learned in the group."

In your experience with cancer, you may never completely extinguish the feelings of powerlessness and confusion that wash over you occasionally. The "dark cloud of unknowing," to use Robert Chernin Cantor's phrase, is something cancer patients can't dispel quickly and easily. However, as you undergo treatment, your active participation, and your expression and sharing of feelings, will help to prevent you from lapsing into helplessness.

NINETY DAYS AFTER TREATMENT—THE NEED FOR SUPPORT

The real ups and downs for the cancer patient come during the three months following completion of cancer therapy. You're out of the hospital, back home, back in the real world. You may be bedridden for a time, or thrust quickly back into your normal routine. (Although your life may continue to be disrupted by additional chemotherapy or radiation treatments.) But you are no longer receiving visitors, no longer the object of so much doting concern on the part of your family. Your shock, and perhaps your denial, are beginning to wear off, and you're feeling the sting of your physical and psychological wounds. You may be wondering, Why me? Many patients are struck in rapid succession by feelings of loneliness, a sense of imminent mortality, and a need to reevaluate work and relationships.

During these three months, you may wish for solitude, which can foster healing. You may have to ask well-meaning friends and family for time on your own, and, as Anthony Storr points out in his book *Solitude,* ". . . it is sometimes difficult to persuade well-meaning helpers that solitude can be as therapeutic as emotional support." Ideally, you will be able to strike a balance between solitude and human connection, because you'll need both. For Type C individuals, however, making meaningful connections is often (though not always) harder than finding solitude.

SOCIAL SUPPORT FOR TYPE C's

The literature of mind-body refers constantly to the beneficial effects of social support. The message is: Get social support and your immune system and health will be enhanced. For Type C copers, this is easier said than done.

Those of you who are Type C often don't get the right quantity or quality of support. Why? Because you're afraid to ask for it, or because you're restricted by the roles you habitually play with your loved ones. Often, you've been the caretaker for members of your family. You've listened, helped, and doled out support in a continuous stream. You don't want to "burden" others with your problems, to "lay" your depression on friends. You think these are "inappropriate" behaviors. Underneath, you want to express your desire for support but you fear that friends and family will have no use for you. Like many Type C individuals, you lack a strong sense of self-worth. You probably have internalized a personal psychological myth: If I express my true self, I'll be rejected out of hand. This myth, and the isolation it breeds, can be hazardous to your health.

It is the *quality* of your social support that contributes to physical recovery from cancer. Perhaps your family and friends are there for you, but you have trouble accepting their care because you feel guilty about being "indulged." In other instances, your support is lacking because your loved ones are made uncomfortable by your illness. They are faced, as if in a mirror, with their own mortality and anxious feelings they can't tolerate. They might maintain a cool distance during visits or even disappear for weeks—until the "worst" is over.

Other members of your family may be *too* available. And certain people may dump their feelings about your illness on you—the last thing you need. Perhaps you want them to listen to *your* problems for a change. However, you may still be expected to play the draining role of caretaker, when you need every ounce of energy for getting well. You'll have to make a shift from caregiver to care-receiver in order to get your needs met by these friends and family members.

Framing Feelings

All these contingencies call upon your will to procure the kind of support that's genuinely nurturing. In *The Road Back to Health,* Dr. Neil Fiore provides a series of communication skills cancer patients can apply with their loved ones. He teaches patients how to "frame" their difficult feelings. Fiore offers this example:

> When you frame difficult feelings, you include all the feelings, the initial anger as well as the fear of hurting someone. Here is an example of how one might frame this patient's feelings: "This is difficult for me to say because I'm afraid you'll misunderstand and get hurt, but I'm really *angry* at you for not coming to visit me in the hospital." This patient has communicated several feelings: how difficult it is for him to bring up the topic, his fear of hurting the other person, and his anger.
>
> To say "I'm angry" wouldn't communicate the entire feeling, might be almost impossible to say, and the listener would be trying to understand why you're having so much difficulty speaking to him. Placing the feeling of anger within the framework of the other emotions makes it easier to express, and lessens the chance that the listener will misinterpret the otherwise unexplained nonverbal signs of nervousness.

Fiore's technique is useful for Type C patients in a wide range of interpersonal binds. When in doubt, remember: reassure the other person that your intention is to improve, not undermine, your relationship and he or she is less likely to react defensively. When you let the person in on your discomfort, she'll know that you are taking a risk in the name of honesty. When you use these techniques, it is more likely that your anger, disappointment, or need will be heard and understood.

Kenneth, one of my cancer patients, was a man in his forties who had always nurtured his mother. She visited him in the hospital, and wept to him about her fears. His impulse was to let her cry on his shoulder. In our work together, Kenneth suddenly realized that he'd fathered her for years. Now house-bound with a life-threatening illness, he needed *her* support, but he was still taking care of her! He wanted to change this pattern but didn't know how. I helped him work out an approach with which he was comfortable. Here's what Kenneth eventually told his mother:

> Mom, I know you are upset. Please don't take this the wrong way and think I don't want your visits. But I just can't hear about your fears at the moment. I have my own distress and right now I'm not able to help you. If I did, I'd be going through the motions. You see, I have to conserve my energy in every way possible for my recovery. I realize that I've always been the one to get you through hard times, but it would be good for us if that changed. It would take the stress out of our relationship. And I know you have a good support system—there are many people who'd be right there for you if you simply asked them. I know you want to help me, and you can. Just let me tell you my fears for a change.

Kenneth was able to stop taking care of his mother and, in turn, got more support from her than he could ever remember. This approach usually works because it communicates on several levels at once. The mother was able to understand:

1) What Kenneth was feeling about his illness and its effect on his energy.
2) What Kenneth needed from her—i.e., to refrain from sharing her emotional upset about his illness.
3) That Kenneth was not telling her to repress her needs. He reminded her that she had real alternatives for support.

4) That the purpose of Kenneth's communication was to make their relationship stronger, not weaker.

You can utilize this type of communication any time a role shift is required from care-giving to care-receiving. The same method works when you endeavor to change the ground rules of any relationship—whether you desire more, less, or a different quality of support.

On rare occasions, the person to whom you are expressing needs will be highly reactive or unresponsive. Depending on the nature and significance of the relationship, this can be a distressing experience for you. You have several options. You can emphasize your desire for a positive resolution and say, "We can deal with this better when I'm well." Or, if his reactions cause you to suffer emotionally, you can ask him to refrain from visiting until you have recuperated.

When you frame your feelings, and respect the vulnerability of the other person, he or she will seldom respond in an irrational manner. For Type C's, this will elicit a surprising discovery: you can express difficult emotions in appropriate ways that not only *don't* cause rejection, but solidify and deepen the bond between you and others.

The Art of Listening

I have come upon a very useful and deceptively simple technique for patients who wish to be better understood by loved ones. In any situation in which you need to express sensitive or painful feelings, preface the talk with a single request. Ask the friend or family member to be completely quiet until you finish having your say. This includes no "I understands," "That's rights," or "Uh-huhs." You are asking them just to listen for as long as it takes for you to express the feeling. This can last anywhere from one minute to a half hour. The results can be astonishing. This method eliminates defensiveness, hyperreactivity, pretend listening, and mutual frustration. The other person doesn't have a chance to "make it better" before you've had a chance to say what's wrong. Often, it puts you more deeply in touch with your feelings and reaches the heart of the other person in surprising ways—for both of you. I will elaborate on this technique in Chapter 16.

Many patients find that, for the first time, they really *want* to let their defenses down with the people they care about. May Sarton, the poet and novelist, was recovering from a mastectomy when she put her desire into words:

> What I long for with those I love is not so much to be understood as to be accepted warts and all, to feel safe to be fully myself even when there are great temperamental differences. What I mean by feeling "safe" is to know that I shall not be cast out when I cry or am angry, to be in the deep sense acceptable because it has been understood that the violence has its positive side.

THE FIRST YEAR: NEW PATTERNS AND PRIORITIES

Over the course of a year, Karola had one series of strange illnesses after another. First there was an ulcer. Then there was a growth in her colon, which had to be removed surgically. Finally, she had to have exploratory surgery for fibroids in her uterus. That's when her surgeon discovered uterine cancer, which had spread to her bladder. To give Karola a chance for survival, he performed a radical hysterectomy and removed fully half her bladder.

Karola, thirty-seven at the time, was in the prime of life, yet she'd lost her child-bearing capacity and now she was in a battle to save herself. She didn't know it until much later, but one of her cancer specialists had estimated that she had three months to live. She did know, however, that she had to change her life in order to win her struggle with cancer.

Karola stayed in the hospital for three weeks. She started on a seven-month-long regimen of powerful chemotherapy drugs and lost all of her long wavy red hair. Karola said that her diagnosis, and the events which followed, was a "cosmic shaking." The message she got from her illness was "Wake up!" In the months that followed, Karola would make major changes in every important area of her life. Now, she describes her life as "B.C." (Before Cancer) and "A.C." (After Cancer).

Karola told me her entire story during a lengthy interview. She had been a wealthy, respected art dealer and gallery owner. Her husband was a successful corporate executive. In retrospect, she felt she was on a fast track to nowhere. She enjoyed the prestige, and certain aspects, of her work, but it had become a treadmill. "I was leading twenty-hour days," she told me, "and I had to achieve more, I had to make more money, I had to go to more parties. It wasn't really me." Karola felt driven to live up to the role of a contemporary "superwoman," as presented by magazines, popular fiction, TV, and movies. "I know that my life looked perfect and glamorous to my friends. That was the irony. Because I felt a deep dissatisfaction. Something was wrong. That's why I was afraid to look at it, to open it up. Then, after all that happened with my cancer, I knew I had *better* open it up."

Karola's realization motivated her to change. She was also motivated to fight, partly because she glimpsed a brighter future, and partly because she didn't want to follow in her father's footsteps. Eight years earlier, he had died of colon cancer. His prognosis was poor from the start, and he never went through the normal stages of coping and grieving. He got stuck in anger, Karola said, which turned to bitterness as he closed down and isolated himself from his family. He was never able to resolve his relationship with them, nor they with him. Karola was left feeling both angry and sorrowful for what her father had done to himself and his family.

With that memory burned in her consciousness, Karola vowed to herself to be different. She was going to reach out to her friends and family and make the changes necessary to stay alive—in every sense of the word.

"I just took on an incredibly positive mantle," she remarked. She read books on the mind-body connection, changed her diet, and found an oncologist who respected and supported her choices. She meditated to help her through the hard times of chemotherapy. She clipped and saved every newspaper or magazine story about someone overcoming incredible odds—and started a file called "inspirational stories." She read these stories over and over to keep her hope alive.

After her hospital phase, Karola began to address the larger life issues that cancer had caused her to "open up." Karola quit being an art dealer and gave up her gallery. She felt some regrets but a great deal more liberation as she became a free-lance writer and art critic. She hopped off the treadmill, gave up the social whirl, the status, and the additional money, but her new priorities—namely, her health and inner peace—made these losses relatively easy to bear.

Karola had been in psychotherapy for years but felt that her therapist wasn't helping and challenging her enough. She made the hard decision to find another therapist to work with her on the new issues and feelings that were fast emerging after her diagnosis. She also entered a group for cancer patients led by Warren Berland, a noted cancer psychotherapist. The new therapist, and her group, helped her to stop playing the roles of "nice lady" and "super-woman." Gradually, she was learning to express her needs and her anger in a healthy way. Karola was developing emotional flexibility.

"Superwomen don't ask for things," she said. "They just have to appear perfect. Therapy and the group helped me examine and overturn that. I started asking for things from people. I became very active and aggressive in trying to find and meet my needs."

During her months of chemotherapy, she asked herself the stark question, What do I want to be doing? Every cancer patient who undergoes a life transformation has his or her own answer. For some, it's a new career path. For others, it's finding romantic love or starting a family. For Karola, it was quite simple: she just wanted to spend more time with her close friends.

Day in and day out, several friends would pick her up and take her to lunch and to art galleries. "It was very wonderful because people gave to me. That was what I wanted, to be with these friends. Prior to the illness, I was always afraid of what they were thinking of me. Afterward, I really didn't care what they were thinking of me. I just wanted to enjoy their company."

That was a crucial shift for Karola. The paradox is this: when we care too much about what people think of us, we care less about spending time with them. When we stop trying to please them, we start wanting to be with them. That's when joy enters our relationships. Karola abandoned her social mask with these friends, and the relationships deepened. "It made them more real," she said. "It made them closer."

Her relationship with her husband also changed. Karola discovered that, for a long time, the two of them had conspired to keep her needs suppressed. She was afraid to admit them, and he was afraid to hear them. Over several years, a transformation occurred:

she began expressing her needs more openly and he began respond-ing. That made *him* feel freer to express *his* needs. Despite incred-ible stresses, their twenty-one-year marriage got stronger.

When I met Karola—four years after her diagnosis—she was completely free of disease. All her red wavy hair had grown back. She had a vibrant energy and a wholehearted enthusiasm for life. Every year, she told me, she sends all her doctors New Year's cards saying "I'm still here!"

I saw her as a person with nothing to hide. She was thoroughly honest with herself yet also forgiving of herself. These qualities were apparent as she faced yet another ordeal. She and her husband were adopting a child, which triggered in her a grieving process over the loss of her capacity to have children of her own. She looked back with great sadness at a period prior to her illness when she and her husband had considered having children and decided against it. At the same time, she knew they'd made their decision for good rea-sons—they just weren't ready. The consequences of premature par-enthood, she said, could have been bad for their child *and* their marriage. Karola's realism saved her from undue suffering beyond her grieving process.

Karola also had been asked to be the chairperson of a major fund-raising event for an art museum. It was a year-long job, which she described as lucrative and prestigious. She weighed the offer carefully, considering the social rewards that would be bestowed upon her. Finally, she decided to turn it down because it was an enormous amount of work and "wasn't what I really wanted to be doing." It was hard to say no, but Karola's experience with cancer had fully realigned her priorities. Before, she'd have jumped at the opportunity. Now, she balked and decided to take care of her deeper needs.

"That good-girl syndrome doesn't change overnight," she said. "You handle it one instance at a time. You take a little baby step forward. It's a slow but steady change." In one year, Karola had taken many small *and* big steps forward, and achieved many victories. Her story exemplifies the kind of gradual metamorphosis experienced by many cancer survivors. You may not have to make the big changes so quickly, but you can reorder your priorities, develop emotional flexibility, and take the small steps.

We don't have to be "exceptional" to change our patterns a day at a time. Knowing that change is possible, and understanding the spiritual rewards, is sometimes all we need. I'm reminded of a quote from Franz Kafka. He wrote this in his diary on October 18, 1921:

> It is entirely conceivable that life's splendor forever lies in wait about each one of us in all its fullness, but veiled from view, deep down, invisible, far off. It *is* there, though, not hostile, not reluctant, not deaf. If you summon it by its right name, it will come.

Karola had summoned life's splendor "by its right name." What is that "right name?" Psychotherapist Robert Chernin Cantor provides an answer, one with which I agree, one which is the basis for Type C transformation: it is faith in one's own personal experience. "Feeling, any and all feeling," he wrote, "must be acknowledged and welcomed if we are to derive from our personal experience the affirming and life-sustaining visions which are an intimate part of our human endowment."

SECURING YOUR LEGITIMATE RIGHTS

I've seen several lists of cancer patient's rights, published by cancer support groups. Patients are encouraged to secure their rights to dignity, privacy, and control over their medical care. Each "bill of rights" is intended to empower patients in every area of their lives, but most especially in their medical treatment.

In my view, securing your legitimate rights as a cancer patient—and a person—is more than empowering; it is healing.

When you secure your legitimate rights, you are automatically transforming your Type C pattern. You're moving from acquiescence to assertiveness, from self-neglect to self-care. This shift, in and of itself, can contribute to immunological vigor, a critical aspect of your recovery.

I've developed a list of rights specifically for Type C cancer patients. This list can become your guidebook, for any behavior aimed at securing these ten rights is an antidote to passivity, helplessness, and hopelessness. Viewing these rights simply *as rights* is itself a major step toward self-expression and fighting spirit.

1) The right to harbor hope for your recovery
2) The right to make decisions about your medical care
3) The right to pursue complementary medical and mind-body alternatives
4) The right to receive humane treatment from doctors and nurses
5) The right to be heard
6) The right to privacy
7) The right to express all your needs—emotional, spiritual, physical
8) The right to express all your emotions—positive and negative
9) The right to seek and experience pleasure
10) The right to receive support from loved ones

With rights, of course, come responsibilities. To exercise your right to control your medical care, you'll have to take responsibility for gathering information on your disease and its treatment. To exercise your rights of expression, you'll have to hone your communication skills so that you preserve integrity and mutual respect in your relationships. To exercise your right for support, you'll have to find the courage to ask for what you need. To grasp your right to hope, you'll have to fend off messages to the contrary, whether they come from medical books or careless doctors.

The world around the cancer patient is so complicated, with the buzzings of high-tech medical care and the suddenly changed relationships, that the natural flow is often *against* your needs and rights being fulfilled. Therefore, taking responsibility for securing your rights requires some work. But in the process, you win for yourself more energy, support, control, dignity, and hope. All of these rewards can be used in your fight for life.

CHAPTER 13

Perhaps all the dragons of our lives
are princesses who are only waiting to
see us once, beautiful and brave.
Perhaps everything terrible is in
its deepest being something
that needs our love.

—Rainer Maria Rilke

Cancer can be seen as a limitation of story, a limitation
in the relationship between cells, so that one limited
but imperialistic story proliferates. On the simplest
level, the cure is the burning or cutting out of the
imperialistic story. The more complex cure is the
finding of ways for the richer, deeper stories
to rise within the organism.

—Jean Houston

What does not destroy me strengthens me.

—Friedrich Nietzsche

Stories of Hope, Change, and Survival

Six years ago, Rachel had a mastectomy. Distressed but not derailed, she adjusted to the situation and got on with her life. Then, three years later, Rachel had a terrifying experience that occurs all too frequently among women with breast cancer: she found out that her cancer had returned with a vengeance—it had spread to one of her lungs. This is always considered a grave medical situation, but in Rachel's case, it was as bad as it could be. Her new tumor was so large and bulky that her lung collapsed under its weight. Her doctors told her she had one year to live.

Rachel reacted differently to this second bout of cancer than to her first. This time she was far more frightened, depressed, and she knew she needed help. And this time, she got the help she needed. Rachel was referred to Dr. Steven Greer at the Royal Marsden Hospital in London, whose work I discussed in Chapter 7. Dr. Greer had developed a treatment for cancer patients called Adjuvant Psychological Therapy, or APT for short. He had designed his therapy to engender fighting spirit in patients who felt hopeless, helpless, or otherwise lacked a healthy sense of control in their struggle with cancer. Rachel became part of the study Greer was conducting to test the effectiveness of APT.

Rachel embraced Greer's notion of fighting spirit. His program helped her overcome her resignation, and gave her faith that her active participation in treatment, and her creative embrace of life's possibilities, would bolster her recovery. She developed a blazing determination that, no matter what her doctors said, she would beat the disease. She orchestrated her medical care, which included ongoing chemotherapy treatments. She would no longer passively submit to any medical prescription without understanding its purpose, side effects, and expected results.

"I think you're crazy if you don't use conventional drug treatment," commented Rachel. "My goodness, it works! And it's worked in my case. But I don't think that you are a machine. You've got a body and a soul and a spirit, and you've got to use all of them. If you're cutting off the mind, which is a very powerful instrument within your body, you're losing a whole spectrum of possibilities for healing."

Dr. Greer encouraged Rachel to make the most of every moment of her life. Many patients adopt a philosophy of "make every day count," a phrase which, to healthy people, can seem like a Hallmark card cliché. But for cancer patients, it's not. The shock of diagnosis gives meaning to this simple sentiment, and it becomes a way of life. A person will never "make every day count" because a guru or therapist tells her to; she'll do it when she's shaken to the core and knows it's time to reorder her priorities. That's what Rachel did. With Greer's guidance, she began to fulfil her long-cherished dream of teaching school. At the same time, she took up a vigorous regimen of biking and other sports that not only energized her but also reinforced her sense of taking control of her life and health.

With her new mind-set, Dr. Greer's therapy, and chemotherapy, Rachel's lung tumor regressed. Though in the last three years she's had two more recurrences involving metastatic tumors in both lungs, they have not diminished her fighting spirit or curtailed her activities. Most recently, Rachel's diagnostic X rays showed that the lung tumors are still present but significantly smaller. Their growth is under control, and her doctors are surprised and encouraged. She's not yet cured, but she has come a long way toward overcoming advanced cancer.

In Chapter 5, I told you about Dr. Greer's discovery that patients with fighting spirit had a better chance of survival than those who were stoic or hopeless. Greer's APT therapy is designed to inspire fighting spirit by giving patients hope, a sense of control, and the tools to work through depression, grief, and anger. Already, Greer has preliminary findings from a study of 156 patients, showing that patients who begin therapy feeling hopeless end with lower test scores on scales of depression and distress, as compared with patients who also felt hopeless but did not receive therapy.

How does Dr. Greer cultivate fighting spirit in his patients? He uses behavior therapy to modify behaviors, cognitive therapy to change thoughts, and some aspects of traditional psychotherapy to help patients express emotions. APT consists of individual sessions—often including the patient's spouse—once a week for six to twelve weeks. Greer believes that the patient's emotional reaction to cancer will depend on his appraisal of the threat posed by the disease. The APT therapist challenges ideas—such as "there's nothing I can do to bring about my recovery"—that cause the person to feel hopeless. At the same time, he gives patients the freedom and understanding they need to express grief and anger openly. In a sense, he nudges the patient from one stage of coping to the next, so that they don't get stuck in depression or rage. Moving through these stages, it seems, is a powerful way to overcome or prevent hopelessness.

Dr. Greer's program has much in common with Type C transformation. My approach has a different emphasis than Greer's—namely, on changing the Type C pattern as a means to empower the cancer patient. But our goals are similar and our methods overlap.

You may ask yourself, If fighting spirit is going to help me recover, how can I develop it? A good question because, as I discussed in Chapter 5, fighting spirit is a difficult concept to grasp. And it isn't enough to say to a patient, "You can beat this thing." One reason I stress Type C transformation is that it sparks fighting spirit. In order to have hope, one must work through and express one's grief, anger, and fear. In order to take charge of one's medical care, one must alter one's lifelong pattern of acquiescence and accommodation.

So often I hear therapists preach the gospel, "Live your life to the fullest." That's not easy for Type C individuals! For them, the questions arise: What changes must I make—what difficult, demanding changes—in order to live my life fully? What hurdles must I overcome in order to assert my needs, find my own sense of meaning, and make my mark in the world? Why haven't I had fighting spirit in *life,* let alone in response to cancer?

In this chapter, I'm going to tell you about patients who developed fighting spirit. I'm afraid that there's no ten-point plan for developing fighting spirit, but in my experience we learn about spirit from stories, not manifestos. I've seen these stories unfold in my work as a therapist, and reported several of them in previous chapters. My experience has been confirmed by other therapists. Even years ago, before scientists were examining the effects of emotions on illness, similar case histories were recorded. The following stories are drawn from my informal research, from interviews I've conducted with cancer patients who have worked with other therapists I have known, and (in two instances) from the literature of cancer psychotherapy.

I've studied these patients in order to learn more about healing transformations. Their stories illustrate principles of change, self-expression, and renewal. They tell us about the intangibles of healing and give us a glimpse into the processes of psychological, spiritual, and physical regeneration.

WORKING THROUGH HOPELESSNESS

The most dramatic case I have ever heard of a cancer patient working through hopelessness in therapy—and coming out the other side with fighting spirit—was told to me by Dr. Greer. He encountered this client in his study of APT therapy for cancer patients.

Jim, a man in his late forties, entered therapy with Greer in the worst possible condition. He had a malignant sarcoma on his leg, an extremely aggressive cancer. He had to have his leg amputated at midthigh, and even then his cancer still spread to his lungs and brain. The doctors determined that the metastases in his brain had not affected his thinking, but they held out no hope for his recovery. Jim was not expected to live more than six months to a year.

He was understandably extremely depressed. But worse than that, Jim had completely given up on everything. "He was lying in bed, not doing anything, not eating, literally waiting to die," said Greer.

Jim had been depressed long before the metastases or the amputation—indeed, prior to his contracting cancer. He had not made love with his wife, Janet, for years. Jim and Janet had owned an antiques shop, which they ran together, but Jim decided to close the shop after they were robbed by gunmen. That was five years before his diagnosis, and it marked the beginning of Jim's sense of hopelessness. He still owned this lovely store, with its collection of fine antique furniture and ornaments, but kept it boarded up, seemingly for good.

Dr. Greer began to sense a great well of anger in Jim. He told Jim that he thought he was angry—about his cancer, his life, the loss of the antiques shop—and encouraged him to talk about it. Jim refused. Greer let it go, but returned to it again and again over the next few sessions. Finally, Jim opened up, and when he did, out came an almost gothic story of soul-destroying psychological and physical trauma.

Jim, it should be said, was a very big muscular man who had always taken great pride in his physical strength. He was an excellent athlete and accepted the cultural images that equate physical power with manliness. His trauma occurred the day he and Janet were robbed in their antiques shop. Three masked gunmen broke into the shop in broad daylight. They grabbed Jim, trussed him up "like a chicken," and proceeded to throw antique valuables into a bag. Then, to thoroughly humiliate both of them, the thieves began to sexually assault Janet. At this point, Jim managed to free himself from the binding and attacked one of the men molesting her. The robber pulled out his gun and shot Jim twice, once in his lung and once in his leg. He and the other two ran, and Jim, bleeding profusely, chased after them.

Meanwhile, Janet called the police, who quickly entered the chase and eventually apprehended the criminals. Jim recovered from his wounds, but the shot in his leg had entered his groin, damaging one of his testicles, which had to be removed surgically.

When Dr. Greer finally got him to tell his story, Jim did so with blind fury. He had suppressed the anger since that day five years earlier, and now it erupted with near-volcanic force. These men had shamed him, humiliated his wife, and forced him into a state of helplessness he could not endure. Not only had they psychologically emasculated him, they had also done the job physically. From that day on, Jim no longer felt he was a man. Now, in Greer's office, he screamed and cried with murderous rage over the memory. He wanted to kill them all. Jim vented his hatred over the course of several therapy sessions.

Up until that moment, Jim knew he was angry, but he had never felt or expressed it before. Instead, he blamed himself. He thought: *I shouldn't have let them tie me up. I could have fought them more fiercely. If I'd been stronger, I would have prevented the attack on my wife. I should have avoided being shot.* Despite the fact that there was nothing more he could have done, that, in truth, he had acted heroically, to him it still added up to one thing: *He hadn't been man enough.* After the robbery, he could no longer make love to his wife. He was physically capable, but not psychologically able. And he could no longer work in the shop, the scene of this devastating trauma. The next five years were hell. He became emotionally removed and found little joy in life. Eventually, he developed a tumor on the same leg where he had been shot by the robbers. This may not have been sheer coincidence. Greer believes that Jim's cancer was a result, in part, of the terrible psychic and physical wounds he suffered.

Once Jim released his rage, his despair began to lift like dark clouds dispersing after a cleansing thunderstorm. He felt terribly relieved, as if a strangulating force had been removed from his body. And he no longer blamed himself. Dr. Greer was now able to reach Jim, to help him understand that he had done everything a human being could be expected to do and more. In fact, he had prevented his wife from being raped and, by chasing the robbers, contributed to their capture. Jim never saw that reality before; he had turned his anger against himself. Once he expressed the rage, the focus of his hatred was off himself and back where it belonged—on his attackers.

The changes in Jim were startling. He became less depressed, less hopeless, and more interested in making the rest of his time pleasurable and worth living. Janet, who attended many of the therapy sessions, was enormously supportive and loving. Jim had previously refused to deal with the issue of their lovemaking. Now, he was ready to try. Within a matter of weeks, Jim and his wife were able to make love again.

Jim decided he wanted to reopen his antiques shop. Janet was thrilled; for years, she had wished they would return to their life before the accident. They started buying antiques to make up for the lost items. They dusted off the old pieces that were still intact. By Christmas of that year—a few months after beginning ther-apy—Jim and Janet held a grand reopening of their shop. The event mirrored Jim's own reopening of himself to life's possibilities, to memories, and to the polarities of pain and pleasure.

"It was an extraordinary change over a short period of time," commented Dr. Greer. "I believe it was largely related to getting that awfulness, the murderous feelings he had suppressed for so long, out of his system."

Jim had no illusions about being "cured." His cancer was well beyond the point where any form of therapy—medical or psychological—could trigger a complete remission. However, his fighting spirit began to rally, and he wished to try anything that gave him a chance—even if only to live a bit longer. Greer reminded him of what the doctors had said, that there was nothing more they could do for him, but Jim asked if there were any experimental treatments. Greer found out that there was a new drug regimen being tried on a few select patients with terminal cancer. Without hesitation, Jim enrolled in the program and began receiving chemotherapy treatments again.

Dr. Greer's most recent report has Jim responding well to the experimental drug. He has returned to the antiques shop full-time and is seizing the opportunity to enjoy life. It has been slightly over a year since he was told he had only a matter of months to live. Neither the doctors, nor Jim, expect this to last forever.

"He is living longer than expected," said Greer. "And no matter how much longer that is, he'll certainly have lived more happily."

Jim's case shows that, for cancer patients in psychotherapy, spiritual recovery is as worthy a goal as physical recovery. It also shows that fighting spirit helps not only through its presumed positive effect on the body's natural defenses, it also spurs positive behaviors: Jim would never have asked for the experimental drug in his previous state of mind.

The seeds of hopelessness are planted long before cancer. Many so-called "terminal" patients don't lapse into total resignation. But those who do give up, it seems, are those who've felt hopeless—consciously or not—for a long time. Jim's case is exceptional in that one incident from the past was the turning point. For most of us, the cause of long-term hopelessness isn't a single dramatic event but a series of small events over a lifetime, or several "bad years" that wear down our defenses and energy.

If you are a cancer patient who feels hopeless, then psychotherapy can help you address the past and present issues that have contributed to your loss of hope. You may not experience the dramatic catharsis that Jim did—few patients have so singular a trauma and so discreet a resolution—but you can whittle away at the minor insults and major stressors that led to your unhappiness. In the process, you will discover the reasons why you withdrew from both the pains and joys of living. You can lighten your load and rediscover the zest for life you lost somewhere along the way. This will give you more energy with which to fight your illness.

Some cancer patients also suffer from clinical depression or other psychiatric illnesses. If you are experiencing constant symptoms of depression or anxiety (which can include loss of appetite, insomnia, and an inability to function in daily life), you should seek an evaluation by a psychiatrist. The hospital where you are (or were) being treated can refer you to one of its attending psychiatrists. If necessary, he or she can prescribe medical treatment in addition to regular psychotherapy.

CATHARSIS AND RADICAL CHANGE

Jim's psychological renewal also demonstrates how people, physically ill or not, can undergo a catharsis in psychotherapy. Jim was able to burst through the dam of his pent-up rage by reliving the painful event that caused it, and by releasing a cluster of feelings associated with that event. This doesn't always happen to patients in psychotherapy, but for some people, especially for Type C cancer patients who have held in their feelings for decades, catharsis can be the beginning or the apex of a fundamental transformation.

I found another similarly remarkable example of catharsis, this time reported by Lawrence LeShan, Ph.D., and Marthe L. Gassmann, M.D., in a 1957 issue of the *American Journal of Psychotherapy*. They told of a patient (whom I'll call Thomas), a thirty-two-year-old man with extensive metastases from malignant melanoma, who in early adolescence had witnessed his father prepare to murder the only adult who had ever been warm and kind to him. The murder was committed. For a long time, he was overwhelmed by fear that he'd be called in to court, in which case he might feel compelled to testify against his father. Subsequently, "he repressed the entire incident and consciously believed that his father was innocent and 'framed.' " Here is the doctor's description of what happened to Thomas many years later:

> During the course of psychotherapy, recurrent dreams and associations indicated that tension over his relationship to his father's guilt in the murder was mobilized. At the same time, he began to complain of pain in his throat and increasing difficulty in swallowing. Examination revealed a rapidly growing neoplasm [cancer] in the right tonsillar and right glosso-epiglottic area. Preparations were made to remove it surgically so that he could continue to eat. In a psychotherapy session on the day before the operation was scheduled, he recalled the entire incident with all the emotion he had felt at the time. He recounted it in detail, weeping and trembling. Four hours later, he told the therapist that he had just finished the first meal he had been able to eat in a week without pain in his throat. Twenty-four hours later, it was even smaller; and within four days, it had disappeared. The surgical procedure was not carried out.

The paper describing Thomas's case includes excerpts from the surgeon's report confirming the tumor and its disappearance.

Thomas's cathartic recollection of his traumatic experience regarding his father prompted a sudden, seemingly spontaneous regression of his tumor. By all accounts, this kind of occurrence is extremely rare. I would not suggest that cancer patients can cure their cancers by reliving traumatic events in their past. However, remarkable cases such as Thomas's can't be dismissed as flukes— they should teach us something. Undoubtedly, his repression of painful memories, searing conflict, fear, and grief had contributed to his illness. Remembering the events *with the emotions he felt but never expressed at the time* alleviated his condition. Catharsis is one way—albeit a dramatic, extraordinary one—that people can break through barriers to emotional expression. And, in my view, emotional expression can stimulate healing processes, both psychological and immunological.

DREAM LEOPARDS: THE IMAGERY OF
TRANSFORMATION

I return to the case of Leah, the self-blaming cancer patient I told you about in Chapter 10. Leah was thirty-one when she first noticed tingling sensations in her arms and legs. Thinking it was wrong to complain about such symptoms, she ignored them until she actually began to lose movement and sensation. Her doctor performed exploratory surgery, and a tumor (an intramedullary epinoma), which had penetrated her spinal cord and brain stem, was discovered. Two long and complex surgeries were required to remove the cancer. During her strenuous rehabilitation, she still had partial paralysis in her hands and feet, and she fell into a dark depression characterized by intense feelings of self-blame.

That's when Leah entered therapy with Dr. Roger Dafter, who later reported her case. He described Leah as a classic Type C coper who never expressed anger. She also fit the pattern of patients who lapse into hopelessness after their diagnosis: Leah was plagued by fears at night and weighed down by distress in her waking hours.

Dr. Dafter helped Leah to work through her depression, and he used a variety of creative techniques to enable her to contact her deeper self. One of these methods was dream analysis. After two months of therapy, Leah had a breakthrough dream. She dreamed that a murder had been committed next door. The murderer, who emitted an evil green light from his head and eyes, had left a clue—a radio with the batteries taken out. In her dream Leah recognized evil in other people by this same green light, and she was afraid of people who had a lot of green light, because they could harm her just by getting close. The day after the murder, Leah came home, and the radio was in her house with the batteries removed. The murderer was now stalking her. She searched for people to tell this to, but she had to be careful to share this information only with those who did not emit green light.

The dream setting shifted and Leah found herself in a lush jungle. Seven leopards leaped out of the underbrush. Everyone with the evil green light ran from the leopards. "I hold still, sitting, covering my eyes and thinking *peace*," wrote Leah of the dream's denouement. "The leopards run past me after the other people, leaving me alone."

Dr. Dafter helped Leah to interpret the dream. The murderer

with the green light was the grim reaper, who "killed by taking out batteries, or vital life functions." She had to avoid others with the green light to stay away from "death" influences and move toward life influences. It was a vivid, symbolic drama that allowed Leah to mobilize her will to live. In Dafter's interpretation, Leah's leopards were "classic inner allies and advisors." They represented her life force and its fierce protectors. In a later dream, Leah experienced her*self* as being a "vigorous, energized leopard of white light."

Leah worked with these images in therapy, and they provided relief from her self-condemnation and fear of death. They freed her and enabled her to face the changes she would need to make to find herself and recover from her illness. Here's how Dr. Dafter described her progress:

> The energy of the leopards was a compensation for her current physical illness as well as for years as a victim of others' needs rather than her own. The leopards helped her to overcome these limitations by leading her to look within herself to care for her own needs, even when others had different expectations for her.
>
> Gradually, Leah learned to integrate these new ways of being and relating into her relationships with her husband and parents. In essence, she transformed the core experience of herself as inferior and invisible to being worthy of taking up space in this world.

Leah eventually returned to full-time work, which her doctors predicted she would never do. After five years of remission—considered cure—she conceived her first child and has been able to be an effective, nurturing mother.

Images can be powerful means for self-transformation. Leah's dream images were telling her what she needed to understand; they were like divining rods that helped her to locate and mine her own inner resources. With her therapist's help, she used the dream leopards to tap into a well of fighting spirit that had been buried underneath the sediment of self-doubt and denial.

Beginning in the 1970s, innovators such as Jeanne Achterberg, Carl and Stephanie Simonton, and Bernie Siegel introduced visualization for cancer patients. They would guide subjects into a relaxed, meditative state and instruct them to visualize their cancer-fighting immune cells attacking tumor cells. A potpourri of images have been used to personify immune cells as fighters: man-eating sharks, jaw-snapping Pac-Men, vicious attack dogs, Star Wars weapons, and noble white knights astride their horses. By contrast, cancer cells are viewed as weak and confused. The exercise culminates with the cancer fighters effectively destroying cancer cells and flushing them from the body. Many patients have been helped by these techniques, though the question of whether they prolong survival remains a source of sometimes bitter debate.

Visualization techniques may help to mobilize aggressive energies in otherwise passive Type C cancer patients. Many patients report a renewed vitality and sense of well-being from these exercises. I don't believe that you can simply "visualize" cancer away, but I do believe you can use imagery the way Leah did, to bring about transformation and to generate fighting spirit. These changes, in turn, may stimulate physiological healing.

Leah's dream leopards were heroic (though nonviolent) defenders that sprang from her own unconscious. Thus they were images that spoke to her in a profoundly personal way, and she could work with them and draw strength from them.

For patients who feel fatigued and overwhelmed by their illness, aggressive imagery can perhaps mobilize reserves of energy and spirit that have lain dormant for years. But the lesson to be learned is that images shouldn't be imposed from the outside—the most effective ones spring from the unconscious. I know many people who can't relate to their immune cells as either killers or white knights. And, paradoxically, I've found that aggressive images don't always spark fighting spirit. Many patients can't connect with warlike imagery. Dr. George Solomon told me of an AIDS patient, a pacifist who could not comfortably "promote killing" in his own body. Instead, he visualized "the good white blood cells very politely requesting that the infected cells just leave." Some patients may need to wage war on their tumors; others may need to engage in "peaceful" civil disobedience; still others may need to accept the reality of their tumors.

I recently met a colon cancer patient, Felicia, who imagined her tumor as a red sponge ball. In her mind's eye, the ball was stuck in a dark dry place. Through deep breathing and imagery, she sent waves of light and blue water down into her lower abdomen. The water splashed over the red ball like ocean waves rushing onto shore. The gentle active waves picked up the ball and tossed it playfully on their spreading surface. Then Felicia's own energy, in the form of blue light, enveloped and animated the ball, causing it to roll away from the water's edge and onto the beach. Finally, she summoned the energy of the sun to merge with her energy. Together, they loved and surrounded the ball, which melted into a creamy red puddle on the sand.

Only you can know what images will summon forth your fighting spirit. Over time, your tactics may change—shifting between aggressive and accepting imagery or searching for images that work best for you. Trust your impulses.

THE INTEGRITY OF THE SELF, OR LEAVING THE SPIDER'S WEB

Barbara Genest, a psychotherapist who has survived "terminal" cancer of the lymph system, is a fighter whose fight has never been *against* her tumor. Her fight has always been about overcoming obstacles to finding, developing, and honoring her self.

And that may be why she has survived.

I learned about Barbara's struggles, and her successes, when I interviewed her at length for this book. Barbara was first diagnosed in 1978, after lying on the beach on her stomach, and thinking that she was lying on a volleyball. She went to her doctor, and after the usual spate of tests, she was diagnosed with lymphoma. A surgeon opened her up and discovered a grapefruit-sized tumor in her abdomen, which he could not remove. Her doctors recommended forty-eight months of chemotherapy, but they held out little if any hope for her survival.

From the start, Barbara was terrified. "I thought I was going to die, and could not protect myself from the terror." She also blamed herself, thinking "what a monster I must be to give myself cancer." While she was still in the hospital, though, she had close contact with a male friend who helped her begin her transformation. The friend said, "You couldn't give yourself cancer if you tried."

"He was taking me down to a deeper level, to a soul level, where I could accept this as a learning experience, not a punishment," she explained. "Then I began to see cancer as having had everything to do with my experience in life. Not that I was to blame, but it had something to do with me, as opposed to being some hideous thing that had visited me out of the blue. That made sense, and it meant I wasn't a helpless victim. It empowered me."

I wanted to know what in her experience was related to her illness. "I didn't have names for it, but all my life I felt hopelessly bleak and tried to keep that down. I just didn't feel there was anything I could do about it."

Barbara kept her despair from others because, in Type C fashion, she thought that it would not please them. "You certainly can't please yourself because, at some point, there isn't any self to please. Just a big black hole. You have to please others because that means you exist. You know you exist because you just made somebody smile."

Her image of herself throughout her precancer life was of someone completely tuned into what others thought of her:

> I had eyes in the backs of my legs, on top of my head, everywhere. I didn't know I was doing that. But my image was of being a spider in the center of my web, and the web was perched over an abyss. I spent my entire life making sure that the tendrils of that web were securely attached to the edges of the abyss so that I wouldn't fall into oblivion. That was what I did all the time. It's hard to develop a full, mature personality when you're busy saving your life every minute.

Cancer, it seemed, had pulled the web out from under her and, for a short time, left her hanging over the abyss. But instead of plunging, she began to float, until she realized that she was faced not only with the possibility of death but also with the possibility of freedom.

As Barbara lay in the hospital, she began hearing a different voice in her head. It was not a voice of doom and despair, but one that beseeched her to be true to herself completely for the first time, to "live with integrity so that the day I died I would be proud of myself." It wasn't a bargain, a deal struck between two sides of herself that guaranteed "victory" if she kept her word. It was just a commitment to live with integrity for whatever time she had left.

This commitment allowed Barbara to be guided by her inner voice through each phase of her life after her diagnosis. She would take care of herself in every way possible and develop her emotional, spiritual side, which she'd long neglected in favor of an existence "all in her head." She began by tending to her physical self. She turned to meditation, imagery, nutritional programs, brush massages, and hot and cold showers. She never thought that any one of these—or even the whole package—would cure her. She saw them as an expression of her steadfast conviction to honor her needs. Barbara read one book that theorized that cancer cells don't survive well in a healthy cellular environment, and that guided her approach. "I realized that I didn't have to kill off the tumor," she remarked. "I had to get healthy. That was extremely empowering, because few people in the world know how to directly dissolve cancer, but there's a lot known about how to get healthy."

Barbara had gotten the message that she felt her illness was sending her: to end her self-neglect and begin finding and developing her real self. That process would include psychotherapy, in addition to all the changes she made to improve her physical health. Only two months after her diagnosis, having had only two of the proposed forty-eight chemotherapy treatments, Barbara went in for an exam and her doctors discovered that her tumor was gone. It had literally disappeared. Her doctors were stunned, and they pulled other specialists in to study her case.

In reality, and in Barbara's mind, the miraculous regression of her cancer was only the beginning of her transformative journey. That journey has lasted seven years and continues today. While she remains totally free of cancer, she has not stopped honoring her commitment to herself. Along the way, she's learned that her despair was caused by a profound disconnection between head and heart, ego and id, social mask and inner reality. Over time, she repaired that rift, until one day she woke up and felt that she was integrated, whole. "There weren't two mes anymore, the real me versus the other one who beat me, hated me, obstructed everything, closed me down, defended me, and shut out reality."

How did she heal her inner split? With her psychotherapist, who used imagery and bodywork (involving massage and physical manipulations to "open up" the body), she began to recall moments in her childhood when her needs and feelings went underground. She went progressively back through the layers of psychic defense erected over many years and gradually dismantled them, until she hit upon certain key "decision points." These were painful events that had led her to believe that her emotional needs were unacceptable and couldn't be met, so she simply cut them off.

"Later in life, there was nothing that could ever make me need or want again. When I was in the hospital, people asked, 'What do you need?' and I literally had no idea what they were talking about. I'd studied psychology for years, but I had no experiential awareness of what it meant to need. But by the end of my analysis, I got back to those decision points. I began to undo the damage, and I was able to express needs again."

Barbara went back to school to study psychology, got her degree, and began working with other cancer patients to shepherd them through the same kind of transformative journey she had undertaken. She believes that this path requires the utmost energy and conviction, and a capacity to tolerate both the pain and joy that one encounters along the way. In her view, it's an inner journey with outer manifestations and consequences. For Barbara, that meant changes in her relationship to others and to the world.

"Every year, my mother used to take creative and clever photos of our family for Christmas cards," Barbara said. "Looking back at them, I was struck by the fact that I was always retracted, in the shadows. My mother would come into a room where I was and not see me, because I had so recessed myself from the world that I was virtually invisible. In the seven years since my diagnosis, you can always see me in those pictures, standing out."

Barbara doesn't work much with cancer patients anymore, because she says it takes too much energy out of her. She currently sees a small group of patients, most of whom are physically well and wish to change. And she continues to keep her promise to herself. "I've gotten physically healthier than I've ever been," she told me. "But the most important benefit has been the peace of knowing that, for the first time, I have my ground—a self I can count on."

The battles worth fighting are the ones *for* something—an ideal, a cherished goal, self-preservation, the protection of loved ones. When the fight is strictly against a feared and despised enemy, in this case a tumor, then the motivating principle is hatred. From the beginning, Barbara's fight was focused not against her tumor but against any force limiting or constraining her knowledge of— and compassion for—her real self, a self that had been hidden since childhood. More important, she fought *for* that self, to defend that self, to become one again with that self. That is why Barbara's struggle generated in her a broad spectrum of feelings—anger, joy, fear, sadness, exhilaration—which formed the wellspring of motivation she needed to keep going in the face of terrifying odds.

Had it not been for her illness, Barbara might never have left her spider's web, a psychological safety net that kept her from falling into an abyss of insecurity, but also confined her. When cancer strikes, many people like Barbara are able to leave their webs, because they're faced with the reality of death and they're not afraid anymore of the abyss. They can finally let go and, in the process, discover parts of themselves held in abeyance as they struggled simply to survive in their webs. Those self-discoveries, and their ability to finally show those sides of themselves in the world, appear to have an uncanny, stimulating effect on their body's healing systems.

CARPE DIEM

I've said that Type C behavior is a defense we use to adapt to painful circumstances in our families and society. I've also called Type C a fragile accommodation to the world, because the ways in which we hide and restrict ourselves eventually leave us in a quietly unhappy or imperceptibly imbalanced psychological state. In addition to all this, Type C behavior can be a rut, plain and simple. It's a pattern of coping that leaves us few options, that tends to keep us in the same, often stultifying jobs, roles, or relationships for decades.

Which brings me to the story of Irwin, a man who, in his mid-twenties, found himself stuck in a rut. He had devoted his life to becoming an Episcopal minister, but while attending seminary he was plagued with doubts and angers that caused an aversion to the church. Abruptly, he dropped out. Instead of sending Irwin into a period of creative flowering, leaving the seminary sent him headlong into several years of ambivalence and inertia. During that time he lived with his girlfriend, but the relationship couldn't solve all his problems.

In 1959—three years after leaving the seminary—Irwin was diagnosed with testicular cancer. The cancer had spread to his lymph nodes, chest, and lungs. One tumor on his neck had grown so large that he was forced to keep his head at an odd tilt. His doctors told him he had three to four months to live. "They said I had essentially zero chance of survival," he said. The testicle was removed, and he was given radiation, cobalt treatments, and nitrogen mustard—the best medical therapy available at the time. But this was done mainly to reduce his discomfort and the size of his tumors.

Irwin's diagnosis startled him out of his inertia. He sought the help of an unconventional psychoanalyst, a woman named Lotte, who used hypnosis along with traditional analysis to help Irwin not only cope with cancer but work on his long-term life goals. "I wasn't digging my grave," Irwin told me. "I was doing things that weren't terribly appropriate for someone who was supposed to die."

Lotte helped Irwin discover that abandoning the church, though his decision, had been a real loss—a loss of his vocation, his sense of meaning, and his faith. With her help, he broke out of his ambivalence and returned to the seminary to complete his studies. He also decided to marry his girlfriend.

Within a month of his marriage—and on the very day Irwin was ordained as an Episcopal priest—he got the news that his follow-up X rays showed no more evidence of cancer. His lymph nodes and lungs were completely clear. This seeming miracle occurred six months after his original diagnosis.

Irwin's medical treatments may have contributed to his cure. But his doctors had not expected Irwin to achieve complete remission—a result unheard of at that time.

Today, thirty-three years later, Irwin is alive, well, and cancer-free. His case has been studied and written about. Lotte published an article in a psychiatric journal which described his entire case, including her therapeutic methods and the details of his medical condition. I spoke with Irwin recently, and asked him to what he attributed his unexpected recovery.

"It's hard for me to pinpoint one thing," he said. "I was working with the right therapist at the right time. Without her, I believe I would have floundered. Also, I assume that having one of the more humane doctors in this world helped. I assume that getting married helped. I assume that getting ordained helped. And I assume that my cooperation with the cobalt machine helped." (Irwin was referring to the fact that during his treatments, instead of lying passively he exhorted the cobalt machine to do its best and imagined his cancer cells running for cover. It was an early, self-styled version of the kind of visualization technique that became popular fifteen years later.)

As Irwin related his entire story—what happened both before and after his diagnosis—I began to make sense of his transformation. He had broken out of his Type C rut and reentered life with the courage to make transitions and move on to new phases. This involved a deeper exploration of his feelings, an opening to love, and an ongoing dynamic search for meaning.

Irwin had found Lotte just before his diagnosis, and in group therapy he began to express anger fully for the first time. This loosened his psychological armor. Once diagnosed, Irwin was ready for Lotte's novel approach. He was open to the healing suggestions she made while he was under hypnosis. He was open to overcoming blocks in his capacity to love and be loved. More in touch with his gut instincts, Irwin began asking the larger questions: What do I want to do with my life? What is my relationship to God? How can I rediscover my faith?

To use my term, Irwin developed emotional flexibility. This allowed him to approach life's turning points with curiosity and creativity. After his ordination, he became the vicar of a small mission, but after four years he once again experienced doubts about the church. This time, instead of withdrawing, he sought meaning in a new way: he got his graduate degree in psychology and began working as a psychologist. As a therapist, he learned more about himself and the human condition. Irwin was drawn to humanistic psychology and soon to transpersonal psychology, in an attempt to bring together his psychological insights and his hunger for spiritual development. Years later, he returned to the church. But now, his quest reflected a greater maturity. Irwin was still fascinated by Christian tradition, but he wanted to synthesize his work in psychology, meditation, and hypnosis with Christian practices. "My new interests don't quite fit in with conventional religion, but I am trying to bring my sense of spirituality back to the church," he remarked.

I don't know whether spirituality per se was the key to Irwin's healing. From my experience, the path to healing does not have to be either religious or secular. Irwin's story implies that it's healing to open up our emotions, to search for meaning, to become willing to make passages from one life phase to the next. When Irwin responded to an inner call of carpe diem (Latin for "seize the day"), his disease reacted as if it had no proper place in his body.

"Everybody wanted to lay claim to being the healer," said Irwin to a journalist who wrote an article about him. His therapist, his radiologist, and his bishop, who attributed his remission to "divine grace," all credited their own approaches. I credit Irwin, who seized life and began a three-decades-long journey that continues to this day.

THE RESISTANCE-SURRENDER CYCLE

What do the patients in this chapter have in common? All of them overcame blocks to feeling. They began to act on their feelings rather than their intellectual decisions or the desire to please others. Each one embarked on a process of change and self-realization. They all lived as if they were going to *live,* not as if they were going to die. As extraordinary as these patients are, none of them could have done it alone. They all needed the guidance and support of a skilled therapist in order to make their transformations.

They had another thing in common: they all had to contend with psychological and physical ups and downs, whether in the form of relapses, periods of despair, moments of self-blame, times of anxiety and confusion, or sudden alterations in life plans and goals. This teaches us something important about fighting spirit: to have fighting spirit doesn't require that you become a fearless warrior who never lets his guard down. You can be a part-time warrior who also suffers, has doubts, stumbles, and needs help. That requires acceptance of your vulnerability.

Robert Chernin Cantor describes this phenomenon precisely in his book, *And A Time To Live.* He calls it the resistance-surrender cycle:

> For many of us the surrender to powerful forces acting upon our lives is in violent conflict with our defiant fighting instincts. It is not at all uncommon to want to give oneself over, to trust in one's fate, to surrender control and responsibility and then a short time later to reverse oneself and want to fight, while yet again, still later, to return to a desire for

release and passive acceptance. The *resistance-surrender cycle* is profoundly human. One woman expressed the conflict with poignant clarity: "I have cancer and I have to overcome it. I want to overcome it very badly. [But] sometimes when I'm in pain, I feel like . . . why can't I just wake up dead? That's a very funny thing to say." It is a paradoxical emotion and yet it captures the ambivalence perfectly; I want to surrender (in this case to die) *and* I want to wake up triumphant.

A dynamic life contains both the inner force of heroic resistance and the inner force of acceptance and surrender. When we feel beaten, we would do well to reach out for our fighting spirit, and when we find ourselves unproductively thrashing against an irreversible reality, we would profit from a greater ability to surrender and accept it. The crucial judgment rests upon an intuitive understanding of when fighting is appropriate and when surrender seems the wisest course.

By working through feelings of sadness and even hopelessness, you are respecting your need to surrender and freeing your pendulum to swing back toward heroic resistance.

Another aspect of surrender is allowing yourself to relax. Generals, boxers, activists, and unrequited lovers all need time to rest, reflect, and regroup before reappearing on their respective battlefields. Alexander Lowen, M.D., a psychoanalyst and author of many books on mind-body therapy, put it another way:

> One has to let down to renew oneself. One has to lie down to recover one's strength. Unless one lets go of the day, one can't enjoy the sleep of the night. Symbolically, we die each night, but we are reborn the next day. Without death there can be no rebirth. Unless we go down, we cannot rise.

We all know intuitively that sleep is healing. How many times have you gone to bed with a chronic symptom—like a headache, backache, or incipient cold—and after a particularly deep sleep awakened to discover that your pains had vanished? Irwin, the patient whose cancer disappeared after he got married and was ordained, told me that his therapist regularly put him into a deep hypnotic state that was essentially a healing form of sleep. I'm not saying that sleep is an answer to cancer—rather, that one's willingness to "let down" or "let be" is an important aspect of recovery from any illness.

Type C transformation is not a smooth, straight line from diagnosis to recovery. Transformations like the ones I've described in this chapter are bumpy, arduous, and take work. Moreover, they don't guarantee recovery. Full recovery is certainly possible—and even more likely—when transformation is one aspect of a broader program of wellness that includes medical treatment. The stories in this chapter are undeniable examples of that. But regardless of your physical outcome, the transformation is worthwhile, because the life it ushers in is one worth living.

PART V

TYPE C TRANSFORMATION— FOR PREVENTION

CHAPTER 14

Speak now, I said to myself, release your true feelings
before it's too late. Be yourself. Take your place in the
world. You are not a cosmic orphan. You have no reason
to be timid. Respond as you feel. Awkwardly, crudely . . .
but respond. Leave your throat open. You can have
anything the world has to offer, but the thing you need
most and perhaps want most is to be yourself. Stop being
anonymous. The anonymity you believed would protect
you from pain and humiliation, shame and rejection,
doesn't work. Admit rejection, admit pain, admit
frustration, admit pettiness, even that; admit shame,
admit outrage, admit anything and everything that
happens to you, respond with your true, uncalculated
response, your emotions. The best and most human
parts of you are those that you have inhibited
and hidden from the world.

—Elia Kazan

Type C Transformation in Everyday Life

The purpose of Chinese medicine is radically different from that of the West. In ancient China it was established that the primary function of medicine should be *prevention*. Only recently has Western medicine begun to speak the language of prevention, and we are still far from fluent. The Chinese physician reads the subtle signs of "dis-ease" in his patient's mind-body; senses a change in his voice, breath, or emotional tone; and determines his dietary, hygenic, and sexual practices. These diagnostic procedures enable him to detect imbalances, and apply the correct treatment to nourish and strengthen the natural state of health. Traditionally, doctors who treated patients with a full-blown illness were considered failures, since they had been unable to ward off clinical disease. This statement of the Yellow Emperor's chief medical advisor, from the *Internal Book of Huang Di*, sums up the Chinese perspective:

> To administer medicines to diseases which have already developed . . . is comparable to the behavior of those persons who begin to dig a well after they have become thirsty, and of those who begin to make their weapons after they have already engaged in battle. Would these actions not be too late?

The purpose of this section of the book, metaphorically speaking, is to help you dig a well before you become thirsty and to make weapons before you engage in battle. More to the point, I offer some new weapons in your internal battle with cancer cells, to prevent war from breaking out with a full-blown tumor. If we keep our immune defenses in fighting trim, we increase the probability that we will vanquish any malignant cells in our bodies before they proliferate out of control. In this way, we avoid a potentially life-threatening confrontation with the clinical reality of cancer.

There are many ways to strengthen immunity. Nutritional changes, such as lowering the fat in your diet and adding certain foods and nutrients to it, are excellent ways to enhance and fine-tune your immune responses. Avoiding toxic chemical agents will protect your immune system from damage. In recent years, meditation and imagery have been offered as mind-body therapies with potential immune-balancing effects.

When I found in my research that the melanoma patients who expressed emotions had more lymphocytes surrounding their tumors, as compared with patients who inhibited emotions, I realized that helping cancer patients express their feelings could improve their chance for recovery. Now I believe that healthy people can bolster and balance their immune system and, quite possibly, ward off cancer—by making long-term changes in their Type C behavior.

In this chapter and the following two chapters, I will describe Type C transformation for healthy people. As compared with the program for cancer patients, this program entails slower, broader, and deeper changes in the way you relate to yourself and others. It addresses issues of everyday life: ways to express emotion; become more assertive in your relationships; manage anger effectively; and tend to the needs of your mind-body.

THE SCIENCE OF CANCER PREVENTION

Human behavior is one of many factors that contribute to malignant disease. External habits like smoking, certain dietary practices, and excessive alcohol intake can increase our risk of developing certain cancers. These behaviors are risky because they bring us in direct contact with carcinogenic agents. If everyone quit smoking and modified their diets to reduce fat and increase fiber, then occurrence of lung, throat, colon, breast, prostate, and oral cancers would radically diminish. Air, water, and food pollution must be reduced or eliminated in order to banish cancers caused largely by environmental agents. I support wholeheartedly these crucial actions. But my goal here is to stress the power we have to reduce risk from our internal environment—the potential risk caused by Type C behavior.

Type C behavior may increase cancer risks by upsetting our biological homeostasis and diminishing the power of our immune defenses. Just as Chinese doctors, in accord with their medical model, can sense changes in their patients' state of health by examining the body and taking the pulse, so must we take our own psychological pulse and use the information and insight gained to fine-tune our behavior in the quest for health.

Scientific proof that mind-body therapy (or transformation) could actually prevent cancer is hard to come by. We need long-term intervention studies, in which a group of healthy people who undergo mind-body treatment is followed for many years and compared with a similar group who receives no such treatment. Researchers could then determine whether the treated group develops less cancer over a long period of time.

In the absence of such studies, no one can make surefire claims that mind-body therapy prevents cancer. However, I have cited a wealth of data in this book suggesting that Type C's, who lack quality social support, internalize stress, and inhibit emotions, suffer biologically as a consequence of their pattern. In addition, several studies have shown that *people who reverse these behaviors and trends increase their resistance to disease.* Scientifically sound research has correlated emotional expression, relaxation, and social support with better immune functioning or more positive disease outcomes. I'll describe research on relaxation and social support in Chapter 16; here, I'll tell you how sharing emotions can boost immunity.

THE IMMUNE BENEFITS OF OPENING UP

Dr. James W. Pennebaker, the psychologist at Southern Methodist University whose research was discussed in Chapter 12, has conducted a series of fascinating studies that show that expressing emotions and confiding past traumas boosts immunity and improves overall health. Pennebaker and his colleague Sandra Beall compared several groups of Southern Methodist University students who were asked to write about different experiences over the course of four days. One group was told to write about trivial matters, like the layout of their dorm room. Another was told to write about traumas they experienced in the past—but only the facts involved, not the feelings. A third group was asked to tell the whole story of a trauma, facts *and* feelings.

This final group was referred to as "emotional disclosers." Here is how Pennebaker described their experiences:

> For the students, the immediate impact of the study was far more powerful than we had ever imagined. Several of the students cried while writing about traumas. Many reported dreaming or continually thinking about their writing topics over the four days of the study. Most telling, however, were the writing samples themselves. Essay after essay revealed people's deepest feelings and most intimate sides. Many of the stories depicted profound human tragedies.

> Pennebaker and Beall were amazed that eighteen-year-old students attending an upper-middle-class college had been through so many traumas: family abuse, alcoholism, suicide attempts, divorce of parents, and public humiliation were frequently reported.

The researchers obtained physiological readings for all forty-six subjects, including heart rate and blood pressure. After the four days, the emotional disclosers had increased blood pressure and said they felt more upset. But six months later, the emotional disclosers had experienced less illness, and made far fewer visits to the student health center, when compared with students in the other groups. They also were asked to reflect on the experiment, and the disclosers said it had a positive effect: they had more insight, less anxiety, and a sense of resolution about the traumas they revealed.

But Pennbaker wondered, Could these remarkable results have been a one-time fluke? And what explained the better health of the emotional disclosers? In search of answers, Pennebaker collaborated with psychologist Janice Kiecolt-Glaser, Ph.D., and immunologist Ronald Glaser, M.D., on a similar study with a new dimension. They evaluated the immune status of students who confided past traumas, and compared them with others who completed only trivial writing exercises. The subjects who disclosed their traumas had much livelier T-cells after the exercise and six weeks later; the control subjects did not. The disclosers also had far fewer visits to the health center than the people who wrote only about trivial subjects.

Pennebaker asked the disclosers to indicate whether they were revealing experiences and feelings that they had previously kept secret from others. He then divided them into two groups: the ones who confided suppressed facts and emotions were the *high disclosers;* the others were termed *low disclosers.* The high disclosers showed a more rapid rise in immune-cell strength than did the low disclosers.

Pennebaker has shown that acknowledging painful experiences—and expressing feelings about these traumas—reduces stress, enhances certain aspects of immune functioning, and wards off illness. The psychological benefits are similar to those people can achieve in psychotherapy—peace of mind, a sense of resolution, and relief from emotional tension. We now have evidence for the physical benefits as well.

Pennebaker gave the example of one woman in his study, who had written about her sexual abuse:

> One woman, who had been molested at the age of 9 years by a boy 3 years older, initially emphasized her feelings of embarrassment and guilt. By the third day of writing, she expressed anger at the boy who victimized her. By the last day, she had begun to put it in perspective. On the follow-up survey six weeks after the experiment, she reported, "Before when I thought about it, I'd lie to myself. . . . Now, I don't feel like I even have to think about it because I got it off my chest. I finally admitted that it happened. . . . I really know the truth and won't have to lie to myself anymore."

Healing our alienation from ourselves involves admitting our pains first to ourselves and then to others. Pennebaker's disclosers did both. Writing down their traumas was both an act of coming to terms with memories and feelings held inside, and an act of confiding those memories and feelings. Pennebaker's work is extraordinary validation that such acts have a demonstrable positive effect on our health and immunity.

THREE LEVELS OF TRANSFORMATION

James Pennebaker's subjects participated in a writing exercise that enabled them, if only briefly, to recover and express parts of themselves lost in the "bag" (Robert Bly's metaphor for that invisible repository of repressed feelings and memories). Type C transformation in everyday life involves similar elements—recovering lost shards of the self, confiding inner truths, and also acting to assert one's needs.

Type C is a cognitive, emotional, and behavioral pattern. For this reason, transforming Type C involves changes on all three levels. The leaders of the cognitive movement in psychology theorize that negative emotions stem from negative thought patterns. Change the thoughts, they say, and you'll change the emotions. Proponents of more traditional psychotherapy, and many neo-Freudian schools, view pathological thoughts and behaviors as stemming from unresolved emotions. Get to the emotions, they claim, and you'll change the thoughts and behaviors. Behaviorists downplay the role of emotions, and believe that modifying behavior takes care of other levels of consciousness. (I am simplifying a bit; there are some cognitive therapists, traditional psychotherapists, and behaviorists who work on multiple, complex levels.)

The arguments between these factions often comes down to this: which comes first, the thought or the feeling? It's a classic chicken-or-the-egg question. I take the view that thoughts don't *cause* feelings and feelings don't *cause* thoughts. There is a two-way flow between levels of consciousness, a continuous back-and-forth interrelationship between what we think and how we feel. That's why, as a therapist, I work to help the individual change on several levels at once. In my view, overreliance on one narrow set of techniques can be unnecessarily limiting, and therapy should involve cognitive, emotional, and behavioral dimensions.

Evelyn, a physically healthy therapy patient, came to me with marital problems. She was a Type C coper who never expressed her needs or anger to her "difficult" husband. She thought he would reject her if she demanded more quality time with him. From my work with Evelyn, it seemed clear that her husband, whatever his problems, loved her and would not have rejected her for becoming more assertive. A strict cognitive therapist might have said, "Her thoughts are causing her fear and timidity. She has to learn that he won't reject her if she stands up for herself. Then, her fear will diminish and her behavior will change." True, up to a point. If she *could* be made to believe that he would not walk out on her, her fear *would* subside. But many Type C's have a deeply held belief that they will be rejected for asserting themselves. Sometimes, no amount of rational talk can change their mind.

In this case, Evelyn needed to explore and express her fears of abandonment, to discover where they originated. It turned out that she'd been conditioned by an old-fashioned father to behave in a ladylike fashion at all times. She recalled being severely disciplined as a child for behaviors he considered "rude" and "aggressive." Over time, she learned to play the role of the sweet, refined, and always responsive woman to the men in her life. She never got angry, because she feared a similarly harsh response. Her belief that her husband would reject her for being too "uppity" was based on a bedrock of past fears. In therapy, she discovered that her fears were deeply rooted in her relationship with her father. Evelyn didn't require ten years of psychoanalysis to accomplish this—only a few therapy sessions. Once expressed, the fear didn't go away, as if drained from some inner pool—but she *had* located its source.

Evelyn then was open to cognitive reframing. She no longer saw her husband as a projection of her father. I said to her, "From everything you've said about your husband, I don't think he'll walk out on you if you assert your needs more forcefully." She could begin to *believe* this, from the inside out, not from the outside in. I wasn't *training* her, I was guiding her to make discoveries on her own. Evelyn accepted that her husband would not reject her, because she had distinguished him from her father, the present from the past, her current feelings from her old feelings. She had a better grasp of reality and a good deal more courage to face him with her needs. Then, without much prodding from me, she made behavior changes. Over the course of a year, Evelyn began to ask more of her husband. For a while, they fought more than usual. But they struggled through this period and eventually, both came to feel that their marriage was more exciting. They began to spend more quality time together. Even their love-making improved.

Of course, we are all unique creatures. In the case of Evelyn, the emotional work came first, then the cognitive, then the behavioral. For other women in the same situation, cognitive or behavioral approaches might have been a better initial choice. The main point is this: Type C transformation is a "whole person" approach, requiring changes on the levels of thought, feeling, and behavior.

How can you apply this flexible approach? If you're changing through psychotherapy, select a therapist who does not rely upon one limited technique but rather, one who responds to you as a whole person. You can "interview" prospective therapists, and inquire about their background, beliefs, and methods. Feel free to ask them if they rely on a technique that addresses one or several levels of human experience. If you are changing without formal therapy, then read this chapter carefully. It will help you deal with the cognitive, emotional, and behavioral levels in a dynamic way that is right for your distinct personality.

BALANCING INNER/OUTER TRANSACTIONS

Every moment of every day of our lives involves transactions with our outer environment. The vital balance of health depends on transactions that retain the integrity and balance of our inner environment. Eating and breathing are transactions with our environment, and if our food or air is tainted with germs, viruses, or chemicals, our body must overcome them (via its immune system). Otherwise, these foreign agents would overwhelm us and destroy our integrity. In the same manner, if our social environment places inordinate demands on us, and our psychological system can't handle these demands effectively, our integrity is again threatened. That is the real meaning of stress: an external reality that our mind-body cannot accommodate and cope with effectively.

Consider the example of a woebegone midlevel executive, whom I'll call Calvin. One Friday, Calvin's employer demands that he finish a big report over the weekend. If not, his boss slyly implies, he may be fired. The problem is, the report requires two weeks of work instead of two days. Calvin immediately feels the grip of viselike inner stress. How can he respond emotionally and behaviorally in a way that restores balance with his environment—namely his boss and his work?

Everyone has his own unique coping style, and there is no single correct way for Calvin to respond. Multiple contingencies come into play, such as the boss's personality and the degree of importance Calvin attaches to keeping his job. However, one thing is sure: if he doesn't take action in his own defense and behave in a way that moderates his mind-body stress and reduces the threat to his livelihood, he'll be left in a state of disequilibrium that will damage his health.

That's where Type C coping comes into play. Type C is a style of handling inner-outer transactions that maintained balance in an early stage of life but fosters imbalance in later stages. Calvin, a classic Type C coper, will tell his boss he'll have the report first thing Monday. He won't say, "This can't be done," for fear that his boss will fly off the handle. So he goes home and spends an excruciating weekend trying to accomplish an impossible task. He returns Monday morning, fatigued and frightened, to face his boss with his half-completed, hastily prepared report. Predictably, his boss explodes. Calvin sits and takes it, hoping this will all blow over. Relations are further strained, and even though he doesn't get fired, he knows he's walking a fine line. From that point on, Calvin's job stress only gets worse.

Calvin's Type C response creates further mind-body disorder in three ways. On a low level of consciousness, he is holding emotions of anger and anxiety. These feelings are never resolved. Not only can't he express them to his boss, which might not be appropriate anyway, but he can't share them with people in his support system because he's not sufficiently aware of them. As we know, there is a physiological price to be paid for chronically repressing emotions. Second, Calvin takes no assertive action to change his environment. The stressful transactions continue, unmitigated, because he hasn't insisted that his boss come up with a more realistic deadline. Third, Calvin tries to do work that can't be done, and exhausts himself physically in the process. This puts pressure on all his biological systems—nervous, cardiovascular, and immune.

Calvin had two choices: he could have calmly but firmly explained that he needed more time to complete the project, giving his boss every opportunity to either respond well or blow off steam.

Even if he did explode at Calvin, as long as the boss granted him extra time, Calvin would have gotten his need met and would simply have had to endure one more of his boss's tantrums. Alternatively, Calvin could have reached the decision that his boss made his job (and life) far too stressful, and begun looking for a new position.

Type C coping breeds imbalance in a person's inner-outer transactions. There has to be "give" somewhere, and for the Type C coper, the "give" is somatic: the immune system falters, leaving the person more vulnerable to a variety of illnesses.

AUTONOMY: CHANGING TYPE C RELATIONSHIPS

In his fine book *The Betrayal of the Self,* Arno Gruen gives a cogent definition of autonomy: "Autonomy is that state of integration in which one lives in full harmony with one's feelings and needs." The goals implied by this statement are as broad as they are difficult to attain. They are especially hard to reach—but equally essential— for Type C individuals. For autonomy—which entails knowing one's self and honoring that self in human relationships—represents the opposite of passivity, conformity, and compliance.

One way to develop autonomy is to focus on your important relationships with relentless honesty and specificity. Ask yourself these questions about any significant relationship:

1) Do I try to perceive how this person wants me to behave, and then behave that way?
2) Am I often afraid of behaving in ways this person will find unacceptable?
3) Do I suppress my real needs with this person?
4) Do I express needs with this person, but find myself constantly frustrated by him or her?
5) Am I frightened of expressing anger, fear, or sadness with this person?
6) Do I take care of this person to a large extent?
7) Is his or her love and approval dependent on my caretaking?
8) Is his or her love and approval dependent on my obedience?

9) Do I feel victimized by this person?
10) Is my sense of self-love and self-confidence dependent on the approval of this person or of my superior(s) at work?

If you answered yes to many of these questions, then lack of autonomy is a central feature of your Type C behavior. Relationships based on the suppression of autonomy are inherently unfulfilling. The self that is loved is not your real self. It is, to use D. W. Winnicott's term, a "false self," one that you learned to present from earliest childhood in order to hold the approval of your parents. A Type C individual believes that he can't be loved for his real self, which was buried long ago with needs and feelings deemed "unacceptable." When these emotions emerge in consciousness, they are threatening because the person associates them with early rejections or humiliations. As he grows, he develops longings—sometimes secret—to let these feelings out of the bag. For this reason, relationships based on the struggle to please are never really stable—no matter how stable they appear. The person's yearning to express his hidden real self, and the repressed feelings held there, never really dies.

When you ask the questions I've presented here, be completely honest. You'll discover the desires and feelings that remain unexpressed in your relationship. You may realize that you've been playing a role, one you've played for many others in your life. This doesn't mean your relationship lacks value. It means that you need to reintegrate vital parts of yourself into the relationship. In some instances, the relationship is based upon domination or abuse, and you will be able to detach from it as you undergo transformation.

The Type C person views himself as loyal, responsive, supportive, and loving. He is all these things, but he has taken these positive qualities too far at the expense of his own self. Often, when I encourage people in therapy to focus on their needs, they become confused, thinking that I am asking them to stop being the helpful, wonderful people they are. I tell them: you can be loyal without being obedient. You can be responsive without being a compulsive people pleaser. You can be supportive without being servile.

Many Type C's never grant validity to inner voices that say, "I'm frustrated!" "I'm bored!" "I struggle and struggle—for what?" "I can't be myself with him/her!" These are like screams muffled for years by a suffocating pillow of psychic self-protection. If you allow yourself to hear these voices, you can begin to change the relationship.

The first question that arises is, Do I abandon the problematic relationship? or Do I try to make it better? There is no formulaic answer. However, one key distinction can help you decide: is the relationship simply frustrating, or is it abusive? The healthiest thing you can do upon discovering that you are in an abusive relationship—whether it involves sexual, physical, or emotional abuse—is to find your way out. If the relationship is merely frustrating, you'll need to do a great deal of introspection as well as "field-testing" to find the right road.

OLD RELATIONSHIPS, NEW SONGS

Here's what I mean by "field-testing." As you change your Type C pattern, your spouse, family members, or friends may be taken aback by your new, more expressive behaviors. It's your responsibility to communicate your needs and feelings, but it's not their responsibility to approve and accept every new move you make. Learn to expect uncomfortable responses, especially when you show more assertiveness. The more autonomy you develop, the less important it will be for people to embrace every newly discovered facet of yourself. What will be important is whether they hang in with you over a long period. In time, you'll find out the answer.

The patterns in long-term relationships can become like deeply worn grooves in an old vinyl record. You and your partner have played the same "song" hundreds of times, and every bar has a comforting predictability. If one person suddenly wishes to sing a different song—to put on a new record—the other person may protest: "What are you doing! I don't know that song. Put that old Beatles record back on!" He'll be disturbed at first, but with a little trust and imagination he may come to hear the new song, even if at first it seems abrasive or challenging. What you need to carry off the change is a little persistence and a lot of patience. If he never likes the song, so be it. You can still be friends (or lovers). He doesn't *have* to like the song. On the other hand, if he attacks you verbally and expresses hostility that you dared to play this weird new music and abandon the old, then you need to reevaluate the relationship.

Very often, Type C persons get into relationships in which the currency of every interaction is *struggle.* You find someone who is both attractive and frustrating, and expend all your energy trying to win his/her love and approval.* The self-help movements for psychological and spiritual growth have helped many people to extricate themselves from such destructive relationships and find their way into nourishing ones. This is a promising trend. For the purpose of changing Type C behavior, there is a specific relationship trap that can be avoided.

In therapy, one of the comments I've heard from Type C patients in such relationships is "But I'm expressing my needs! I'm acknowledging my real feelings and he/she just can't accept them. I'm being myself, but that isn't working." The circumstances these people find themselves in are often the same. They can't be themselves in most of their roles or relationships, so they find one person on whom to hang their hopes for self-actualization. They enact—or more accurately, reenact—the drama of the search for self-acceptance. Tellingly, these individuals never find someone who is capable of accepting their needs, idiosyncracies, anger, and vulnerability. They find others who are distressed by these parts of themselves, who withdraw love and approval whenever they act too angry or needy. Thus, a circular pattern is set in motion—of pursuit and withdrawal, fighting and forgiving, blame and retaliation. To return to my vinyl analogy, this person puts on a new song but there's a skip right at the beginning of the record! The same screechy bar of music repeats over and over, and neither of them ever hears any new music. The Type C person constantly struggles to have his/her inner self accepted but is continually, painfully disappointed.

What I tell such patients is this: you are re-creating the conditions of the original loss of your real self. You have found a parent substitute who behaves in much the same manner as your parent(s) did in your childhood: he or she simply cannot accept your authentic needs and emotions. Now, on the stage of this relationship, in

---

*Countless self-help books have been written, many for women, on this type of relationship. Whether it is *Women Who Love Too Much* or *Codependent No More,* the pattern described is a treacherous psychological trap for both men and women.

340 THE TYPE C CONNECTION

the theater of adult life, you are trying to win the unconditional love you never got. Unfortunately, this is a futile effort, because you needed it *then,* not now. No person in your present can make up for the losses of your past. Furthermore, you have selected an individual who doesn't accept you, so that you can play your part to the hilt. The inherent frustration could keep you going for a lifetime, forever struggling to find that elusive early acceptance.

If, through therapy or your own introspection, you can recognize the early origins of this behavior, you've made a breakthrough toward autonomy. Know that your struggle is a valiant one, even though it is misplaced. You have an "inner child" who is still trying to express him/herself and win love. The struggle relationship is a derailed attempt to rediscover your real self. It is crucial to recognize the futility of getting someone to make up for past losses. On the other hand, it is liberating to accept those early losses, to grieve for the unconditional acceptance you did not have as a child. Once this occurs, the drive to replay the past over and over diminishes. You're no longer magnetically attracted to those who frustrate you, who offer opportunities for you to act out your early drama. You begin to gravitate toward people who really do accept you for who you are. Before, such individuals seemed to offer no excitement. How can you play a dramatic scene with someone who doesn't oppose your true self?

Part of expressing your needs is finding people who can listen and respond. If you are constantly finding people who can't or won't, then you are re-creating the past, not expressing your real needs in the present. Realizing this is one way to clarify confusion about needs and their expression in healthy relationships. However, it's also helpful for you to recognize that an ongoing pattern of struggle relationships won't change overnight. The conflicts underlying this aspect of your Type C behavior are powerful. I recommend you seek the help of a counselor, support group, or individual therapist to help you change this tenacious pattern.

CHAPTER 15

We only become what we are by the radical and
deep-seated refusal of that which others have made of us.

—*Jean-Paul Sartre*

I was angry with my friend:
I told my wrath, my wrath did end.
I was angry with my foe:
I told it not, my wrath did grow.

—*William Blake*

Notice how—in your past—every time you were angry
you were frightened. You have a right to anger. You
don't have to earn it. Take it. Anger saves.

—*Elia Kazan*

Our anger empowers us in the struggle against destiny. As
Beethoven cried, "I will seize my fate by the throat!"
And out of that came the Fifth Symphony.

—*Rollo May*

Expressing Anger: What's Effective?

When anger becomes the phantom emotion, it gets lost in the mind's shadows. There it lurks as a force beyond our reckoning, and there its potential for destructiveness grows. Removed from the shadows, seen and felt and experienced in the light of day, investigated, expressed, and sometimes shared, anger evaporates. The cycle recurs: anger will arise again and once more be discharged. We never rid ourselves of anger, since it is part of our emotional repertoire. But we can stop anger from festering, blinding our perceptions, making us meek, crippling our capacity for love, or making us physically sick.

As I've shown, our defense against cancer and other diseases may be protected, in part, when we are able to express our anger. In order to realize the health benefits, we must learn how to accept, manage, and communicate anger appropriately and effectively. Where do we begin? Harriet Goldhor Lerner, Ph.D., in one of the best books on the subject, *The Dance of Anger,* provides an answer:

> Anger is a signal, and one worth listening to. Our anger may be a message that we are being hurt, that our rights are being violated, that our needs or wants are not being adequately met, or simply that something is not right. Our anger may tell us that we are not addressing an important emotional

issue in our lives, or that too much of our self—our beliefs, values, desires, or ambitions—is being compromised in a relationship. Our anger may be a signal that we are doing more and giving more than we can comfortably do or give. Or our anger may warn us that others are doing too much for us, at the expense of our own competence and growth. Just as physical pain tells us to take our hand off the hot stove, the pain of our anger preserves the very integrity of our self. Our anger can motivate us to say "no" to the ways in which we are defined by others and "yes" to the dictates of our inner self.

Once you become aware of your anger, there are choices you make about how to express it. Some choices are healthier and more effective than others. In her book, which is addressed primarily to women, Lerner describes two types of women who handle anger in opposite ways. There are the "nice ladies," who are always sweet, helpful, and often play the role of "peace-keeper." And there are the "bitchy women," who are often described as "nagging," "complaining," and "unfeminine." According to Lerner, these two styles, while radically different, have something crucial in common: both are ineffective means of managing anger (although it's important to remember that some women who *appropriately* express anger are still called "bitches," particularly by men who can't accept women's anger).

I can compare Lerner's idea of two opposite, extreme, and ineffective ways of expressing anger with my Type A-Type C continuum. At one pole is the Type A person, who vents anger in a compulsive, unhealthy manner. At the other pole is the Type C person, who never expresses anger or asserts him/herself. These tendencies appear in slightly different forms in men and women, and are perceived differently based on social and cultural conditioning. In fact, "nice lady" describes the Type C woman in our culture—she is passive, sweet, and serves the needs of the people in her life, especially the men. When corresponding qualities are seen in men, they are enacted—and perceived by others—in a slightly different way. The Type C man might be described as "wimpy" "henpecked," or "withdrawn." (Notice how perjorative these cultural definitions are.)

The Type A woman is comparable with Lerner's "bitchy woman." We tend to think of Type A men as businessmen or workaholics, who are always pumped up, often nasty, and engage in cutthroat behavior on the job. We see Type A women exhibiting similar tendencies at work, but in relationships this behavior is described as "aggressive," "demanding," or "castrating."

Whether someone is described as a Type A man or a son of a bitch, a Type A woman or a bitchy woman, his or her expression of anger is distorted. This style involves fighting, blaming, and hostility (not clean anger) that leads nowhere. These displays do not resolve anger, but often make it worse for the person who is venting. Though "letting off steam" can sometimes be useful, it almost never is for people stuck in a broken-record pattern of venting rage. The conditions that cause the anger—both internal and external— are hardly changed through this mode of expression.

Whether someone is called a Type C man or a nice guy, a Type C woman or a nice lady, he or she ignores or misinterprets the inner signals of anger. The inability to feel one's anger, to pay attention to its meaning, and to take appropriate action to change the circumstances that caused it lead to a growing—and often silent— sense of powerlessness.

When I encourage Type C individuals to express their anger, I am not telling them to become cantankerous Type A's. Obviously, healthy expression of anger does not mean indulging in indiscriminate explosions in front of other people. Type A's who dump their hostility on others suffer on three counts. They alienate others and can permanently jeopardize work or social relationships; they never achieve psychological well-being; and their pent-up rage produces dangerous physiological results—including high blood pressure and heart rate, increased cholesterol levels, and increased risk of heart disease.

When Type C individuals contact their anger and find constructive ways to express it, they rarely swing to the other Type A extreme. However, there are potential pitfalls for Type C's who are learning to express anger for the first time in their lives. It is an extremely difficult task that requires the development of new communication skills. When we learn these skills, we are able to stretch out into the world and assert ourselves in a healthy way. Without these skills, our fears about expressing legitimate anger might be confirmed and send us reeling back into our Type C shells. These fears are internal—"I'll blow up and lose control"—and external— "The person will hate me or abandon me." When we learn appropriate expression, we minimize the chances that our worst-case scenarios will become reality.

What is healthy expression of anger? Stephen Levine provides a description of its purpose in his book *Healing into Life and Death:* "In the Tibetan Buddhist tradition, they speak of taking anger and turning it around to motivate practice, because in anger are qualities like straightforwardness and resoluteness which can be turned into commitment. . . . Anger too has the quality of an unwillingness to allow things to remain as they are."

Levine's last statement sums up the healthy focus for anger—the "unwillingness to allow things to remain as they are." To the extent that we use anger as a constructive agent of internal and external change, then this emotion can be a remarkably and often surprisingly positive force in our lives.

In his book *Freedom and Destiny,* Rollo May distinguishes distorted expressions of anger from those that are clean, and captures the healthy functions of anger:

> In our society we confuse anger with resentment, a form of repressed anger that eats away at our innards. . . . Or we confuse anger with temper, which is generally an explosion of repressed anger; with rage, which may be a pathological anger; with petulance, which is childish resentment; or with hostility, which is anger absorbed into our character structure until it infects every act of ours. I am not referring to these kinds of hostility or resentment. I am speaking, rather, of the anger that pulls the diverse parts of the self together, that integrates the self, keeps the whole self alive and present, energizes us, sharpens our vision, and stimulates us to think more clearly.

SKILLS OF ANGER EXPRESSION

When any situation spurs in you even the slightest flicker of anger, ask yourself two very simple questions: Why am I angry? and What do I want? Even in a fleeting moment, you can tune in to your mind-body and ascertain the reason for your anger. Then, in the seconds, minutes, hours, or weeks before you take action, find out what you need: What is my purpose? How can I express my anger to bring about a desired result?

Anger can be stimulated by a verbal or physical attack on yourself; an attack on your integrity; an attack on someone you care about; an injustice committed against you, your family, or another person; an attempt by others to take something that belongs to you, whether it is a personal possession or a human right. In any of these situations, anger represents both a physiological arousal that stimulates action and an opportunity to exercise choice: "How can I rectify this situation?" Some schools of thought argue, "Follow your angry impulses, they tell you the truth and should guide your actions." Other experts say, "Anger should only be expressed—if at all—after careful consideration, in rational terms, with due respect for any and all consequences."

Each side of the argument possesses only half the truth. Taken together, they point to a middle ground of healthy expression. You must allow yourself to *have your anger*. This means respecting the emotion in its raw form, accepting its validity—*even if it seems irrational*—and allowing yourself to experience the feeling. Does that mean you should fire off every angry impulse you feel? Absolutely not. When you are in a sticky interpersonal situation, and your anger builds, it's best to give yourself time to consider the best course of action. That doesn't mean you repress the anger; it means you experience it internally, respect its validity, and then allow yourself time before reacting. (The lag time between feeling and action depends on the circumstances. When someone attacks you verbally, you do well to respond quickly; when your employer devalues your work, you may need more time to consider your reaction.) Sometimes you will need to remove yourself from a situation in order to have your anger, then calm down and determine the most effective response.

The first step, however, is being aware of your anger. Take the hypothetical case of Charlie, a Type C coper. He is driving his Honda down the street when the driver of a Chevy pulls out of a parking space, without looking, and smashes into him. Charlie is unscathed, but there is a cavernous dent in the side of his Honda. Offhand, it looks like at least five hundred dollars worth of repairs, maybe more. The other driver pulls over and Charlie meets him around the Honda. "I guess it doesn't look so bad," says Charlie. "But I better take your information so I can collect an insurance claim."

The offender is high-strung, impatient, and defensive. "Listen, pal, I gotta get moving. I'm late for an important job interview, and I can't take the time. Sorry." He strides back toward his car, and Charlie stands there silently.

Not only has the offender caused damage to Charlie's car, he takes no responsibility for his actions and leaves Charlie in the lurch. What was Charlie thinking when he let the guy return to his car without a confrontation? Based on hundreds of interviews I have conducted with Type C copers, here is a list of thoughts that Charlie really might have had:

"If I was more careful, I could have avoided this."

"How do I get myself into these things?"

"It probably won't cost that much."

"That guy was really in a hurry. It must have been an important interview."

"Maybe the guy's had trouble with the law and was worried."

"He seemed pretty aggressive. He might have hauled off and punched me if I gave him any trouble."

"I'm just lucky to be alive."

"Maybe the insurance company will accept my claim without information from the offender."

Whether Charlie has one or more of these thoughts, they all serve the same function: to block his awareness of anger. And it was his anger that could have spurred him to action, by stopping the offender and getting the necessary information.

The accident was the other fellow's fault, and Charlie knew it. But Charlie always blamed himself for everything that went wrong. Underneath, he knew the repairs would cost him, but he didn't want to focus on that reality. The fact that Charlie could concern himself for one moment with this stranger's problems shows how far he would go to avoid feeling angry at someone other than himself. Charlie may be lucky to be alive, but that doesn't change the fact that he just got badly manipulated and will have to pay the price. If Charlie had been thinking clearly, he'd have realized instantly that his insurance company won't pay any claim without the proper information.

What derailed Charlie so badly? His Type C pattern, deeply ingrained, made him feel both undeserving of redress and afraid of confrontation. The minute this fast talker said "I've got to run,"

Charlie froze with fear. To stop the guy, he'd have had to oppose him. He'd have had to stand his ground and insist on completing the interaction. For Type C's, this causes instant anxiety. The anxiety made Charlie *forget his own reality.* At that moment, Charlie's reality was "My car is damaged. It's not my fault. I must be covered by insurance, or else I'll have to pay out of pocket. That would not be fair to me."

You can circumvent the paralyzing effects of anxiety in situations in which a confrontation is called for. *Focus on your own reality and purpose.* If Charlie had held on to two thoughts—"I deserve to have my car fixed," and "I must get his information to do so"—he would have transcended his fear of confrontation. His own reality and purpose would have propelled him into action. A starving man will be altogether fearless in his pursuit of food unless he's so numb to his own hunger that he doesn't even try.

Focusing on your own reality and purpose also brings your emotions into clear relief. Had Charlie felt he deserved redress, he would have been angered by this fellow's cagey attempt to duck responsibility. That anger would have sparked Charlie to insist, in no uncertain terms, that he stay put and provide the necessary information. If Charlie were at the other extreme—a Type A person—he would have been filled with rage and focused on nothing else. He might have started a fistfight with the fleeing offender and would have accomplished nothing. *The most effective expression of anger is the one that most properly redresses the problem at hand.*

Everyone, no matter how Type C, has an inner source of self-love and self-protection. For Type C's who allow themselves to be taken advantage of, this source is well hidden. Such individuals usually need psychotherapy to work through feelings of worthlessness and develop genuine self-esteem. However, for the purposes of here-and-now Type C transformation, it is possible to tap that hidden source of self-esteem.

The following guide will help you get healthy anger back into your emotional repertoire, and develop a self-esteem that will move you to assertive action.

A GUIDE TO ANGER AND ASSERTIVENESS

Tune in and Take Time. Tune in to your bodily sensations when you're upset over an interpersonal conflict or environmental stressor. Is sadness there? Is fear there? Or is anger there? When and if you feel slighted for any reason, pay careful attention to the feeling. You'll hear voices in your head trying to talk you out of your distress. For the moment, push these voices aside and simply contact the emotions associated with being slighted. Before you have a chance to explain, rationalize, or assuage the feeling, ask yourself these questions:

- Why am I angry (or upset)?
- What feels wrong, unfair, or cruel about what has happened?
- What are my needs in this situation?
- What can I do to right this wrong?

No matter how Type C you may be, you can clear your mind of anger-blocking cognitive clutter and focus on your own reality and purpose. This taps your hidden well of self-protective impulses (which we all have), and guides you through situations that would otherwise derail your sense of yourself and your rights. It's a bit like becoming the hero in your own adventure movie, instead of just an extra. Have you ever seen an action/adventure film in which the hero forgets, even for a split second, his or her overriding purpose?

This advice does not apply to Type A individuals. They are stuck in a feeling of being constantly attacked and wounded by the world, and hence the changes they need to make are quite different from what I suggest for Type C's. Remember, throughout this section *I am primarily addressing people for whom anger is the phantom emotion.*

Stake Your Claim—Don't Blame. Once you know why you are angry and what it is you wish to change in your environment or relationship, you can express anger appropriately. But there is one very common pitfall to avoid—blaming the other person for your discontent. Blame implies "If only *you* would change, everything would be fine." Blaming comes from a sense of powerlessness, because the blamer believes that his/her well-being depends solely upon a change in the other person. Even if this person has behaved terribly, blame is an ineffective tool for change. It reinforces the blamer's sense of victimization and often causes the blamed to become defensive or inflamed by a reactive anger.

We all have been on the receiving end of blaming accusations, and it's never pleasant. It's only natural for people to defend themselves when their character is being directly impugned. We don't become introspective when someone puts us down—we reflexively fight back. All too often such blaming arguments deteriorate into pointless shouting matches.

Many experts on anger, including Harriet Goldhor Lerner, have advocated a simple, pragmatic approach to effective expression. Instead of making blaming "you" statements—such as "You never listen to a word I say"—make "I" statements—like "I need you to hear me out." Tell the person how his or her behavior makes *you* feel, and what it is *you* want from him or her. Clear, direct declarations of your needs, wants, feelings, and perceptions are honest, nonblaming, and have the best chance of being heard. The following are examples of blaming "you" statements, followed by alternative "I" statements:

"You never do anything around this house," *or* "I work incredibly hard around this house. I wish you would share this responsibility with me."

"You're totally incompetent when it comes to our finances," *or* "I'm really worried about our financial situation, and I wish you would sit down with me and discuss it."

"All you care about is your buddies," *or* "I wish you'd make more time for us."

"You never want to make love," *or* "I'd really love to make love more often."

"You can't be trusted to take care of your little brother," *or* "I want to feel safe about leaving you with your little brother."

When you use "you" statements, you force the other person into a defensive stance. When you use "I" statements, you invite the other person to listen and understand your anger. None of this involves a watering down of your feelings. It's a matter of sharpening your focus and staking your claim. Even with "I" statements, some people may be threatened by your anger, but at least you have taken responsibility for your emotions and minimized the chance of misunderstanding and irrational retaliation. You have demonstrated respect for yourself, made your position clear, and given the other person a chance to respond to rational but heartfelt arguments, not accusations.

Don't Try to Change the Other Person. Blaming and ineffective fighting are often based on attempts to change the other person in a relationship. No matter how "correct" we believe our critique is, it is an illusion to think we can alter substantially another person's basic personality or modus operandi. A real change has to come from within them, not from our efforts. Indeed, the more we try to control them, often the more resistant they become. This cycle leads to relationship stagnation instead of renewal. As Harriet Goldhor Lerner points out in *The Dance of Anger,* If we maintain our focus on our needs, rights, and beliefs, *things automatically change.* Lerner uses the metaphor of couples in a dance: you can't force someone to change his steps, but if you change *your* steps, "the dance no longer can continue in the same predictable pattern."

"It is our job to state our thoughts and feelings clearly and to make responsible decisions that are congruent with our values and beliefs," writes Lerner. "It is not our job to make another person think and feel the way we do or the way we want them to. If we try, we can end up in a relationship in which a lot of personal pain and emotional intensity are being expended and nothing is changing."

Avoid Passive Aggression. When Type C individuals suddenly become aware of anger, they also discover within themselves an underdeveloped sense of self-worth. There's a feeling of "Hey, wait a minute! What about *me!*" But there's still a lag time before most Type C persons are able to develop effective skills of anger expression. Until they do, they often act out their sense of entitlement—and their anger—in indirect ways. This is often referred to as "passive-aggressive" behavior.

Norman, one of my therapy patients, complained constantly about his girlfriend. She "made" him drive her to work every day, even though he could barely afford the extra time it took. "She refuses to learn to drive," he muttered. Norman would do little things to act out his resentment, such as not being ready to leave on time, thus causing his girlfriend to be late for work. The tension this dispute caused was so painful, he finally broke off the relationship.

I asked Norman, "What was it about your way of handling your anger that sustained the problem, instead of resolving it?" After much introspection, Norman realized that he had been afraid to say what he really wanted and needed to say: "I don't have time to take you to work every day. You will have to find another way." Norman was scared of taking this clear stand because he was sure she'd reject him for no longer taking care of her need. In fact, despite his inner resentment, he felt more in control of the relationship when he dutifully took her to work. She'd keep loving him for his good-guy behavior, he thought. But the price of this illusory sense of control was far too great: his passive aggression kept surfacing, and tore the fabric of the relationship.

Norman recognized his own contribution to the problem and began to express his needs and his anger more directly. There's an interesting postscript to Norman's story. Soon after the breakup of the relationship, his ex-girlfriend got into an accident in her home in which her leg was badly injured. Norman visited her in the hospital and began running some errands for her. This time, he was doing it out of choice, because he really wished to help during her recuperation. They reestablished a close friendship, and he occasionally drove her to work again. After a few months, her leg was back to normal. One day, on the way to work, Norman said, "You're really better now. I'm not going to drive you to work anymore." His tone was calm, clear, and firm. She knew he really meant it, and no fight ensued. A week later, she started driving lessons and now drives herself to work. She and Norman are still friends.

Because Type C individuals have so few outlets for anger, the dammed-up feelings find expression elsewhere. Sometimes the only manifestation is physical symptoms. In other cases, a Type C secretly harbors feelings of entitlement, bitterness, and resentment, causing him to feel like a wounded martyr: "Look at all I've done for them, and what do I get in return!"

The passive-aggressive individual has been wounded, but the wounds were almost always delivered in childhood. If he can discover the original wounds, he can stop projecting anger and frustration on those around him.

But you can also take here-and-now measures to reduce passive-aggressive behavior. As in the case of Norman, it's crucial to define and communicate your real feelings. Norman wished to stop driving his girlfriend to work. Because he was afraid to assert this desire, he let it go underground, where it festered and became resentment. Discover your need, confront your own fear of assertion, and then take action, using the nonblaming skills already described. This is one way to stop passively acting out your anger.

Dealing with Double-decker Anger. When you begin to accept inner signals of anger, you may be mad at people for reasons that seem dubious at best. You yourself may not understand the reasons, and begin to experience your anger as a bottomless pit of irrational impulses. You feel rage that you know is unjustified. Or, quite commonly, you get caught in a vicious "knot" with someone in a close relationship. You find his or her behavior intolerable and get ensnared in terrible fights. This is a particularly tricky situation, because you may not know that your anger is unjustified.

In these situations, you are usually employing the psychic defense mechanism known as "projection." Put simply, you take old feelings toward someone from the past, or current feelings toward someone (or something) in your present, and project them onto the wrong target—an unsuspecting person currently in your path. You almost never realize you are doing this, and obviously, the results can be damaging.

The most problematic form of projection occurs when you shift old anger toward a parent onto a current target. I call this "double-decker" anger, because there is a "top layer" of anger in the present, which sits upon a "bottom layer" of unresolved anger from the past. I use this image to show that sometimes there is real, justified anger in the present, and other times there is not. One has to separate carefully the top from the bottom layer to determine, "Do I have a reason to be angry now, or are all my feelings from the past?"

In cases of double-decker anger, you will often have good reason to feel angry in the present *and* you are acting on the basis of old feelings. Let's take the example of a woman who is furious at her husband for being late to the theater. She starts a heated fight with him: "You're *always* late!" He admits his error and says he will try hard to change. But she can't let go of her rage, and the fight continues. Their evening at the theater is ruined, supper is ruined, and the fight spills over into the weekend. What causes this? In her therapy session the following week, the woman realizes that her father always came home from work hours later than he said he would. He routinely broke promises to his daughter to spend time with her in the evenings. Her anger, along with deep hurt, remained powerfully lodged in her unconscious.

She had every right to be angry with her husband for his chronic lateness. But her rage exceeded reasonable bounds because it was fueled by past anger triggered by her husband's behavior. Here, the top layer is contaminated by emotions rising up from the bottom layer.

Double-decker anger explains why so much fighting is fruitless. A person gets his feelings off his chest and, instead of feeling better, he feels worse. Type A individuals who vent and vent and vent their anger still don't feel relieved—not only because their acting-out worsens the current situation, but because they are replaying old tapes without knowing it. They never discover the true source of their rage and hence, they never find peace and resolution.

It's really not hard to diagnose double-decker anger. What's hard is distinguishing the two layers and dealing with each separately. Your anger is probably double-decker if:

- you are in a relationship characterized by relentless, ineffective fighting.
- you compulsively blame the other person for all problems in a relationship.
- you feel waves of anger that you know are unjustified in the present.
- you experience "free-floating hostility"—intense anger or hatred that is triggered by everyday occurrences, like waiting in line.

In all these instances, your task at hand is to locate the sources of your anger in both the past and the present. If gut intuition tells you that your rage has a component from the past, then explore its sources. The best way to do this is in psychotherapy: ferreting out old anger is slow and painstaking and requires the help of a skilled and properly trained professional. Often, therapy is a safe place to release the energy of past anger in its raw form. And repressed anger is invariably bound together with other feelings, memories, and realizations, which a skilled therapist can enable you to process. He or she can then collaborate with you on the delicate procedure of peeling apart reality from your projections—an important step toward appropriate expression of anger in the here and now.

When to Act Decisively. There are times in life when threatening circumstances leave you no time for reflection. When you, or someone else, is being abused emotionally, physically, or sexually, swift action is required. What is abuse? When your physical or sexual boundaries are violated, when your dignity or integrity is assailed, when you become the object of another person's irrational rage. Gabrielle Roth, in her book on ritual healing, *Maps to Ecstasy,* defines anger that is an immediate response to violation:

> Anger is an integrity-protecting response to the invasion of your personal boundaries. It is "no" to a wrong, a violation. It draws lines and throws up barricades. Proper anger cuts like a knife through water. It is quick, clear, needs no explanation. It's the bared teeth of a bitch protecting her litter, the arched back and hiss of a cat threatened by a coyote. There's nothing cleaner, more effective than appropriate anger. Authentic anger is specific and justified, and its direct expression exposes impropriety and defends integrity in a way that benefits everyone.

Certain other circumstances outside of frank abuse also call for a sharp immediate response. We all have had the experience of dealing with bureaucracies in which the personnel are cogs in an impersonal, oversized, dysfunctional machine. Often, meeting vital needs depends on your capacity to cut through red tape, confront authority figures, and stand your ground. Whether you're dealing with a corporation, hospital, insurance company, or government agency; whether your goal is to obtain crucial benefits, medical treatment, or redress from discrimination, there are times when you have to take the bull by the horns. After other approaches have been exhausted, the time comes to use your anger as a clarion call.

A scene from the movie *Terms of Endearment* illustrates my point. You may recall the hospital scene in which Debra Winger, who is dying of cancer, complains to her mother, Shirley MacLaine, that she's in dire need of more pain medication. The nurse had refused because Winger had already received her prescribed dose for the day. MacLaine is livid, goes out to the nurses' station, and proceeds to throw a wild-eyed yet perfectly coherent temper tantrum of such incendiary force that the nurses don't even bother to argue with her. Winger gets her medication seconds later. The movie audience erupts in cheers of vicarious identification—it's what we all wish we had the guts to do when our voices have been disregarded for too long.

Obviously there is no formula for knowing when such action is appropriate. But when you start paying attention to your own physiological responses, you will know. Your heart beats hard, your face gets flushed, you may even break into a sweat. Apply your beliefs about justice to your own situation: if I were someone *else* going through this, would I root for him/her to act, and act decisively? If so, it is time for you to speak up, to use your anger to cut through indifference or injustice.

Learn to Say No. For Type C's, *no* is a four letter word. *No* is the word that draws boundaries between you and another, that sets you apart and confirms your autonomy. *No* is a stand on your own behalf, and while it's true that others rarely like to hear *no,* your ability to accept their discomfort is your ticket to a stronger sense of self.

I've told you about my findings with long-term survivors of AIDS. They differed from their counterparts who succumbed early to the disease on several counts, one most notably: the survivors said they would refuse to do a favor for a friend if they did not really wish to do that favor. Their own needs came before doing deeds in order to be liked.

For Type C's especially, the simple act of uttering no is an anxiety-provoking moment. You have believed that you will be liked—and loved—insofar as you please and appease others. What happens when you cease to please and appease? In your mind, you're certain to be rejected. What purpose do you serve now?

Learning to say no takes a great deal of patience with and compassion for yourself. It's a learned skill, but it also depends on a fresh outlook on your relationships. Specifically, ask yourself, Is it really true that I will be abandoned by this person if I say no to his/her requests or needs? You assume it's true, but you can't know the outcome until you've tried. Furthermore, if it is true, what does that say about the relationship?

The only way to know whether a friend, lover, family member, or work associate can handle greater assertiveness is to field-test saying no when you don't wish to comply with a request or fulfill a need. You'll be changing an old dance step, so don't expect a fluid reaction. The other person may be taken aback, appalled, anxious, angry, tense, or bewildered. This is normal. For you, the trick is to tolerate the anxiety this causes in *you*. If you can, you've won a victory on behalf of yourself and your quest for greater autonomy. And once the tension subsides, you'll find that you've brought a new pattern into the relationship. It won't be easy, but altering old patterns in relationships is never tension-free.

If, however, the other person remains continuously angry, feels profoundly betrayed, and never forgives you, then you have a vital new (albeit depressing) piece of information about the relationship. You now know that things went fine as long as you played your nice guy or caretaker role. When you ceased to play that role, she could not look beyond her personal hurt and stick with you. She has a right to feel wounded, annoyed, and angry, but if she withdraws completely, her prior commitment was not to you but to the part you played for her.

When striking out in this new direction, bear this question in mind: Do I want to be loved or esteemed only for a part of me—the part that is "good," nice, and takes care of others? Or, do I want to be loved or esteemed for my whole self, which includes actions such as drawing boundaries, standing my ground, and expressing my *own* needs?

BRINGING ANGER OUT OF THE SHADOWS

When we split off, dissociate, repress, and otherwise obliterate anger from our emotional repertoire, we cut off a source of our strength and self-esteem. Why does this happen? It is due partly to harsh early conditioning, and partly to our fear of the potential destructiveness of our anger. That's why reintegrating anger is so difficult for so many of us.

Therefore, when we begin to work on our awareness of our anger, we must recognize that years of repressing anger has indeed turned it into a potentially harmful force. This is all the more reason why we have to find a safe place in which to explore the irrational side of anger, with compassion for ourselves. Those of us with a great well of anger can benefit the most from work with a psychotherapist. We can discover the origins of repressed anger, defuse its explosive inner force, and gradually rid ourselves of the need to block all awareness and expression of it. The paradox is this: once we have taken anger out of the shadows, it loses its hidden negative power over us. Then we can use the energy of anger for constructive purposes, as when we take assertive action on our own behalf.

One of the first steps we can take is to stop judging our innermost angry feelings and fantasies. We can explore them with a therapist or through creative means: drawings, paintings, keeping a journal, wild dancing, pillow smashing, exercise, singing, or even solitary tantrums. There are ways to separate out the irrational aspect of anger and allow it to live and breathe without judgment from ourselves or potential harm to others.

Once we've made that separation, then our present anger, whether toward a friend, work associate, spouse, child, or parent, is no longer profoundly tainted by old angers previously banished to our unconscious mind. We now can find constructive ways to communicate anger. We can learn the skills of expression and apply them in the present—by learning to say no, staking our claim, and acting decisively. This allows us to stand our ground without fear that we are enacting some old drama on the current stage of a relationship. We can stop pushing our anger into the shadows where, over time, it exerts its toxic effects on mind and body.

CHAPTER 16

We must reserve a little back-shop, all our own, entirely
free, wherein to establish our true liberty and principal
retreat and solitude.

—*Michel Eyquem de Montaigne*

We do not like to look at the shadow-side of ourselves;
therefore there are many people in our civilized society
who have lost their shadow altogether, have lost the
third dimension, and with it they have usually
lost the body.

—*Carl Jung*

Too often the therapist with too narrow a view of
emotion sees it as an abortive transformation,
and rushes in with relief. One could expect
Job's friends or the companions of Jesus
in Gethsemane today to step forward
with a tranquilizer.

—*James Hillman*

Every child is an artist. The problem is how to
remain an artist when he grows up.

—*Pablo Picasso*

Tending the Mind,
Trusting the Body

Because Type C's are other-directed, they often have highly developed skills of sensitivity and perception. They are experts at reading other people's feelings; they easily intuit other people's needs. This enables them to modify their own behavior to win love and approval. Type C's are often brilliant in their roles as caretakers, rescuers, or enablers. This "brilliance" is no meager talent to be downgraded—it includes qualities of keen insight and empathy. The only problem is, the Type C person applies *too much* nurturing attention to others and far *too little* to him or herself.

Type C transformation involves better ways to tend your mind and trust your body. In this chapter, I will discuss methods that redirect that nurturing energy back toward your self. This is not a throwback to the "me" decade philosophy of the seventies and eighties because I'm not suggesting that this applies to everyone. Type C's are a select group (albeit a very large one) with a marked tendency toward selflessness—not selfishness. And the needs that require more tending are not material; they are psychological and spiritual. The person whose needs have been met also has a great capacity for giving. The only difference is, his or her giving is not at the expense of the self.

I will describe mind-body techniques like meditation, mind-body mechanisms like laughing and crying, the importance of social support, and fundamental issues of self-development and creative expression. Each of these approaches and issues has direct relevance to changing Type C behavior *and* enhancing immunity and health.

RELAXATION AS IMMUNE REGULATOR

Relaxation by any name is still the same—it yields measurable benefits to your health and well-being. Whether it is transcendental meditation, yoga, relaxation response, biofeedback, or Zen, when you find a relaxing and centering technique and use it regularly, you reduce the harmful effects of stress on your body.

Drs. Janice Kiecolt-Glaser and Ronald Glaser of Ohio State University recruited a group of elderly people from retirement homes and assigned them to one of three groups: relaxation training, brief social contact, or no intervention. One month later, the patients who practiced relaxation three times a week had higher natural killer cell activity and more antibodies to the herpes simplex virus—another sign of vigorous immune-cell activity. Kiecolt-Glaser and Glaser also explored the benefits of relaxation in medical students who were in the throes of exam-related stress. The researchers drew blood from the students one month before exams and on the last day of exams. Half the students received relaxation training in the interval between blood draws, while the other half did not. The students who practiced relaxation on a frequent basis had more helper T-cells than all others in the study.

"These data provide further evidence that relaxation may be able to enhance at least some components of cellular immunity," the Glasers wrote, "and thus . . . might be useful in influencing the incidence and course of disease."

For many, meditation conjures up the image of high-stress, hyperactive go-getters stealing away for twenty minutes each day in order to breathe deeply and slow down their racing vital functions. But people who seem to be low-gear—including Type C copers— can benefit in a different way. Type C's may not be high-strung, but their inattention to their mind-body state can cause them to suffer creeping cases of fatigue. Type C individuals who practice meditation discover that they are more tense and tired than they thought, and their efforts to relax will yield surprising benefits.

Meditation can be a time to contact your feelings. While meditating, you may become aware of inner states just below the surface: "I've been depressed for days—I must find out why." "I'm harboring constant anger at work—it's this current project." "I'm chronically holding my breath because I'm so tense." "My throat is tight because I want to cry." For some, meditation can even awaken a spirituality that deepens your sense of self, your connection to others, and your relationship to a "higher power." For those interested in meditation as part of your Type C transformation, I recommend a number of excellent books in Appendix II, page 418.

BODY AWARENESS

Because we are often out of touch with bodily sensations, and therefore miss crucial signals, developing body awareness is an important aspect of Type C transformation. There are many ways to go about this: exercise, biofeedback, body-oriented therapies, and meditation/relaxation.

I've told you about meditation for relaxation and awareness, but meditation is also a powerful way to specifically enhance body consciousness. In *The Power of Myth,* Joseph Campbell reminds us that consciousness is not confined to mental processes:

It is part of the Cartesian mode to think of consciousness as being somewhat peculiar to the head, that the head is the organ originating consciousness. It isn't. The head is an organ that inflects consciousness in a certain direction, or to a certain set of purposes. But there is a consciousness here in the body. The whole living world is informed by consciousness.

There is a meditative practice used in the southern Buddhist tradition known as "sweeping the body." Stephen Levine, who utilizes this practice, wrote, "In the course of this meditation, one may discover unknown pains and joys—areas of tension as well as areas of high receptivity and openness. As one teacher pointed out, 'It is not so difficult to be out of the body as it is to be in it.' . . . This meditation allows awareness to meet the body not as idea but as the direct experience of the field of sensation."

Once you become aware of body states like tension, loneliness, restlessness, fatigue, and frustration, you can identify causes of these states in your environment and make the necessary changes. Perhaps you will seek more social contact, pursue new creative projects, alter the course of your career, get more physical exercise, eat more healthfully, have sex more often. The changes required become self-evident when you have a pipeline to your mind-body's deepest needs, and meditation can provide that pipeline.

Use meditation to develop body awareness. You can add visualization to your practice, but stay open to the flow of images in your mind. This enables you to learn what your mind-body needs, rather than having your mind (ego) telling your mind-body what it needs. Here's a brief example of meditation as an inner probe of mind-body sensations:

Meditation for Body Awareness

Sit comfortably or lie on a flat surface. Begin by breathing deeply and relaxing the tensions in your body. As you breathe, focus your awareness at the top of your head. Inhale, become aware of the sensations and feelings there, then exhale, and relax the area. Awareness as you inhale; relaxation as you exhale.

With awareness, ask yourself, What do I feel at the top of my head? Tension? Hardness? Softness? Tingling? Feel the area, receive the sensations. When you exhale, relax the area. But don't force a change. Relaxing means sensing, feeling. Awareness and relaxation are two sides of the same coin. Both are moving deeply into the area—bringing mind, heart, and energy there.

When you're ready, move gradually down to your eyes. Scan for any tension in the eye muscles. Don't force relaxation, just open to the sensations. Keep breathing deeply into your lower body. Keep an open channel.

Move to the jaw. Is there tension? Holding? Anger? Relax the jaw on the outbreath; become aware of any changes.

Now the throat. Is there constriction? Pain? Pleasure? Relax, open the channel that is your throat, and receive sensations. Are there any emotions there? Sadness? Fear? Desire?

Sweep the rest of your body, moving slowly, making

discoveries as you go. Don't push or force change; softly receive sensations. Caress each part of your body with awareness: face, chest, arms, abdomen, pelvis, legs, and feet. Find what's there: pain, pleasure, constriction, hardness, softness, rigidity, flexibility, heaviness, lightness, warmth, coldness, tingling. Are specific emotions held in these areas? Do you sense anger, fear, longing, anxiety, sadness, rage, or sexual desire? Let these feelings enter your awareness. Don't push them into mind or out of body; let them live and breathe. Become one with them and they will move through your mind-body. When you do this, you don't have to change them. Change unfolds by itself.

Any method that helps you enhance sensory awareness is worthwhile. Of course, you can go too far and become hypervigilant about sensations of pain or tension, and ultrasensitive to feelings of sadness, anger, and fear. For those of you who have long been insensitive to your body's messages, a swing may occur to the opposite extreme of sensitivity. This can be part of a normal progression before you return to a simple awareness of bodily needs and sensations.

I like the metaphor of the smoke detector for body awareness. If it's insensitive or the battery's low, fire is going to overtake our house before enough smoke is generated to set off the alarm. If it's oversensitive, we simply light a cigarette or turn on the stove to boil water and that screeching alarm sounds. Our relationship to bodily signals of pain, fatigue, anger, and emotional stress is similar. Type C's have unresponsive detectors. An internal "fire"—be it fatigue, unmet needs, or an incipient illness—may take over before we realize that we have ignored this threat to mind-body integrity. Others of us have hyperresponsive detectors; we go into a state of total alert at the slightest sign of trouble.

Body awareness—whether achieved through meditation, biofeedback, exercise, massage, or other techniques—is a process of fine-tuning that smoke detector. You'll want to become sensitized to, but not self-consciously engrossed in, the life of your body. In so doing, you achieve a sense of mind-body harmony and restore the natural grace you may have lost through years of stress and inattention.

LAUGHING AND CRYING: THE HEALTH BENEFITS

What better forms of emotional expression are there than laughter and crying? As somatic forms of expression, they have proven health benefits.

Most of the publicity about healing effects has focused on laughter, but crying has its own function of maintaining mind-body balance. The idea that crying is salutary to health actually dates back to Aristotle, who believed that drama could "cleanse the mind" of suppressed emotions, a process called *catharsis*. The phenomenon is no different today, whether we're at the theater or watching a Hollywood tearjerker.

Dr. William Fry, a biochemist at the St. Paul-Ramsey Medical Center in St. Paul, Minnesota, has led research on crying. He has theorized that emotional distress produces toxic substances in the body, and crying helps to eliminate them. He organized a study to find out whether tears produced by emotional crying differed from tears caused by a physical irritant. A group of test subjects watched a surefire tearjerker, and Fry collected their tears. The same group returned a few days later, when he exposed them to fresh-cut onions and again collected their tears. After chemical analysis, Fry discovered important differences between the tears caused by sorrow and those caused by the irritant. Emotional tears contained much more protein, which confirmed Fry's theory that crying serves a biochemical-balancing function.

"What we are now looking for in emotional tears are certain chemicals released during emotional stress," said Fry. He already has found evidence that emotional tears contain stress hormones such as adrenaline and, possibly, higher concentrations of endorphins.

Crying serves many marvelous functions. It communicates, telling others what you are feeling in an undeniable way. It both expresses and releases feelings of grief and sadness. Crying is an essential part of any grieving process, the free flow of painful emotions that helps clear the mind-body from the grip of despair. In fact, for anyone who has endured a loss, the blocked expression of crying is a sign that grieving has been derailed. The result, all too often, is depression.

Dr. Alexander Lowen refers to depression as a suppression of feeling, most often feelings of sadness and loss. "When a person sobs deeply, the feeling of despair is always lessened," wrote Lowen. "Sometimes, if the crying is deep enough, the person breaks through into feelings of gladness and joy." Lowen describes the struggle of some depressed patients who, afraid to "let down" into the depth of their sadness, try to stay "above" their feelings. This misplaced effort only keeps them in a depressed state.

Type C individuals try to rise above pain and despair. They are afraid that grief will overtake them, and they work hard to keep on a happy face for the world. And Type C caretakers often don't allow themselves the indulgence of tears. Many lost the capacity for crying in childhood, when parents either prohibited, ignored, punished, or disapproved of this behavior. Very often, psychotherapy—whether individual or group—is an arena where people relearn the natural function of crying.

When Norman Cousins sang the praises of laughter in his book *Anatomy of an Illness,* there was little scientific evidence to support laughter's healing potential. Now, there is. Dr. Kathleen M. Dillon of Western New England College measured serum IgA (Immunoglobulin A)—antibodies that protect against viral invasion—in student volunteers after watching a humorous videotape. Dr. Dillon detected an increase in IgA concentrations but found no such increase after the same students watched a nonhumorous tape. She also found that students who said they used humor as a way of coping with stress had higher levels of protective antibodies to begin with. In another study, Dr. Lee S. Berk of Loma Linda University Medical Center in California found a significant boost in immune-cell proliferation in subjects who had just watched an hour-long humorous film. They also showed a marked decrease in cortisol, an immune-suppressing hormone.

In a recent *New York Times* article, health writer Jane Brody referred to "the growing number of physicians, nurses, psychologists, and patients who have used the uniquely human expression of mirth to reduce stress, ease pain, foster recovery, and generally brighten one's outlook on life, regardless of how grim the reality."

Health writers, holistic healers, and now even doctors are recommending funny films, joke-fests, and a humorous outlook for people with serious illnesses. What about laughter for prevention? It makes sense, but there are no data yet to support this novel idea. I suppose we'll just have to wait for long-term studies of thousands of people made to laugh constantly day in and day out for about twenty years, who can then be compared with a control group of people consigned to a jokeless existence. The problem, of course, is that such a study would be about as practical and ethical as assigning one group of people to eat lobster for dinner for the rest of their lives, and the other group to eating Spam. In all seriousness, perhaps someday a research group will actually develop a way to study laughter's preventive powers.

HEALING OUR ISOLATION

Prevention of and recovery from all variety of illnesses are enhanced when we have the support we need. A number of population studies have shown increases in cancer mortality among widowed, divorced, and single individuals, when compared with married people. As mentioned, in their study of more than sixty-eight hundred people in Alameda County, Drs. George Kaplan and Peggy Reynolds found that women who were socially isolated had a significant increase in their risk of dying of cancer. And isolated women who said they *felt* alone had a far greater likelihood of contracting cancer.

Type C's often bear their loneliness in silence. They are afraid to ask for help because they believe it is their job to give, not receive. Caretakers "give in order to get," but what they get is connections based on role-playing. Hence, the paradox that many Type C's have many so-called friends, i.e., people who depend on them for support and favors. But unless they have others they can turn to with their needs, problems, and emotions, they remain lonely. Some are aware of feeling isolated; others are not. Only by conducting careful interviews, as I did in my research, was I able to uncover the isolation common among Type C's.

As you embark on Type C transformation, the people close to you will react, in some way, to your behavior changes. Some will welcome your newfound assertiveness or self-expression; others will be threatened. There may be times of loneliness, but you are looking to improve the quality of your support, and with an enduring sense of commitment, you will develop stronger relationships. You are seeking greater honesty, spontaneity, and acceptance from family and friends. In order to get there, be prepared to ride some choppy waves.

When your behavior changes have a profound effect on close family relationships, causing conflict or misunderstanding, I suggest that you discuss the possibility of family therapy with your family members. Often, one person will take responsibility for changing his or her own behavior, and—knowingly or not—expose an unhealthy pattern within the entire family. If you find yourself in this position, gently approach each person and discuss your awareness of problems within the family. If you can get your family into treatment with you, you will have initiated a process with the potential to change all your lives, and relationships, for the better.

THE LISTENING TECHNIQUE

I encourage one simple approach to improve the quality of your support, which I call *the listening technique.*

I had one patient, Karen, who had a great deal of stress at her job as a research assistant. She came home from work every day to her husband, and her stress level would get even worse. He would ask, "How was your day?" and she would proceed to tell him about her anger toward her egocentric supervisor. He'd say, "Don't get upset with me!" or "I didn't do that to you!" or "Don't bring your problems home with you." Karen's husband felt assaulted by her anger, even though it was clearly not aimed at him, but rather was Karen's attempt to deal with pent-up feelings. She'd say, "I'm not angry at you, I'm telling you what happened that upset me." But he couldn't hear anger without being personally threatened.

Another patient, Helen, had terrible problems with her boss at the social-services agency where she worked. His autocratic behavior made her feel worthless. She would come home to her boyfriend and cry out her sadness. Right away, he would rush in to make it better, saying, "Oh, don't cry. It's not really that bad." He'd also say, "I know you can deal with this."

Karen's husband was fearful and defensive, while Helen's boyfriend couldn't handle her sadness, so he had to salve her feelings. In both instances, the women needed simply to be heard. Listening is the highest form of validation. People need to discuss their options with loved ones, to get advice, but there is a natural rhythm to human communication, and *the first beat is one person's uninterrupted expression.* After a pause, the second beat is response. The third beat is exchange. If the first beat is interrupted, the second and third are based not on a full sharing of feelings but on a frustrated effort by the subject to get his or her emotions across to the other.

I advised both Karen and Helen to ask the men in their lives to practice the listening technique. It goes like this:

> When I'm very upset, here's what I'd like for you to do. Just listen to me. Let me tell you my problem, and express my feelings, for however long it takes. Please don't interrupt. I know this will sound strange, but don't even say "right" or "uh-huh" or "I understand." Be as quiet as you can. Look at me—I need to see your response—but don't rush in to offer comfort or advice. Wait until I'm completely finished. It may take five minutes or twenty-five. I'll let you know when I'm done. After I am through, I'd love to talk with you about the problem. Until then, the most wonderful thing you can do for me is to listen.

The listening technique can be used for any problem or emotion, including conflicts with the individual whom you are asking to listen. When we have relationship difficulties, this technique can sometimes trigger a healing, because we break the old patterns. When one person only listens, he or she can't fall back on old habits like defensiveness or rescuing. What we really want is neither to be dismissed nor saved, but rather to be simply heard and understood.

This technique also helps you, the talker, get in touch with your feelings and express them more fully. You don't have to maneuver strenuously to be heard. And most often, you *are* more well understood. The other person has to lay his or her agenda aside and experience the totality and depth of *your* experience.

Type C's also do well to apply the listening technique to others. It's a way to be there for the other person without rescuing, saving, or making it all better. And it's another way to communicate that you'd like the same in return.

FIND YOUR BACKSTAGE AREA

The famed sociologist Erving Goffman created a rich theatrical metaphor for our social existence. In his view, we all give "performances" on a variety of "stages," ranging from the small, insular stage of our homes to the grand stages of our social institutions. As such, every place where we interact has a "frontstage" region and a "backstage" region. Frontstage behavior represents the performance proper, while backstage is where suppressed facts, information, and expressions make their appearance. The performers show their true selves only when backstage.

There are many examples of backstage regions. Every service organization or facility has a backstage region where workers relax, let their hair down, vent their hostility, gossip, and in general allow themselves a free rein of behavior that would be totally unacceptable on the public stage. In his book *The Presentation of Self in Everyday Life,* Goffman cites examples of backstage regions in every imaginable setting and institution, from palaces to housing projects, from schools to cathedrals.

For the people involved, backstage regions serve a vital social and psychological purpose. As Goffman wrote, "Here the performer can relax; he can drop his front, forgo speaking his lines, and step out of character."

Many Type C copers have grave difficulty invoking a "backstage style," to use Goffman's term. Type C's have been so conditioned to exhibit only socially acceptable behavior that they rarely relax their guard. They are afraid of being seen as "sullen," "angry," "impudent," "depressed," "profane," "sloppy," "giddy," "selfish," "irrational," or any behavior that doesn't fit the accepted social norm. Type C's have internalized social taboos to such an extent that they've lost touch with these parts of themselves. When they reach a backstage "area," they can't use it as a place to let it all hang out, because they've long since lost the habit.

It's a tremendous strain on mind and body to play roles without surcease. To an extent, we are all forced to play roles, especially in certain work and social situations. When we cannot escape the pressure to perform, at least we can find some space to unwind and express parts of ourselves proscribed on the public stage.

Your mind-body has no opportunity to renew itself unless you offset work with recess, performance with play, selflessness with selfishness, restraint with abandonment. Alexander Lowen captured this eloquently in his book, *Fear of Life:*

So much energy is required to maintain a role or facade that little is left for pleasure or creativity. Imagine an actor playing a role constantly, both offstage and on, and you will get some idea of the energy it takes to do that. Being is effortless because it is spontaneous and natural. That is why children can be so creative. However, most people do not sense the effort or the energetic drain of the role they play. What they do feel is chronic fatigue, irritability, and frustration. When one plays a role, the end result is always depression.

Lowen has described the Type C trap perfectly. Perhaps you have been to a large social gathering—a party or a wedding—and recall that afterward your face hurt from the effort of maintaining a smile. In fact, your entire body was exhausted from hours of performing for countless relatives and acquaintances. Some of us subject ourselves to that kind of pressure constantly, on a day-to-day basis, frontstage and back. Hence the fatigue, irritability, and frustration.

You can move away from ceaseless role-playing by finding a backstage style, backstage friends, a backstage space—which is anywhere you can take off your social mask. Eventually, with time, you can remove the mask onstage as well. But you have to start "shedding skins" somewhere, and for Type C's, it's wherever you feel most comfortable. In the long run, you need to be able to show your true face to those people who are important in your life. For some, that's the place to start—with your spouse, close friend, or parents. For others—especially those of you who've settled into fixed roles in relationships—it can be invaluable to find another backstage to "rehearse" new ways of being and behaving.

Your backstage space could be a bowling alley where you meet a group of friends once a week. It could be the back table at your work cafeteria or any meeting place for a particular crew of colleagues. It might be the garage of your home, where you can be alone with your woodworking. Perhaps you've discovered certain women in the laundromat of your apartment building who have no inhibitions about discussing topics from the sublime to the ridiculous. You find them so refreshing that you can't wait the two weeks until your next load needs washing. Or you may have a side room in your house where you can practice meditation, or just sit and think about what you'd *really* like to do, say, or be in various phases of your life. Sometimes, a place for solitude is the best of all backstages.

It is often said that the truly great actors are not actors at all. When they step on stage, they're not acting, they are *being*. If you have ever been startled—truly moved—by an actor's performance in the theater or on film, you know you were not watching a simulation of human experience—you were watching the real thing. We all have the capacity to be "great actors" on our own front-stages by bringing more of ourselves and less of our "act" into work and relationships; more of our bodies and less of our costumes; more of our *real* expressions and less of our masks. The beauty of backstage is that it is a place where we can discover who we are, practice new ways of being, and experiment with expression before we take the brave and risky step of moving front and center to reveal our previously hidden selves to the world.

THE SEARCH FOR CREATIVE EXPRESSION

In his many years of therapeutic work with cancer patients, Lawrence LeShan uncovered a common dilemma among them. They saw life as a stark choice between two roads, and both seemed to be psychological dead ends. There appeared to be no third road, no alternative to despair.

The first road, the one most well traveled, was to be conformist (Type C), and as such, to follow a course in their career and creative pursuits that pleased family and friends. To veer off this safe, predictable path would be to shake the foundations of familial harmony and peer acceptance. And there was always enormous social and economic pressure to maintain the status quo, especially if status quo paid the bills. The second road was to find their own unique form of expression. This meant pursuing work they loved— activities that brought meaning and energy to life—instead of work that served primarily to win status and approval. But the patients saw this path as fraught with certain danger. They believed, "If I follow my desires—if I express myself emotionally and creatively—I will lose the love and approval of those who matter most."

Theirs was a Faustian take on life: give up your soul and win the riches of affection and stability, or keep your soul and forfeit love and human connection. Obviously, both roads are unacceptable. LeShan's patients saw no possibility of a third road, no escape from this no-win situation. So they long ago chose the seeming lesser of two evils: the safe road of conformity. Hence, LeShan noted that the vast majority of his patients were well liked but lacked meaning, zest, and validity in their work and creative pursuits.

I noted similar tendencies among the Type C melanoma patients I studied. When it came to their life's work, many had followed the path of least resistance. Why pursue a life course that cut against the grain of others' expectations and risk losing their esteem? This held true whether the others were parents, spouses, children, associates, friends, or all of the above.

Many of my therapy patients have awakened to a sense of disappointment in their work and creative activities. Creative pursuits *are* expression, and the creative impulse is an alchemical mix of feeling, perception, intellectual delight, and imaginative powers. Anyone who rediscovers repressed emotions is also likely to jog loose the creative impulses left behind at the crossroads between conformity and authenticity.

LeShan's message, and mine, is that the third road is possible. But it's a hard road, and one must accept risk, loss, and compromise in order to stay the course. Unlike the negative fantasy of the second road, however, it doesn't mean giving up the love of friends and family. You will have to accept the growing pains that occur when your relationships are redefined. Or you may face financial instability when you make a career change. But the romanticized notion of the starving artist, or the stereotype of the over-the-edge iconoclast, doesn't have to apply.

I have a group of friends from college whom I call the "frozen hippies." I don't use the term perjoratively, because the aspect of counterculture they freeze-dried was a healthy idealism about self-expression. All of them wanted to write poetry or fiction, play music, make films, or paint paintings. By the mid-1970s, they each had realized that they would forfeit a social existence—including family life and certain modest amenities—if they were to write, play music, film, or paint all day. So they stayed in the same close-knit community and got jobs as waiters, carpenters, proofreaders, etc. In the evenings, they pursued their respective arts and supported each other in doing so.

By the mid-1980s, many of them realized that they were leading schizoid lives. This approach served its purpose, but now many felt stifled in their day jobs. One of my female friends once said to me, "No matter how many paintings I make on my days off, I can't be a waitress anymore!"

They began to search for ways to find common ground between their money-generating and creative activities. One friend, Thomas, was a painter who worked in a garage as a mechanic. His boss asked him to do a mural for the garage to make the environment more pleasant. For two weeks, he went to work and painted this mural, while another mechanic took over his workload. Thomas enjoyed this so much he decided he could no longer come to work to fix cars. It was time to merge his double life as much as possible. He sought work as a creative sign painter, which engaged his special skills to a large extent and which he enjoyed much more than replacing mufflers. He wasn't getting paid a lot for his sign painting, but he felt he had healed a split in his life. And he kept on painting canvases at night.

The inability to see a third road is caused by narrow, black-and-white thinking. Thomas might have said, "I'll be a mechanic my whole life and be resigned to painting only at midnight." But with keen desire and sufficient imagination, Thomas found a livable compromise. Next year, he many find another, even more livable compromise. It's ceaselessly difficult to live out the dream of a creative life, so many people blame themselves when they can't pull it off perfectly, thinking, "I must be a terrible painter." At the other extreme, some people blame everyone else: "The world won't allow me to make a living as a painter."

In our culture, we are told to follow our dreams. The downside is when our expectations become blown out of proportion because our dream has been shaped by unrealistic parental or media influences. I'm thinking of the actor who feels worthless because he has yet to be cast in a Hollywood blockbuster, despite good work in film and theater. Or the painter who thinks she's a failure because her canvases have never hung in the Museum of Modern Art. One of my therapy patients, referring to her search for creativity, said, "I must not be very good at this, because I haven't succeeded in making my life a paradise." I replied, "Don't shoot for paradise, shoot for pleasure." If you expect a dream to be fulfilled absolutely, you set yourself up for disappointment and self-blame. If you follow the naked impulse to create, cleansed of material considerations and ruminations about the future, your work will take on a life of its own. I'm reminded of a passage from the *Tao-te-ching,* by Lao-tzu:

> Act without doing;
> work without effort.
> Think of the small as large
> and the few as many.
> Confront the difficult
> while it is still easy;
> accomplish the great task
> by a series of small acts.
>
> The Master never reaches for the great;
> thus she achieves greatness.

In order to follow through on creative impulses, you often need to clear out the doubting and self-deprecating voices in your head. These voices are usually internalized from parents or society, who have transmitted messages to follow a safe course. Their intentions may have been good, but the legacy of these voices limits and constricts your freedom to create. How can you replace them with a nurturing voice, one that cultivates and supports your creative efforts? Psychologist Neil Fiore suggests one way to tap a higher self, a nurturing voice that holds your best interests at heart. Replace the "parent" voice—the questioning superego—with the "grandparent" voice, the harbinger of unconditional love. For many of us, our grandparents were the most nurturing adults of our childhoods. They didn't take on the role of socializer as our parents did. They delighted in our behavior, were thrilled with every crayon drawing and surprised when any new word tumbled out of our mouths. They showered us with affection—no strings attached. Fiore encourages his patients to find that voice in themselves, whether it is modeled on an actual grandparent, a teacher, an aunt or uncle, or simply conjured in one's imagination.

THE EXPERIENCE OF HEALTH

Because the Type C person has blotted memories, emotions, and sensations out of consciousness, he has a blind spot in his capacity for unalloyed experience. This blind spot constricts and impoverishes his experience of health. Here is how Larry Dossey, M.D., describes this state of affairs in his book, *Beyond Illness:*

> Many of us feel we have become inured to health. We have lost what we once knew how to feel, what we once sensed with exuberance, what we early on knew in keen purity, excitement, fulfillment. We are numb to the *experience* of health. . . .
>
> We feel, as [D. H.] Lawrence described, only what we allow ourselves to feel. We allow only a piteous counterfeit of the real thing to creep in from time to time. We mistake the map for the territory, in the semanticist Alfred Korzybski's words, mistakenly supposing that lab tests and physical examinations are the same thing as health.
>
> To allow more than objects to enter our experience— *really* enter—would entail a painful reassessment of who we are. It would mandate a redefinition of our relationship with the world. . . . It would entail an immersion in the "organic system of life," from which "we shall produce such real blossoms of life and being," as Lawrence put it.

Type C transformation for healthy people involves a "redefinition of [your] relationship with the world." The goal is to restore the balance in your inner/outer transactions, and the desired result is to become alive again to the experience of health. I mean health in the broadest sense: psychological, spiritual, and physical. The more alive you are to the experience of health, the more well protected you are from disease.

Of course, no matter how healthy we are, we're never invulnerable. We can never extinguish the possibility of disease and death. As Larry Dossey has pointed out, health and illness are inextricably bound—we can't know one without the other. We can't banish illness from our consciousness or our world, nor should we try. We *can* develop immune power, but no one has ever attained immune omnipotence. The search for health shouldn't become a veiled war against death. Such a war can't be won. The search for health can, however, be a passionate embrace of life.

In our age of cholesterol-counting, fiber-foraging, and workout mania, it is time to reevaluate our priorities. Health is not simply a matter of what you do right or wrong, of keeping up with an endless series of brand-new products and practices prescribed by media health advocates. Health, and disease prevention, has more to do with achieving a dynamic balance. The health of our inner environment is not dependent only on proper fuel, lubrication, and tune-ups, as if our tissues and organs were parts of a well-oiled machine, but on an organic harmony within and between overlapping systems. Since we cannot separate our "mental" systems from our "physical" systems, the vital balance we seek involves not only what we eat and how we exercise but how we think, feel, and relate to the world outside.

For prevention, we have to pay attention to the whole of our being, nourish the health of all our "parts." How does this translate into daily life? The same impulse that compels us to take care of our emotional health also inspires us to quit smoking. The same courage it takes to ask others for what we need is also necessary to confront patterns of addiction to alcohol, drugs, or food. The drive to assert ourselves in the world can also be channeled into activism to reduce environmental carcinogens and other threats to our planet. The same fierce concern for ourselves that spurs us to make difficult but needed changes in work or relationships also propels us into the doctor's office for early detection of cancer. Both types of action—inner- and outer-directed—contribute to cancer prevention.

Transforming Type C behavior is like a slow emergence from a protective shell. As a kind of rebirth, it has a natural rhythm. It's a slow rhythm, because meeting the world with a new face— your own—is like coming out into a strange and confusing place.

You need time to make the passage, to adjust to a new environment, to test new responses in the world. Your relationship to yourself has changed, and your relationship to others will also change. The periods of pain and frustration you endure are part of the process, part of your identity formation. These growing pains are far more endurable when you hold fast to the realization that you are nourishing the life of your body, and at the same time, you are opening your mind and heart to all that experience has to offer.

PART VI

THE FUTURE OF THE TYPE C CONNECTION

CHAPTER 17

The true scientist never loses the faculty of amazement. It is the essence of his being.

—*Hans Selye*

Science herself consults her heart when she lays it down that the infinite ascertainment of fact and correction of false belief are the supreme goods for man.

—*William James*

Let knowledge grow from more to more,
Yet more of reverence in us dwell;
That mind and soul, according well,
May make one music as before. . . .

—*Alfred, Lord Tennyson*

The Future of the Type C Connection

As we approach the twenty-first century, the new mind-body medicine is taking root in research labs, clinics, and in people's personal practices. The unity of mind and body is being demonstrated on the molecular level, and the road ahead is wide open for more breakthrough discoveries. As neuroscientist Candace Pert said in a recent article on psychoneuroimmunology, "It's going to be so quickly forgotten how controversial this all was."

Unfortunately, the wide-ranging findings of PNI research still have not reached or been fully accepted by important segments of the medical community. However, as more young scientists enter this burgeoning field, infusing it with fresh ideas and energy, the future is bright with possibilities. By the next century, research that confirms earlier mind-body findings, and studies that forge altogether new connections, will bring about a revolutionary change in medicine.

Cancer is still the most controversial area of mind-body research. Early investigators showed a link between emotions and cancer, but their research lacked the rigor that today's scientists demand. As a result, their work was unfairly branded as scientifically worthless. (I'm thinking of David Kissen and Lawrence LeShan, among others.) Even though their methods were imperfect, many of their theories and findings have stood the test of time.

Recent studies, with more refined and efficient methods, have corroborated their general notion of a behavior pattern peculiar to cancer progression and susceptibility. The main features of Type C behavior—nonexpression of emotion, a passive coping style, and hidden hopelessness—have been substantiated in the past decade by myself, Dr. Steven Greer, Dr. Sandra Levy, Dr. Caroline B. Thomas and Drs. A. H. Schmale and Howard Iker, among many others.

To some, the notion of a mind-cancer connection is heresy, while to others it offers new hope for control of this disease. The biggest fear is that people will blame themselves either for getting or succumbing to cancer. As I've argued, we are responsible only for changing unhealthy behavior when we know it's unhealthy. Even then, modifying deeply ingrained patterns takes not only consciousness but hard work.

The recovery/codependency movement set in motion by twelve-step programs like Alcoholics Anonymous (AA) and Adult Children of Alcoholics (ACOA) has begun to transform our society's view of self-destructive behavior. Type C behavior is not an addiction per se, but many of the issues involved in changing this pattern are similar to those addressed by twelve-step programs. These groups have recognized the role of personal responsibility for change, while removing the harmful specter of blaming the victim. Now we can begin to recognize how early experiences affect many levels of our being—psychological, spiritual, and yes, physical— without stigmatizing ourselves or others.

In a context of complete confidentiality and unconditional support, the addict can begin to take responsibility for his actions. But twelve-step programs never promote the illusory belief that an addict can or should have absolute control over his behavior. The Saint Francis prayer, which is repeated at every twelve-step meeting, points the way: "Grant me the serenity to accept the things I cannot change, the courage to change the things I can, and the wisdom to know the difference."

If we in mind-body science adopt this philosophy, we will advance in leaps and bounds, unafraid to explore the deep recesses of mind-body interactions. We must abandon the antiquated and dangerously distorted idea that people wounded by life inflict their psychological or physical problems on themselves because they are too weak-willed to change. Liberated from our moralistic blinders, we can explore how our pains, struggles, and pleasures affect our bodies without fear of misunderstanding.

There are many pressing research issues for the 1990s. We need more long-term studies following thousands of healthy people, both to confirm and expand the findings of Drs. Caroline B. Thomas, Patrick Dattore, and George Kaplan and Peggy Reynolds on the role of psychological risk factors in cancer. We also need more studies following cancer patients to confirm that the progression of their disease is influenced by emotions and behavior. These studies should also include immune measures, as Dr. Sandra Levy and I have done, as well as other measures of biologic response, to better understand how our defense system is a bridge between mind and cancer.

In the coming years, I will track the melanoma patients I have studied over the past decade. This will enable me to determine to what degree Type C or other psychosocial factors affect long-term survival. Currently I am studying behavioral factors in HIV infection and AIDS, including biological and psychosocial response patterns relevant to the progression of HIV/AIDS. Dr. George Solomon and I will continue to study long-term survivors of AIDS. Thus far, our results suggest that a form of fighting spirit can lengthen the life span of those suffering with this disease.

Right now I view the immune system as one of the crucial links between cancer and the mind. Future study holds the promise of discovering other connecting corridors. More work is needed on the role of the mind in influencing hormones that, in turn, affect malignant growth. But the most far-reaching investigations will examine the mind's effect on molecular processes. Already, Drs. Janice Kiecolt-Glaser and Ronald Glaser have shown a link between stress and inefficient DNA repair. DNA repair is a vital defense mechanism against all mutations—an initial stage of malignant transformation. When DNA repair is faulty, the possibility of cancer development is increased. The Glasers' work suggests that mind-body factors can directly impact the internal machinery of the cell.

There are suggestions in the medical literature that certain groups of genes can be "turned on" or "turned off" by messenger molecules (such as neuropeptides). Recent breakthroughs in molecular biology teach us that, fundamentally, cancer is triggered by genes (oncogenes) within the cell. Might it be possible that messenger molecules—some of which originate in the brain—have a role in triggering or suppressing cancer genes? While this remains pure speculation, it is an area ripe for investigation. If the concept is found to have validity, we will soon be engaged in heated debates about a possible *mind-gene* connection.

Finally, and most important, we need more intervention studies. Dr. David Spiegel's study, which showed that group therapy helped to lengthen the life span of cancer patients, paved the way. Will other studies once again show the same extraordinary effect? We also need studies that shed light on whether psychosocial therapies might *prevent* cancer.

Clearly, much work remains to be done on Type C and cancer. However, the prospect of greater control over cancer via the mind is an exciting one. We are finally developing the scientific sophistication to be able to "see" the mind-body connection at the cellular level. Furthermore, we are developing the psychological sophistication to understand what mind states and transformations actually strengthen our defense against disease.

Our newly refined methods are teaching us what the late Norman Cousins once put so eloquently:

> The life force may be the least understood force on earth. William James said that human beings tend to live too far within self-imposed limits. It is possible that these limits will recede when we respect more fully the natural drive of the human mind and body toward perfectability and regeneration.

The paradox of mind-body science is this: the more precise our instruments, the more powerful our technology, the more clearly we see that many of our strongest weapons against disease lie outside the realm of high-tech medicine. We are learning that the power of the mind can be mobilized to fight almost any disease, including cancer. This idea can no longer be discarded as so much "false hope," because science is demonstrating the mind-body's natural drive "toward perfectability and regeneration." We activate this natural drive when we live out our true identity and embrace our full humanity.

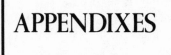

APPENDIXES

Recognizing Your Type C Behavior

Now that I have described the Type C pattern and presented my research findings along with many case histories, you may well recognize Type C behavior or characteristics in yourself. But here is a checklist that you can use as a diagnostic tool to help you identify your own Type C behavior, and pinpoint specific aspects of your pattern that need attention.

Decide whether you agree with each of these statements. When answering, don't consider the implications. Clear your mind and decide your answers as truthfully as you can.

Count how many of these statements you feel are true:

1) I rarely if ever lose my temper.
2) I often feel that I'm one down in personal and work relationships. The other person often has more power than me.
3) I get anxious when I have to ask someone for a raise, a favor, or a helping hand.
4) I would not describe myself as assertive.
5) I tend to focus more on my husband's/wife's/friend's/lover's needs than my own.
6) I'm more concerned with the needs of my family (parents, siblings, children) than my own.

7) If someone I care about asks me to do a favor I'd rather not do, I'll do it anyway.

8) I have a hard time standing up to authority figures.

9) I tend to shy away from competition in work and leisure activities.

10) I'm more low energy than I am high energy.

11) I have felt abused—emotionally or physically—in a number of close relationships.

12) I don't cry very often.

13) It takes a lot to get me upset—I take things in stride.

14) When I feel myself getting too emotional, I try to compose myself as quickly as possible.

15) There are times when I feel my life lacks color, excitement, or meaning.

16) My close relationships are fine, but I sometimes think there is something missing in them.

17) People will reject me if I come on too strong.

18) I think of myself as a very nice person, and other people see me the same way.

19) I don't ever want to be thought of as narcissistic or self-centered.

20) It's best to be positive at all times. I try not to let myself get depressed, sad, or angry when things go wrong.

Most of you will answer yes to a few of these statements. (We all exhibit some of these characteristics at some time in our lives.) However, if you find yourself in broad agreement with many of these statements—ten or more—then you are a Type C coper. If you honestly agree with fifteen or more, you are probably an extreme Type C coper.

In my experience, many people—cancer patients included—find it liberating to recognize and acknowledge their Type C behavior. As in any behavior change, whether from addiction to recovery, from denial to acceptance, or from passivity to action, recognition of the old pattern comes first. Acknowledging Type C behavior means you can say, "Yes, I have had difficulty accepting and expressing my feelings and I have not taken charge in many areas of my life. I know that now, and now I can begin to change. I can stop playing a role that has limited my potential for growth."

Once able to identify and admit your Type C pattern, you can begin the process of transformation I have described in Chapters 11 through 16. Use those chapters to address the issues raised by your answers to this questionnaire.

Being a Type C coper—extreme or otherwise—doesn't mean you're going to get cancer or die from it. It means only that the way you cope with life may slowly undermine your body's natural defenses. That doesn't mean you are fated to become ill. But, like any other risk factor that undermines health—whether smoking, poor eating habits, or drinking too much alcohol—it is something to pay attention to and consider changing. You may cope fairly well with the experiences of everyday life, but if a seriously stressful circumstance should occur, your body's resources may not be up to meeting the challenge.

From a moral standpoint, Type C copers are no different from Type A's, Type B's, or anyone who has a habitual behavior pattern. It's not something to feel guilty about. We all have habits that were originally developed as ways to deal with pain and anxiety. For Type C's, it is being nice and compliant and never acting out or expressing much negative emotion.

It's healthy to understand the downside of this behavior, to take greater responsibility for your psychological and physical well-being. But our goal is not to scare you into change—it's to encourage you to explore new terrain. See the appropriate sections in chapters 11 through 16 for guidance on how to transform your Type C pattern.

APPENDIX II

Notes, References, and Methods

Chapter 1: Introduction

I discuss the origins of my psychoimmunologic research with melanoma patients, and the early development of the Type C behavior pattern, in L. Temoshok and B. H. Fox (1984): "Coping Styles and Other Psychosocial Factors Related to Medical Status and to Prognosis in Patients with Cutaneous Malignant Melanoma." In B. H. Fox and B. H. Newberry (eds.): *Impact of Psychoendocrine Systems in Cancer and Immunity.* C. J. Hogrefe, Toronto.

p. 5 D. Reisman with N. Glazer and R. Denney (1961): *The Lonely Crowd: A Study of the Changing American Character,* Yale University Press, New Haven (abridged edition).

Chapter 2: Portrait of the Type C Individual

p. 20 S. A. Appelbaum (1981): "Exploring the Relationship Between Personality and Cancer." In J. Goldberg (ed.): *Psychotherapeutic Treatment of Cancer Patients.* The Free Press, New York.

p. 23 Rollo May has argued against confusing the healthy aspects of anger and aggression with unhealthy, destructive expressions of hostility, in books such as *Man's Search for Himself* (1953, W. W. Norton, New York), *Power and Innocence* (1972, W. W. Norton, New York), and *Freedom and Destiny* (1981, Delta Books, New York).

Quote from Rollo May (1953): *Man's Search for Himself.* W. W. Norton, New York. Quote from Anthony Storr (1970): *Human Aggression.* Penguin Books, New York.

p. 24 S. Greer and T. Morris (1975): "Psychological attributes of women who develop breast cancer: a controlled study." *Journal of Psychosomatic Research,* 19, pp. 147–53.

p. 25 C. B. Bahnson (1969): "Psychophysical complementarity in malignancies: past work and future vistas." *Annals of the New York Academy of Sciences,* 164, pp. 319–34. C. B. Bahnson and M. B. Bahnson (1966): "Role of the ego defenses: denial and repression in the etiology of malignant neoplasm." *Annals of the New York Academy of Sciences,* 125(3), pp. 827–45. C. B. Bahnson and M. B. Bahnson (1969): "Ego defenses in cancer patients." *Annals of the New York Academy of Sciences,* 164, pp. 546–59.

p. 26 Quote from Boris Pasternak (1959): *Doctor Zhivago.* University of Michigan Press, Ann Arbor.

p. 28 Quote from Karen Horney (1945): *Our Inner Conflicts.* W. W. Norton, New York.

p. 34 Quote from Ralph Linton (1945): *The Cultural Background of Personality.* D. Appleton-Century, New York.

pp. 37–38 M. Friedman and R. H. Rosenman (1974): *Type A Behavior and Your Heart.* Ballantine Books, New York. M. Friedman and D. Ulmer (1984): *Treating Type A Behavior and Your Heart.* Ballantine Books, New York.

p. 40 For an excellent review of research on psychological factors in cancer, focusing on emotional expression, see James Gross (1989): "Emotional expression in cancer onset and progression." *Social Science and Medicine,* 28(12), pp. 1239–248. David Kissen's important work is described in D. M. Kissen (1966): "The significance of personality in lung cancer in men." *Annals of the New York Academy of Sciences,* 125, pp. 820–26. D. M. Kissen and H. J. Eysenck (1962): "Personality in male lung cancer patients." *Journal of Psychosomatic Research,* 6, pp. 123–37. D. M. Kissen, R. I. F. Brown, and M. A. Kissen (1969): "A further report on the personality and psychological factors in lung cancer." *Annals of the New York Academy of Sciences,* 164, pp. 535–45.

Chapter 3: Shared Patterns, Unique Personalities

p. 50 The distinction between suppression and repression is important in understanding Type C behavior and in determining the nature and dynamics of any one individual's Type C pattern.

Freud was the first to discover and fully explicate the various psychic defenses, including repression. "Of the different kinds of inner inhibitions or suppressions, one is especially worthy of our interest because it is the most far-reaching," he wrote. "We designate that form by the term 'repression.' It is characterized by the fact that it excludes from consciousness certain buried emotions and their products." From S. Freud (1938): *The Basic Writings of Sigmund Freud.* Random House, New York.

Alice Miller discusses the long-term toll exacted by severe repression: "When . . . a child must consume all her capability and energy for the required labor of repression; when, in addition, she has never known what it is to be loved and protected by someone, this child will eventually also be incapable of protecting herself and organizing her life in a meaningful and productive manner. . . . The life-saving function of repression in childhood is transformed in adulthood into a life-destroying force." A. Miller (1990): *Banished Knowledge.* Doubleday, New York.

pp. 53–56. I discuss the origins of my theory and research delineating a coping continuum, which posits Type A and Type C as extreme opposites, with Type B representing a healthy middle ground, in L. Temoshok and B. H. Fox (1984): "Coping Styles and Other Psychosocial Factors Related to Medical Status and to Prognosis in Patients with Cutaneous Malignant Melanoma." In B. H. Fox and B. H. Newberry (eds.): *Impact of Psychoendocrine Systems in Cancer and Immunity.* C. J. Hogrefe, Toronto.

In a 1983 book, I developed a theory regarding the biological substrates of various behavior patterns. I hypothesized that different individuals (based on genetic and environmental factors) cope with stress by processing the stress-associated "information" on different levels of mental organization. As discussed, Type A (coronary-prone) individuals are hostile and driven. They accommodate stress at the mental level of "motivation," which has as its biological substrate the autonomic nervous system and endocrine system. I hypothesized that Type C individuals, who cope by blocking awareness of pain and negative emotions, accommodate stress at a lower level of organization—the mental level of perception, which has as its substrate the immune-regulating neuropeptides. For more on this theory, see L. Temoshok (1983): "Emotion, Adaptation, and Disease: a Multidimensional Theory." In L. Temoshok, C. Van Dyke, and L. S. Zegans (eds.): *Emotions in Health and Illness: Theoretical and Research Foundations.* Grune and Stratton, New York, pp. 207–33.

pp. 56–57 Quote from Alice Miller (1983): *For Your Own Good.* Farrar, Straus and Giroux, New York.

Quote from Robert Bly (1988): *A Little Book on the Human Shadow.* Harper & Row, San Francisco.

p. 58 C. B. Thomas (1976): "Precursors of premature disease and death." *Annals of Internal Medicine,* 85, p. 653–58. C. B. Thomas, K. R. Duszynski, and J. W. Shaffer (1979): "Family attitudes reported in youth as potential predictors of cancer." *Psychosomatic Medicine,* 41, pp. 287–302. C. B. Thomas and O. L. McCabe (1980): "Precursors of premature disease and death: habits of nervous tension." *Johns Hopkins Medical Journal,* 147, p. 137–45.

Chapter 4: "Ten Percent Can Make All the Difference in the World"

pp. 65–66 Ken Wilber, in "Do We Make Ourselves Sick?", article/interview in *New Age Journal,* September–October 1988.

pp. 66–67 G. L. Engel (1977): "The need for a new medical model: a challenge for biomedicine." *Science,* 196, pp. 129–36.

pp. 68–69 For a discussion of the causes, natural history, diagnosis, staging, and treatment of malignant melanoma, see S. H. Moseley, F. R. Eilber, and D. L. Morton (1980): "Melanoma. In C. M. Haskell (ed.): *Cancer Treatment.* W. B. Saunders, Philadelphia. pp. 678–94.

pp. 69–72 For a complete description and discussion of my initial study of coping in melanoma patients, see L. Temoshok, B. W. Heller, R. W. Sagebiel, M. S. Blois, D. M. Sweet, R. J. DiClemente, and M. L. Gold (1985): "The relationship of psychosocial factors to prognostic indicators in cutaneous malignant melanoma." *Journal of Psychosomatic Medicine,* 29, pp. 139–54.

In brief, the fifty-nine subjects in this study were patients referred to the malignant melanoma clinics at the University of California and Children's Hospital in San Francisco. Eligibility requirements included, a) eighteen years or older, and b) clinical stage I or II melanoma. Of the fifty-nine subjects, forty-nine were clinical stage I and ten were clinical stage II (regional lymph node involvement). Subjects ranged from eighteen to seventy-two years old, 48 percent fell between thirty and forty-nine. 55 percent were male, 45 percent female. My colleagues and I collected data on tumor thickness and Clark's level of invasion, physical risk factors including skin and hair coloring, patient delay in seeking medical attention, their knowledge of melanoma, and understanding of medical treatment. We conducted our structured interview within one month of biopsy, and all interviews were videotaped. The videotapes were later rated according to a precise coding manual by three master's-level psychologists, all blind to each other's assessments. Interrater reliability (the degree to which our raters agreed on the assignment of subjects to various coping categories) was high, ranging from 87–99 percent. Each subject was rated in the following coping categories:

1) *Catastrophic reaction:* melanoma has disturbed most areas of functioning and provoked dire thoughts.
2) *Coping by avoidance:* copes by action, by avoiding emotional discussions.
3) *Coping by changing:* changing attitudes, relationships, temporal perspective as a result of having melanoma.
4) *Coping by denial:* doesn't want to think, know, or talk about melanoma.
5) *Coping by optimism:* seeing the brighter side of this experience.
6) *Coping with strength:* copes by trying hard to be positive, strong, and stable.
7) *Emotionally expressive*
8) *Faith:* placing faith in external authorities: God and/or physicians.
9) *Minimizes:* minimizes the seriousness of melanoma, in general, or of own condition.
10) *Nonverbal Type C:* mean rating of subjects as more Type C than Type A on seventeen descriptive dimensions.
11) *Stressful changes:* total number of relationship endings, financial loss, major moves, and major changes in personal life during last five years.
12) *Type A:* rated more Type A on the basis of responses to a brief, standardized interview developed to classify subjects as Type A or B.
13) *Type C:* Rated more Type C responses to questions regarding coping with demanding or powerful others; i.e., tries to please others, avoids conflict, does not express negative feelings.

Nonverbal Type C behavior was determined by analysis of the nonverbal behavior of each subject, according to a semantic differential scale of seventeen indices. (See Notes referring to p. 75 for elaboration.)

Each subject was also given the following self-report instruments: Beck's Depression Inventory, the Psychological Distress Scale from the MMPI, McNair's Profile of Mood States (POMS), and Temoshok's Character Style Inventory.

Among the psychosocial variables, significant correlations included: "Faith" with tumor thickness ($p < 0.03$); "Nonverbal Type C" with thickness ($p < 0.05$);

Histrionic Character Style (negative correlation) with thickness ($p < 0.05$); and Narcissistic Character Style (negative correlations) with thickness ($p < 0.5$) and level of invasion ($p < 0.05$). Delay in seeking treatment was correlated with both thickness and level ($p < 0.10$). Less previous knowledge of melanoma and less understanding of treatment were correlated with thickness and level ($p < 0.5$). "At risk" skin coloring was correlated with thickness ($p < 0.5$) and occupational status (less skilled) was correlated with level ($p < 0.5$).

Intercorrelations showed that, in every instance, the psychosocial variable (such as "Nonverbal Type C") retained a significant or near-significant relationship with tumor thickness when any other potentially confounding demographic variable (skin coloring, occupation, knowledge of melanoma or treatment, etc.) was controlled for. The reverse did not hold true. In other words, the psychological factors could not be explained by some other factor(s).

When the population was split into two groups, those younger and those older than fifty-five, the psychological factors were more significantly correlated in younger than in older subjects. For example, in the younger group, "Faith" was associated with thickness and level ($p < 0.02$); "Nonverbal Type C" was correlated with thickness ($p < 0.02$). No significant correlations between these factors and tumor thickness or level were found in the older-than-fifty-five group. "Histrionic Style" was correlated with tumor thickness in the over-fifty-five group.

Dr. Bernard H. Fox discusses the role of age in the relationship of psychosocial factors to cancer in his comprehensive review paper: B. H. Fox (1978): "Premorbid psychological factors as related to cancer incidence." *Journal of Behavioral Medicine,* 1(1), pp. 45–133.

p. 72 C. Darwin (1965): *The Expression of the Emotions in Man and Animals.* University of Chicago Press, Chicago.

p. 74 P. Ekman, W. V. Friesen, and P. Ellsworth (1972): *Emotion in the Human Face: Guidelines for Research and an Integration of Findings.* Pergamon Press, New York. P. Ekman (1984): "Expression and the Nature of Emotion." In K. Scherer and P. Ekman (eds.): *Approaches to Emotion.* Lawrence Erlbaum, Hillsdale, New Jersey.

p. 75 Bruce Heller and I developed a set of nonverbal characteristics enabling us to rate each patient as relatively more "Type C," "Type A," or somewhere in between. Each patient was ranked (numerically from 1 to 7) along a continuum, ranging from more Type C (on the left) to more Type A (on the right) on each of these "semantic differential scales":

down—up
emotionally constricted—emotionally labile
slow—fast
patient—impatient
lethargic—hurried
passive—active
sad—angry
bland—intense
given up—struggling
withdrawn—extended

helpless—in control
hopeless—pursues opportunities world offers
smooth—jerky
appeasing—hostile
accepting—controlling
sincere—guarded
fluid—awkward

The subjects who were rated high in "nonverbal Type C" (and who tended to have thicker tumors) were more emotionally constricted, passive, withdrawn, appeasing, etc., based on analysis of their nonverbal behavior ratings.

p. 80 Quote from G. Sheehy (1982): *Pathfinders,* Bantam Books, New York.

pp. 81–82 M. R. Jensen (1987): "Psychobiological factors predicting the course of cancer." *Journal of Personality,* 55(2), pp. 317–42.

Chapter 5: Emotions and the Mind-Body Bridge

pp. 87–88 For a summary view of research on hostility and cardiovascular disease, see R. Williams (1989): *The Trusting Heart.* Times Books, New York.

pp. 95–97 For a description of my study on the relationship of psychological variables to tumor-host response (including immune response) see L. Temoshok (1985): "Biopsychosocial studies on cutaneous malignant melanoma: psychosocial factors associated with prognostic indicators, progression, psychophysiology, and tumor-host response." *Social Science and Medicine,* 20(8), pp. 833–40.

In brief, each subject's videotaped interview was rated on seven-point scales by an independent coder on the following dimensions of emotional expression: a) verbal articulateness in describing emotion (e.g., vividness of phrase and/or adjectives, use of simile or metaphor); b) consistent nonverbal expressiveness (e.g., looking or sounding angry when describing an anger episode); c) differentiated affective expressiveness (e.g., when relating a sad event, did the subject describe or show sadness or a mix of emotions); d) elaboration of bodily sensations (e.g., flushed face, racing heart for anger; tears, empty feeling in stomach for sadness); and e) cognitive elaboration (e.g., vengeful thoughts during the anger episode). Neither the interviewer nor the rater of the videotape was aware of any aspect of the patient's medical status. Intercorrelations among these emotional expression factors were all positive—patients who did not express anger according to one dimension generally did not express anger according to the other dimensions. As a validity check, a second independent rater, Dr. Neil Fiore, rated subjects on two main dimensions: a) realism (honest confrontation with the seriousness of their condition) vs. denial (minimizing seriousness, being maladaptively positive); and b) expression (using emotional words and gestures) vs. suppression (lack of emotion—fear, anger, anxiety sadness—or flatness of emotion). Dr. Fiore's findings were all positively correlated with our emotional expression findings; the correlations were especially strong and all significant for anger expression. This suggests that the construct of emotional expression/nonexpression is robust—it can be measured from videotaped interviews or from written interview ratings and it can be reliably assessed by different raters or even different scales.

Using factor analysis, my colleages and I were able to "collapse" the various dimensions of emotional expression into one dimension, representing general emotional expression.

The following table shows correlations of emotional expression with prognostic indicators of melanoma, including mitotic rate (rate of multiplication of cancer cells) and lymphocyte infiltration (the number of these key immune cells congregating at the base of the melanoma tumor):

Correlations of Emotional Expression Factor with Prognostic Indicators

Prognostic Indicators	Emotional Expression Factor		
	r (correlation)	p (significance)	N (number of subjects)
Mitotic Rate	−0.48	.008	29
Lymphocyte Infiltration	0.39	.04	29
Clark's Level	−0.15	NS*	40
Tumor Thickness	−0.31	.05	41

*Not significant

All correlations were in the expected direction: emotional expression with positive prognostic indicators, and nonexpression with negative indicators. With the exception of Clark's level, all these correlations were significant. (A low value is "good"; that is $p < .04$ means that these results would occur by chance only four times out of one hundred.)

pp. 97–98 S. M. Levy (1983): "Host differences in neoplastic risk: behavioral and social contributors to disease." *Health Psychology,* 2, pp. 21–44. S. M. Levy (1985): "Behavior as a biological response modifier: the psycho-immunoendocrine network and tumor immunology." *Behavioral Medicine Abstracts,* 6, pp. 1–4. S. M. Levy, R. Herberman, A. Maluish, B. Schlien, and M. Lippman (1985): "Prognostic risk assessment in primary breast cancer by behavioral and immunological parameters." *Health Psychology,* 4, 99–113. S. M. Levy, R. B. Herberman, M. Lipman, and T. D'Angelo (1987): "Correlation of stress factors with sustained depression of natural killer cell activity with predicted prognosis in patients with breast cancer." *Journal of Clinical Oncology,* 5(3), pp. 348–53.

In a recent and most interesting study, Dr. Levy reported that patients with a "perception of high quality social support" had significantly more active natural killer cells. Having a support system isn't enough; believing in your support system is pivotal. See S. M. Levy, R. B. Herberman, T. Whiteside, et al. (1990): "Perceived social support and tumor estrogen/progesterone receptor status as predictors of natural killer cell activity in breast cancer patients." *Psychosomatic Medicine,* 52, pp. 73–85.

Chapter 6: Is Type C a Risk Factor?

p. 101 For a review of research on behavioral and psychosocial factors in cancer incidence, see B. H. Fox, L. Temoshok, with H. Dreher (1988): "Mind-body and behavior in cancer incidence." *Advances,* 5(4), pp. 41–60.

pp. 102–103 Many of the quotes on these pages, including the one attributed to Galen, were discovered and cited by Lawrence LeShan in his historical review paper, L. LeShan (1959): "Psychological states as factors in the development of malignant disease: a critical review." *Journal of the National Cancer Institute,* 22(1), pp. 1–18. Specifically, see C. L. Bacon, R. Renneker, and M. Cutler (1952): "A psychosomatic survey of cancer of the breast." *Psychosomatic Medicine,* 14, pp. 453–60. J. B. Trunnel (1956): "Theories of the origin of cancer." Paper read at the Texas Conference on Psychosomatic Implications in Cancer, Dallas, September 1956. E. M. Blumberg, P. M. West, and F. W. Ellis (1954): "A possible relationship between psychological factors and human cancer." *Psychosomatic Medicine,* 16, pp. 277–86. B. Butler (1954): "The use of hypnosis in the care of the cancer patient." *Cancer,* 7, pp. 1–14.

p. 104 The findings of the Western Collaborative Group Study, which linked Type A behavior to risk of heart disease, was reported in R. H. Rosenman, R. J. Brand, C. D. Jenkins, et al. (1975): "Coronary heart disease in the Western Collaborative Group Study: final follow-up experience of 8½ years." *Journal of the American Medical Association,* 233, pp. 872–77.

pp. 106–107 S. Greer and T. Morris (1975): "Psychological attributes of women who develop breast cancer: a controlled study." *Journal of Psychosomatic Research,* 19, pp. 147–53.

p. 107 H. Scherg (1987): "Psychosocial factors and disease bias in breast cancer patients." *Psychosomatic Medicine,* 49, pp. 302–12. M. Wirsching, H. Stierlin, F. Hoffman, G. Weber, and B. Wirsching (1982): "Psychological identification of breast cancer patients before biopsy." *Journal of Psychosomatic Medicine,* 26, pp. 1–10.

pp. 110–111 For a complete discussion and description of our study of repressive coping in melanoma patients, heart patients, and controls, see A. W. Kneier and L. Temoshok (1984): "Repressive coping reactions in patients with malignant melanoma as compared to cardiovascular disease patients." *Journal of Psychosomatic Medicine,* 28(2), pp. 145–55.

We recruited the three groups from UCSF medical clinics—twenty cancer (melanoma) patients, twenty patients with cardiovascular disease, and twenty people with no health problems. (This latter control group consisted of friends or family members of patients seen in the same outpatient clinics at UCSF.) We matched the three groups by ethnic origin, age, and gender. We also asked the directors of the various clinics to rank their respective patients in terms of estimated survival time. This enabled us to match our cancer and heart patients on prognosis, disease severity, and life expectancy as well. If we ended up finding differences in repressive coping, it wouldn't be because one group or another faced a more grave prognosis.

Studies have shown that emotional responses to stress—anxiety, upset, anger, or fear—have corresponding physiological reactions. One of the physiological measures of internal arousal is called "electrodermal activity." This is a technical phrase for what could loosely be termed "emotional sweating." This phenomenon is caused by the activation of the autonomic nervous system when an individual is subjected to stress. Signals sent from areas of the brain to the sweat glands trigger the secretions, which can be so minimal as to be unnoticeable even to the person who is sweating. But by passing a constant voltage across the skin between two electrodes, the degree of sweating can be measured by the amount of current passed. The more sweating, the greater the current. This is known as the "skin conductance response," or "SCR," and research has demonstrated that an increase of anxiety or emotional arousal is reflected in higher SCR's.

For years, psychophysiologists have looked at skin conductance response as a measure of emotional stress reactions. However, over the past two decades investigators have begun to take note of a particular anomaly in this type of research. Among a minority of subjects, there were discrepancies between their reported reaction to a stressful stimulus and what their SCR reflected. Researchers Joshua Weinstein and colleagues [J. Weinstein, J. R. Averill, E. M. Opton, and R. S. Lazarus (1968): "Defensive style and discrepancy between self-report and physiological indexes of stress." *Journal of Personality and Social Psychology,* 10, pp. 406–13] analyzed six studies where these seeming contradictions abounded. They concentrated on subjects who reported low anxiety in an experimental stress situation but whose SCR readings told a different story. Weinstein et al., found that these same individuals also ranked high on psychological measures of repression and defensiveness. The discrepancies had been neither a fluke nor a mistake. These were people who either did not recognize or did not report their internal emotional reactions. Psychologists Daniel Weinberger and colleagues [D. A. Weinberger, G. E. Schwartz, and R. J. Davidson (1979): "Low-anxious, high-anxious, and repressive coping styles: psychometric patterns and behavioral and physiological responses to stress." *Journal of Abnormal Psychology,* 88, pp. 369–80] also studied subjects who were found, in psychological tests, to be "repressors." The repressors had high electrodermal responses to threatening phrases and sought to avoid their content, while at the same time, they *reported* low anxiety.

Kneier and I designed our experimental procedure for measuring repressive coping based, in part, on these previous efforts. We showed each subject fifty slides with different anxiety-provoking statements. Five categories of emotionally disturbing content were developed, with ten statements in each category: anger, sadness, threats to self-esteem, threats to interpersonal needs, and miscellaneous statements that did not readily fall into one of the above.

Each subject in the procedure would be hooked up to a dermograph that measured the SCR. We used an electrode assembly consisting of three small electrodes attached to the fingertips. As the subjects viewed the slides, we could get an SCR reading to determine the degree of their physiological arousal.

We instructed our subjects as follows: "I am going to show you a series of statements one at a time. These statements say things about you or other people that are generally unpleasant or depressing. People are sometimes bothered by the ideas contained in these statements, and we want to know how much these statements bother you. First read the statement, then ask yourself, 'How much does this bother me?' Then mark your answer on the scale."

This scale ranged from 0, for "not at all," to 10, for "extremely." Each statement was projected on a screen for five seconds, during which time a reading was taken from the dermograph. Immediately after, the subject was asked to mark down his or her reaction.

Because of the anxiety-provoking nature of the procedure, we invited to participate only those melanoma and cardiovascular patients who had been diagnosed many months earlier. (The cancer patients averaged a year and a half since diagnosis; the heart disease patients averaged twenty months.) For the same reason, we did not involve any cancer patients with advanced, metastatic tumors. All our subjects were well beyond the initial shock or distress of coming to terms with their illness.

For each subject, we had two key pieces of information: their physiological response (SCR) to each statement, and their self-report—how much they said each statement "bothered" them. Repressive coping would be determined by discrepancies between the two. Since individual differences had to be reckoned with, we determined the average, or "mean," SCR for each subject and the mean self-report of upset (0–10) for each. For repressive coping, we looked for instances where the subject's SCR was *above* their average, while their self-report was *below* their average. The number of times such discrepancies occurred was the subject's Repressive Coping Score.

We were then able to compare the Repressive Coping Scores among the cancer, heart, and healthy subject groups. As predicted, the cancer patients had the highest Repressive Coping Scores, the heart patients had the lowest, and the healthy subjects had scores right in the middle. (Mean scores: for melanoma patients [8.40 (SD = 4.46)]; for cardiovascular patients [4.84 (SD = 4.84)]; and controls [5.72 (SD = 5.72)].

Most important, the differences between the cancer patients and heart patients on repressive coping were highly statistically significant ($p < 0.01$). The difference between cancer patients and controls, though not as great, was also significant ($p < 0.05$).

Since our approach was relatively novel, we had to double-check its validity. We gave each subject four additional well-validated measures of repressive tendencies (the Byrne Repression-Sensitization Scale, the short form of the Taylor Manifest Anxiety Scale, the Marlowe-Crowne Social Desirability Scale, and the Difficulty in Adjustment to Disease Scale). The melanoma group scored in the more "repressed" direction on three of the four questionnaires, and differed significantly from the heart patients on all three. (Exception—the Marlowe-Crowne Scale.) The differences between cancer and heart patients were just as striking on these questionnaires as they were for our experimental test for repressive coping (i.e., the difference between them on the Byrne Repression-Sensitization Scale was highly statistically significant: $p < 0.001$).

The degree of repressiveness evidenced by the melanoma and heart disease patients had nothing to do with the severity of their diseases, as ranked by the top physicians at their respective clinics. If repression was a defensive strategy used only to cope with a severe illness, then presumably those with more severe disease would be more repressed. However, this was not the case. If repressive coping occurred only as a result of *having* a life-threatening illness, then why would cancer patients be the only ones to use this coping mechanism? Why not heart patients as well, whose illness is equally life-threatening? Our results pointed to a reasonable assumption: repressive coping was not simply a response to illness, it was the characteristic style of most of the cancer patients. Among the cardiovascular patients, expressing anxiety was their characteristic coping style.

Dr. Steven Greer's group at King's College Hospital in London conducted a similar kind of study with thirty breast cancer patients and twenty-seven "healthy" controls. The cancer patients were much more likely than controls to inhibit their emotional reactions (especially anger) while watching emotionally provocative films. See: M. Watson, K. W. Pettingale, and S. Greer (1984): "Emotional control and autonomic arousal in breast cancer patients," *Journal of Psychosomatic Research,* 28(6), pp. 467–74.

pp. 113–117 Relevant references for the studies cited in the chart and discussed subsequently include:

For the Alameda County study conducted by Kaplan and Reynolds: P. Reynolds and G. A. Kaplan (1986): "Social connections and cancer: a prospective study of Alameda County residents." Paper presented at the Society of Behavioral Medicine Meeting, San Francisco, March 1986. G. A. Kaplan and P. Reynolds (1988): "Depression and cancer mortality and morbidity: prospective evidence from the Alameda County study." *Journal of Behavioral Medicine,* 11, pp. 1–13.

For Grossarth-Maticek's prospective research: R. Grossarth-Maticek, D. T. Kanazir, P. Schmidt, and H. Vetter (1982): "Psychosomatic factors in the process of carcinogenesis: theoretical models and empirical results." *Psychotherapy and Psychosomatics,* 38, pp. 284–302. R. Grossarth-Maticek, D. T. Kanazir, H. Vetter, and P. Schmidt (1983): "Psychosomatic factors involved in the process of carcinogenesis: preliminary results of the Yugoslav prospective study." *Psychotherapy and Psychosomatics,* 40, pp. 191–210. H. J. Eysenck (1988): "Personality, stress, and cancer: prediction and prophylaxis." *British Journal of Medical Psychology,* 61, pp. 57–75.

For an extensive, critical review of Grossarth-Maticek's work, see *Psychological Inquiry: An International Journal of Peer Commentary and Review* (1991) volume 2, number 3. The entire issue is devoted to this review; it includes nineteen critical commentaries on an article by Dr. Hans Eysenck on Grossarth-Maticek's cancer research. A commentary by Dr. Temoshok is included: "Assessing the assessment of psychosocial factors."

For Shekelle's twenty-year follow-up of men from the Western Electric study: R. B. Shekelle, W. J. Raynar, A. M. Ostfield, D. C. Garron, L. A. Bielauskas, S. C. Liu, C. Maliza, and O. Paul (1981): "Psychological depression and 17-year risk of death from cancer." *Psychosomatic Medicine,* 43, pp. 117–25. V. W. Persky, J. Kempthorne-Rawson, and R. B. Shekelle (1987): "Personality and risk of cancer: 20-year follow up of the Western Electric Study." *Psychosomatic Medicine,* 49, pp. 435–49.

For Dattore's study: P. J. Dattore, R. C. Shontz, and L. Coyle (1980): "Premorbid personality differentiation of cancer and noncancer groups: a test of the hypothesis of cancer proneness." *Journal of Consulting and Clinical Psychology,* 43, pp. 380–84.

For Caroline Thomas's prospective research: C. B. Thomas (1976): "Precursors of premature disease and death." *Annals of Internal Medicine,* 85, pp. 653–58.

C. B. Thomas, K. R. Duszynski, and J. W. Shaffer (1979): "Family attitudes reported in youth as potential predictors of cancer." *Psychosomatic Medicine,* 41, pp. 287–302. C. B. Thomas and O. L. McCabe (1980): "Precursors of premature disease and death: habits of nervous tension." *Johns Hopkins Medical Journal,* 147, pp. 137–45. P. L. Graves and C. B. Thomas (1981): "Themes of interaction in medical students' Rorschach responses as predictors of midlife health or disease." *Psychosomatic Medicine,* 43, pp. 215–225. P. L. Graves, L. A. Mead, and T. A. Pearson (1986): "The Rorschach interaction scale as a potential predictor of cancer." *Psychosomatic Medicine,* 48, pp. 549–63. J. W. Shaffer, P. L. Graves, R. T. Swank, and T. A. Pearson (1987): "Clustering of personality traits in youth and the subsequent development of cancer among physicians." *Journal of Behavioral Medicine,* 10(5), pp. 441–47.

For Dr. Mara Julius's findings from the "Life Change Event Study," see M. Julius, E. Harburg, A. Schork, et al. (1991): "Sex differences for cause-specific mortality as a function of anger-coping styles (1971–1988)." *American Journal of Epidemiology,* 134(7), pp. 762–63. See also N. Angier (1990): "If anger ruins your day, it can shrink your life." *New York Times,* December 13, 1990.

Chapter 7: Fighting Spirit and Survival

p. 123 B. Siegel (1986): *Love, Medicine, and Miracles.* Harper & Row, New York.

pp. 124–126 The results of Dr. Steven Greer's oft-cited study of psychological coping and survival in breast cancer was first reported at five years after diagnosis in S. Greer, T. Morris, and K. W. Pettingale (1979): "Psychological response to breast cancer: effect on outcome." *Lancet,* 2, pp. 785–87. The ten-year follow-up was reported in S. Greer, K. W. Pettingale, T. Morris, and J. Haybittle (1985): "Mental attitudes to cancer: an additional prognostic factor." *Lancet,* 1, p. 750. The most recent, fifteen-year follow-up was reported in S. Greer, T. Morris, K. W. Pettingale, and J. Haybittle (1990): "Psychological response to breast cancer and fifteen-year outcome." *Lancet,* 1, pp. 49–50.

p. 127 For a description of our replication of Steven Greer's study of psychological response to cancer and outcome, see R. J. DiClemente and L. Temoshok (1985): "Psychological adjustment to having cutaneous malignant melanoma as a predictor of follow-up clinical status." *Psychosomatic Medicine,* 47, p. 81.

By the time DiClemente and I began this effort to replicate Greer's research, twenty-five individuals of our sample population of 117 had either died or suffered recurrences (from an average of one and a half to three years from initial diagnosis). Our goal was to find an accurate way to assess all the initial videotape interviews, in order to determine whether our patients had adjusted to melanoma with fighting spirit, denial, stoic acceptance, or hopelessness/helplessness. Despite some areas of overlap, Dr. Greer's four types of mental adjustment represented a different dimension of psychological responses than the Type C and other coping styles we had defined and studied. We had to review our evidence with a fresh eye trained toward Greer's classifications.

We decided to analyze only the audio and not the video portion of our interviews. (Replicating Greer's approach as closely as possible would prevent any later discrepancies in our findings from being attributed to wide differences in our respective procedures.) Using written transcripts, we pinpointed the portions of the interview dealing specifically with the patients' mental and emotional adjustment to cancer. This enabled our team of psychologists—none of whom had any information about patients' medical outcome—to place each subject in one of Greer's categories.

We also developed a second approach tailor-made for this study. Called a "profile" method, it involved identification of the words and phrases most commonly used by patients in each of Greer's mental adjustment styles. For example, someone with fighting spirit would use such phrases as "I'm determined to beat this disease," and "I'm pretty optimistic." Stoic acceptors often said, "It's just a part of life," or "[that] doesn't bother me." Those exhibiting denial might actually say, "There is no disease," or otherwise deny the existence or gravity of having cancer. Patients who were helpless or hopeless often "thought it was all over for me," saw cancer as "the end of the world," were in "total despair," or were even "prepared to die."

We gave each phrase a numerical rank, based on how strongly it exemplified a particular mental-adjustment style. (For example, the comment "I'm going to beat this disease" ranked high for fighting spirit.) Each patient received a final score in all four categories—fighting spirit, denial, stoic acceptance, or hopelessness/helplessness. We split our patient population by gender, so that we might be able to compare our results with Greer's, whose breast cancer patients were all women.

As noted, among the women we found a significant relationship between psychological adjustment and outcome. (Of the fifty-three women, seven had either died or suffered recurrences. Five of the seven (71 percent) had been stoic in their adjustment to cancer. In our group of sixty-four men, we looked at all the relevant variables, such as age, clinical stage of disease, tumor thickness, and all the patients' psychological adjustment scores (using the new "profile" method described) to find out which factors contributed the most to disease progression. Men who had higher scores of hopelessness/helplessness had a greater likelihood of death or relapse, independent of all the other factors in the mix.

We did not find a connection between hopelessness/helplessness and poor outcome among women, or a link between stoicism and relapse in men. While I cannot fully explain why Greer found such links and we did not, the reasons for these discrepancies may lie in the differences between melanoma and breast cancer, or differences in length of follow-up. (Greer followed patients for over ten years; our study had follow-up reports from one and a half to three years.) Only twenty-five of our group of 117 had died or relapsed at the time of our analysis, and our findings could conceivably be different in another five to ten years.

pp. 129–130 Norman Cousins's story of the defiant survivor was reported in R. Ornstein and D. Sobel (1987): *The Healing Brain.* Fireside, Simon and Schuster, New York.

p. 130 L. R. Derogatis, M. D. Abeloff, and N. Melisaratos (1979): "Psychological coping mechanisms and survival time in metastatic breast cancer." *Journal of the American Medical Association,* 242, pp. 1504–508.

pp. 130–131 K. Stavraky, C. Buck, J. Lott, and J. Wanklin (1968): "Psychological factors in the outcome of human cancer." *Journal of Psychosomatic Research,* 12, pp. 251–59.

p. 131 E. Kübler-Ross (1969): *On Death and Dying.* Macmillan, New York. E. Kübler-Ross (1981): *Living with Death and Dying.* Macmillan, New York. E. Kübler-Ross (1987): *AIDS,* Macmillan, New York.

p. 132 The Richard Lazarus quote is from R. S. Lazarus (1985): "The costs and benefits of denial." In A. Monat and R. S. Lazarus (eds.): *Stress and Coping.* Columbia University Press, New York, p. 160.

pp. 132–133 B. Klopfer (1957): "Psychological factors in human cancer." *Journal of Projective Techniques,* 21, pp. 331–40.

pp. 134–135 For a description of our study of psychosocial variables discriminating patients with disease progression from matched controls, see L. Temoshok (1985): "Biopsychosocial studies on cutaneous malignant melanoma: psychosocial factors associated with prognostic indicators, progression, psychophysiology, and tumor-host response." *Social Science and Medicine,* 20(8), pp. 833–40.

My colleagues and I were able to track the medical progress of all the subjects from both our studies—a total of 117 melanoma patients. After three years of follow-up, twenty patients had either died or suffered metastases to other parts of their bodies (advanced or even terminal cancer).

The purest way to discover differences between the relapsers and the survivors was to match each of the twenty relapsers with another melanoma patient who had remained free of disease. To be able to trust the veracity of the results, we made sure each patient was identical to his or her match in terms of every factor that the medical literature had reported to be important to melanoma progression—including age, sex, and stage of disease. We made sure our matches had tumors that were equally thick, with the same level of invasion into the skin, the same cell type, and a similar location on the body.

Because the psychosocial data from our original interviews was so diversified, we simplified matters by focusing on one set of measures in our comparison of the matched groups. We reviewed how all the patients had initially responded to our pencil-and-paper tests of mood and emotion. These included the Profile of Mood States (POMS), as well as the Taylor Manifest Anxiety Scale and the MMPI Distress Scale. We had also administered the Marlowe-Crowne Social Desirability Scale, which gauges the tendency to give socially appropriate answers on questionnaires. The Marlowe-Crowne picks up an important aspect of Type C behavior—the desire to conform, to be socially accepted.

The poor-outcome group scored higher in tension-anxiety, depression-dejection, anger-hostility, and fatigue-inertia (all from the POMS). On the other tests, they scored higher on depression, anxiety, and distress. The healthy group scored higher only on vigor-activity, a positive-mood state. The matched groups were similar in only two categories: confusion and social desirability.

All of the tests described above were *self-report questionnaires.* The subjects mark down on a piece of paper what they think, feel, or how they behave. An individual may feel distress or anger, and indicate so on a questionnaire. They may—or may not—say so to an interviewer. Also, an individual may report distress on paper, or even to an interviewer, and not openly express the feeling. The point is that a self-report of negative emotion on paper cannot be equated with expressing that emotion.

Had the cancer patients who reported distress on their questionnaires actually *expressed* these feelings? To find out, I pulled together the original findings on emotional expression from our interviews with these same patients. After a careful review, my colleagues and I uncovered striking discrepancies between these patients' self-reports of anger and sadness and our ratings of whether they had actually expressed anger or sadness.

The cancer patients who relapsed or died had indicated negative feelings on their questionnaires, but in general, they had not expressed the same feelings in the interview.

pp. 136–137 A. H. Schmale and H. Iker (1971): "Hopelessness as a mediator of cervical cancer." *Social Science and Medicine,* 5, pp. 95–100. K. Goodkin, M. H. Antoni, and P. H. Blaney (1986): "Stress and hopelessness in the promotion of cervical intraepithelial neoplasia to invasive squamous cell carcinoma of the cervix." *Journal of Psychosomatic Research,* 30, pp. 67–76.

p. 137 For experimental research on stress, helplessness, and tumor growth in animals, see A. A. Amkraut and G. F. Solomon (1972): "Stress and murine sarcoma virus (Moloney)–induced tumors." *Cancer Research,* 32, pp. 1428–33. M. A. Visintainer, J. R. Volpicelli, and M. R. Seligman (1982): "Tumor rejection in rats after inescapable or escapable shock." *Science,* 216, pp. 437–39. M. Laudenslager, S. Ryan, S. Drugan, R. Hyson, and S. Maier (1983): "Coping and immunosuppression: inescapable but not escapable shock suppresses lymphocyte proliferation." *Science,* 221, pp. 568–70. L. S. Sklar and H. Anisman (1980): "Social stress influences tumor growth." *Psychosomatic Medicine,* 42, pp. 347–65. L. Temoshok, H.V.S. Peeke, C. W. Mehard, K. Axelson, and D. M. Sweet (1987): "Stress behavior interactions in hamster tumor growth." *Annals of the New York Academy of Sciences,* 496, pp. 501–509.

p. 138 Quote from R. D. Laing (1969): *The Politics of the Family.* Pantheon Books, New York.

pp. 141–142 Brendan O'Regan quoted from G. Levoy (1989): "Inexplicable recoveries from incurable diseases." *Longevity,* October issue, pp. 34–42.

p. 142 Dr. Charles Weinstock's reports of cases of spontaneous regression of cancer can be found in C. Weinstock (1977): "Notes on spontaneous regression of cancer." *Journal of the American Society of Psychosomatic Dentistry and Medicine,* 24(4), pp. 106–10.

p. 143 R. May (1981): *Freedom and Destiny.* Delta Books, New York.

p. 144 R. C. Cantor (1978): *And a Time To Live.* Harper & Row, New York.

p. 145 Sandra Levy's study wherein she demonstrated that "joy" was a significant factor in survival of breast cancer patients was reported in S. M. Levy, J. Lee, C. Bagley, and M. Lippman (1988): "Survival hazards analysis in first recurrent breast cancer patients: seven year follow-up." *Psychosomatic Medicine,* 50, pp. 520–28.

Chapter 8: The Type C Drama

p. 149 My "process model" of psychosocial factors (primarily Type C behavior, hopelessness, and helplessness) in the development and progression of malignant disease, which I also call the "Type C drama," is fully elaborated in my paper L. Temoshok (1987): "Personality, coping style, emotion, and cancer: toward an integrative model." *Cancer Surveys*, 6(3), pp. 545–67.

p. 150 Quote from Robert Bly (1988): *A Little Book on the Human Shadow.* Harper & Row, San Francisco.

p. 156 H. Kushner (1981): *When Bad Things Happen to Good People.* Schocken Books, New York.

Quote from K. Horney (1950): *Neurosis and Human Growth.* W. W. Norton, New York, p. 197.

p. 157 The quote by Carl Jung is from *Simpson's Contemporary Quotations* (1988). Houghton Mifflin, New York.

p. 159 Dr. William A. Greene's work is described in W. A. Greene (1966): "The psychosocial setting of the development of leukemia and lymphoma." *Annals of the New York Academy of Sciences,* 125, pp. 794–801. W. A. Greene and S. N. Swisher (1969): "Psychological and somatic variables associated with the development and course of monozygotic twins discordant for leukemia." *Annals of the New York Academy of Sciences,* 164, pp. 394–408.

pp. 159–160 D. M. Sweet and L. Temoshok (1988): "Repression of anxiety, breakdown of the repression defense and their relation to the severity of malignant melanoma." Presented at the Society of Behavioral Medicine Annual Meeting, San Francisco, March 1989.

p. 160 Quote from Gary Schwartz from L. Jamner, G. E. Schwartz, and H. Leigh (1988): "The relationship between repressive and defensive coping styles and monocyte, eosinophile, and serum glucose levels: support for the opioid peptide hypothesis of repression." *Psychosomatic Medicine,* 50, pp. 567–75.

pp. 160–161 E. M. Blumberg, P. M. West, and F. W. Ellis (1954): "A possible relationship between psychological factors and human cancer." *Psychosomatic Medicine,* 16, pp. 277–86. H. Leigh, B. Percarpio, C. Opsahl, and J. Ungerer (1987): "Psychological predictors of survival in cancer patients undergoing radiation therapy." *Psychotherapy Psychosomatics,* 47, pp. 65–73.

pp. 176–177 For a comprehensive analysis of the types of studies, trends, and contradictions in mind-cancer research (also known as psychosocial oncology) see the following papers: L. Temoshok (1987): "Personality, coping style, emotion, and cancer: toward an integrative model." *Cancer Surveys,* 6(3), pp. 545–67. L. Temoshok and B. W. Heller (1984): "On Comparing Apples, Oranges, and Fruit Salad: a Methodological Overview of Medical Outcome Studies in Psychosocial Oncology." In C. L. Copper (ed.): *Psychosocial Stress and Cancer.* John Wiley, Chichester, pp. 231–60. B. H. Fox, L. Temoshok, with H. Dreher (1988): "Mind-body and behavior in cancer incidence." *Advances,* 5(4), pp. 41–60.

A. B. Zonderman, P. T. Costa, and R. R. McCrae (1989): "Depression as a risk for cancer morbidity and mortality in a nationally representative sample." *Journal of the American Medical Association,* 262(9), pp. 1191–195. See also the editorial in the same issue: B. H. Fox (1989): "Depressive symptoms and the risk of cancer." *Journal of the American Medical Association,* 262(9), p. 1231.

As I have stated, I don't believe that depression would be readily detected in people long before they develop cancer, and indeed, no relationship was shown between depression and later cancer in this study. I must add, however, that the measures used here can be considered weak. The researchers "detected" depression with a questionnaire including twenty questions asking the subject how he/she felt during the prior week; one other questionnaire, including only four questions, inquired about the subjects' feeling of cheerfulness vs. depression during the prior month. These are not very penetrating psychological instruments.

p. 177 L. LeShan (1977): *You Can Fight For Your Life.* M. Evans, New York.

pp. 177–178 Quote from G. Sheehy (1990): *The Man Who Changed the World.* HarperCollins, New York.

p. 178 Quote from J. Campbell (1988): *The Power of Myth.* Doubleday, New York, p. 124.

Chapter 9: Type C and Mind-Body Science

pp. 183–184 A. Hoffman (1905): *René Descartes.* F. Frommanns verlag, Stuttgart. See also R. Descartes (1958): *Descartes' Philosophical Writings,* Selected and Translated by Norman Kemp. Modern Library, New York.

pp. 184–185 C. B. Pert (1986): "The wisdom of the receptors." *Advances,* 3(3), pp. 8–16.

pp. 185–187 Dr. Ader's original experiments are described in R. Ader and N. Cohen (1975): "Behaviorally conditioned immunosuppression." *Psychosomatic Medicine,* 37, p. 333–40. R. Ader and N. Cohen (1985): "CNS-immune interactions: conditioning phenomena." *Brain and Behavioral Sciences,* 8, pp. 379–426. R. Ader and N. Cohen (1981): "Conditioned Immunopharmacologic Responses." In R. Ader (ed.): *Psychoneuroimmunology.* Academic Press, New York. Dr. Ader's research on conditioning rats with lupus is detailed in R. Ader and N. Cohen (1982): "Behaviorally conditioned immunosuppression and murine systemic lupus erythematosus." *Science,* 215, pp. 1534–536.

p. 186 For a fine, popularly written overview of the development of the field of psychoneuroimmunology, see S. Locke and D. Colligan (1985): *The Healer Within.* E. P. Dutton, New York. For a scientific overview of the field, see R. Ader (ed.) (1981): *Psychoneuroimmunology,* Academic Press, New York, and R. Ader (ed.) (1991): *Psychoneuroimmunology II,* Academic Press, New York.

pp. 187–188 For a review of Soviet, American, and other research on the regulatory effect of the hypothalamus on immune responses, see M. D. Stein, S. J. Schleifer, and S. E. Keller (1981): "Hypothalamic Influences on Immune Responses." In R. Ader (ed.): *Psychoneuroimmunology.* Academic Press, New York. The Swiss researcher Hugo Besedovsky noted the increase in electrical activity in the hypothalamus during immune responses in his study reported in H. O. Besedovsky, E. Sorkin, D. Felix, and H. Haas (1977): "Hypothalamic changes during the immune response." *European Journal of Immunology,* 7, pp. 325–28.

pp. 189–190 S. Mizel and P. Jaret (1985): *In Self Defense.* Harcourt Brace Jovanovich, New York.

pp. 190–191 Drs. Candace Pert and Michael Huff's work on neuropeptides and receptors is reported in C. B. Pert, M. R. Ruff, R. J. Weber, and M. Herkenham (1985): "Neuropeptides and their receptors: a psychosomatic network." *Journal of Immunology,* 35(2). C. B. Pert (1986): "The wisdom of the receptors: neuropeptides, the emotions, and bodymind." *Advances,* 3(3), pp. 8–16. (The latter is also the source for quotes on p. 192.)

For reviews that discuss the presence of receptors on immune cells for a wide variety of neuropeptides and neurotransmitters, see G. F. Solomon (1985): "The emerging field of psychoneuroimmunology." *Advances,* 2(1), pp. 6–19. G. F. Solomon (1987): "Psychoneuroimmunology: interactions between the central nervous system and immune system." *Journal of Neuroscience Research,* 18, pp. 1–9. J. H. Helderman and T. B. Strom (1978): "Specific binding site on T and B lymphocytes as a marker of cell activation." *Nature,* 274, pp. 62–63.

pp. 192–193 Candace Pert discusses immune cells that manufacture neuropeptides in C. B. Pert (1986): "The wisdom of the receptors: neuropeptides, the emotions, and bodymind." *Advances,* 3(3), pp. 8–16. Breakthrough research in this area was conducted by Dr. Edwin J. Blalock, a biochemist at the University of Texas who showed that lymphocytes make substances that are functionally identical to stress-related neurohormones (namely, ACTH, a pituitary gland secretion). See E. M. Smith and E. J. Blalock (1981): "Human lymphocyte production of corticotropin and endorphinlike substances: association with leukocyte interferon." *Proceedings of the National Academy of Sciences USA,* 78, pp. 7530–534.

p. 193 The ability of brain cells to produce an immune system substance, interleukin-1, was reported by Dr. Jean E. Merrill, associate professor in the department of neurology at the UCLA School of Medicine, in a personal communication to Dr. George F. Solomon, described in Solomon's unpublished paper, "Psychoneuroimmunology Revisited," 1988. His findings were also reported in N. Cousins (1989): *Head First: The Biology of Hope.* E. P. Dutton, New York.

Drs. Candace Pert and Francis O. Schmidt are quoted in S. S. Hall (1989): "A molecular code links emotions, mind and health." *Smithsonian,* June issue.

p. 194 For a complete discussion of oncogenes in the development of cancer, see N. Angier (1988): *Natural Obsessions: The Search for the Oncogene.* Houghton Mifflin, New York. Also see C. J. Tabin et al. (1982): "Mechanism of activation of a human oncogene." *Nature,* 300, pp. 143–49.

pp. 194–195 On the relationship between oncogenes and the multiple "assaults" by cancer-causing agents, see H. Land, L. F. Parada, and R. A. Weisberg (1983): "Cellular oncogenes and multistep carcinogenesis." *Science,* 222, pp. 771–78.

pp. 195–196 For a complete discussion of cancer immunology and cancer-specific antigens in animals and humans, see L. J. Old (1981): "Cancer immunology: the search for specificity." *Cancer Research,* 41, pp. 361–75. See also C. M. Chadwick (1986): "Antigens of Normal and Neoplastic Cells." In C. M. Chadwick (ed.): *Receptors in Tumor Biology.* Cambridge University Press, Cambridge.

p. 197 For reviews of the field of "biological response modifiers" ("biologicals") as immunological therapies for human cancer, see R. K. Oldman (ed.) (1987): *Principles of Cancer Biotherapy.* Raven Press, New York. P. F. Torrence (1985): *Biological Response Modifiers: New Approaches to Disease Intervention.* Academic Press, Orlando. W. D. Terry and S. A. Rosenberg (eds.) (1982): *Immunotherapy of Human Cancer.* Excerpta Medica, New York.

For a complete discussion of Dr. Steven A. Rosenberg's cancer therapies using interleukin-2 and tumor-infiltrating lymphocytes (TIL's), see S. A. Rosenberg (1990): "Adoptive immunotherapy for cancer." *Scientific American,* May issue, pp. 62–69.

pp. 197–198 Quote from Dr. Old is from his article about tumor necrosis factor in L. J. Old (1988): "Tumor necrosis factor." *Scientific American,* May issue, pp. 59–75.

pp. 198–199 *New York Times,* December 5, 1989, "Transplant Patients Illuminate Link Between Cancer and Immunity." This article dealing with cancer susceptibility in immunosuppressed transplant patients is also the source for quotes by Drs. Irving Penn, Thomas Starzl, Michael Nalesnik, and Ronald Herberman.

p. 199 Quote from Dr. Lewis Thomas, from a speech delivered in 1983 at the thirtieth anniversary commemoration of the founding of the Cancer Research Institute in New York.

p. 200 *New York Times,* November 11, 1989, "Doctors Closing in on Breakaway Cancer Cells." This article discusses recent developments in scientists' understanding of cancer metastases, and is the source for the quote by Dr. Lance A. Liotta.

pp. 200–201 Dr. Ronald Herberman discovered natural killer (NK) cells in 1972. For a review of this discovery and the role of NK cells in resistance to disease, see R. B. Herberman (ed.) (1980): *Natural Cell-mediated Immunity against Tumors.* Academic Press, New York. See also R. B. Herberman and J. R. Ortaldo (1981): "Natural killer cells: their role in defenses against disease." *Science,* 214, pp. 24–30.

Many animal studies have demonstrated the significant role of NK cells in suppressing tumor growth and especially metastases, as discussed by Dr. Hiserodt. For examples of this work, see E. Gorelik, R. H. Wiltrout, K. Okumura, S. Habu, and R. B. Herberman (1982): "Role of NK cells in the control of metastatic spread and growth of tumor cells in mice." *International Journal of Cancer,* 30, pp. 107–12. K. A. Laybourn, J. C. Hiserodt, L. H. Abruzzo, and J. Varani (1986): "In vitro and in vivo interaction between murine fibrosarcoma cells and natural killer cells." *Cancer Research,* 46, pp. 3407–412. T. Barlozzari, J. Leonhardt, R. H. Wiltrout, R. B. Herberman, and C. W. Reynolds (1985): Direct evidence for the role of LGL in the inhibition of experimental tumor metastases." *The Journal of Immunology,* 134(4), pp. 2783–789. S. Hobo, H. Fukui, K. Shimamura, et al. (1981): "In vivo effects of anti-asialo GM1, I. Reduction of NK activity and enhancement of transplanted tumor growth in nude mice." *Journal of Immunology,* 127, pp. 34–38.

p. 202 S. M. Levy (1983): "Host differences in neoplastic risk: behavioral and social contributors to disease." *Health Psychology,* 2, pp. 21–44. S. M. Levy (1985): "Behavior as a biological response modifier: the psycho-immunoendocrine network and tumor immunology." *Behavioral Medicine Abstracts,* 6, pp. 1–4. S. M. Levy, R. Herberman, A. Maluish, B. Schlien, and M. Lippman (1985): "Prognostic risk assessment in primary breast cancer by behavioral and immunological parameters." *Health Psychology,* 4, pp. 99–113. S. M. Levy (1985): *Behavior and Cancer.* Josey-Bass, San Francisco. S. M. Levy, R. B. Herberman, M. Lippman, and T. D'Angelo (1987): "Correlation of stress factors with sustained depression of natural killer cell activity with predicted prognosis in patients with breast cancer." *Journal of Clinical Oncology,* 5(3), pp. 348–53.

Dr. Levy reported preliminary findings that the breast cancer patients who, from her earlier studies, were passive, helpless copers and had less active NK cells also showed a trend toward earlier recurrences of their tumors. This was reported by Dr. Levy in an interview with H. Dreher, February 6, 1989, and again on September 16, 1991.

pp. 202–203 The study of cancer patients receiving cognitive therapy and relaxation was a collaborative effort of Drs. Levy and Herberman, and psychologists Judith Rodin at Yale University and Martin Seligman at the University of Pennsylvania. Their preliminary findings (showing more NK cell activity in patients who received the treatment as opposed to a control group) were reported in an article in *The New York Times,* "Researchers Find that Optimism Helps the Body's Defense System," April 20, 1989. Their findings were also reported by Dr. Seligman in his book, *Learned Optimism* (1991), Alfred A. Knopf, New York, which is also the source of the quote.

pp. 204–205 The study on exam stress in medical students and the additional effects of loneliness on immunity is described in J. K. Kiecolt-Glaser, W. Garner, C. E. Speicher, et al. (1984): "Psychosocial modifiers of immunocompetence in medical students." *Psychosomatic Medicine,* 46, pp. 7–14. The research on stress and immunity among caregivers of Alzheimer's patients is described in J. K. Kiecolt-Glaser, R. Glaser, E. C. Shuttleworth, et al. (1987): "Chronic stress and immunity in family caregivers of Alzheimer's disease victims." *Psychosomatic Medicine,* 49, pp. 523–35.

pp. 205–206 For a review of Dr. Yehuda Shavit's important animal research on the relationship of stress, helplessness, opioids, immunity, and cancer, see Y. Shavit, G. W. Terman, F. C. Martin, et al. (1985): "Stress, opioid peptides, the immune system, and cancer." *The Journal of Immunology,* 135(2), pp. 834s–837s. See also Y. Shavit, J. Lewis, G. Terman, et al. (1984): "Opioid peptides mediate the suppressive effect of stress on natural killer cell cytotoxicity." *Science,* 223, pp. 188–90.

For a review of the complex role of opiates (and other neuropeptides) in immune regulation, see J. E. Morley, N. E. Kay, G. F. Solomon, and N. P. Plotnikoff (1987): "Neuropeptides: conductors of the immune orchestra." *Life Sciences,* 41, pp. 527–44.

pp. 206–207 Dr. Gary Schwartz's study and theory on repression, opioids, and the immune system was reported in L. Jamner, G. E. Schwartz, and H. Leigh (1988): "The relationship between repressive and defensive coping styles and monocyte, eosinophile, and serum glucose levels: support for the opioid peptide hypothesis of repression." *Psychosomatic Medicine,* 50, pp. 567–75. Dr. Schwartz's study, and several other studies on the negative health effects of repression, were reported in an article in *The New York Times,* March 3, 1988, "New Studies Report Health Dangers of Repressing Emotional Turmoil."

p. 208 A classic study demonstrating that "repressors" experience more inner, physiologic stress (in an experimental stress situation) than people who don't repress was reported in D. A. Weinberger, G. E. Schwartz, and R. J. Davidson (1979): "Low-anxious, high-anxious, and repressive coping styles: psychometric patterns and behavioral and physiological responses to stress." *Journal of Abnormal Psychology,* 88, pp. 369–80. See also C. I. Notariaus and R. W. Levenson (1979): "Expressive tendencies and physiological response to stress." *Journal of Personality and Social Psychology,* 37, pp. 1204–210.

pp. 208–209 Many studies have shown that stress hormones (the two main classes are the catecholamines—such as epinephrine [adrenaline]—and the corticosteroids) can alter and often suppress immunity in animals and humans. See B. Crary, M. Borysenko, D. C. Sutherland, et al. (1983): "Decrease in mitogen responsiveness of mononuclear cells from peripheral blood after epinephrine administration." *Journal of Immunology,* 130, pp. 694–97. A. Depelchin and J. J. Letesson (1981): "Adrenaline influence on the immune response; II—its effects through action on suppressor T-cells." *Immunology Letter,* 3, pp. 207–13. A. S. Fauci (1976): "Mechanisms of corticosteroid action on lymphocyte subpopulations; II—Differential effects of in vivo hydrocortisone, prednisone, and dexamethasone on in vitro expression of lymphocyte function." *Clinical Experimental Immunology,* 24, pp. 54–62. A. S. Fauci (1978–9): "Mechanisms of the immunosuppressive and anti-inflammatory effects of glucocorticosteroids." *Journal of Immunopharmacology,* 1, pp. 1–25. R. H. Gisler and L. Schenkel-Hulliger (1971): "Hormonal regulation of the immune response; II: Influence of pituitary and adrenal activity on immune responsiveness in vitro." Cell Immunology, 2, pp. 646–57.

Much has been written, in this book and elsewhere, about the relationship between emotion- or stress-related neuropeptides and the functioning of T-cells or NK cells. In an excellent study with mice, Drs. Wayne Coff and Mark Dunegan showed that certain neuropeptides have a direct effect on the cancer-killing capacities of macrophages, cells which are crucial anticancer defenders. See W. C. Koff and M. A. Dunegan (1985): "Modulation of macrophage-mediated tumoricidal activity by neuropeptides and neurohormones." *Journal of Immunology,* 135(1), pp. 350–54.

More evidence on the effect of emotional repression on immunity comes from a study showing that repression is associated with increased antibody responses to the Epstein-Barr virus antigen—meaning that the otherwise latent virus is more active. See B. A. Esterling, M. H. Antoni, M. Kumar, and N. Schneiderman (1990): "Emotional repression, stress disclosure responses, and Epstein-Barr viral capsid antigen titers." *Psychosomatic Medicine,* 52, pp. 397–410.

p. 209 Dr. George F. Solomon's pioneering work on the personalities of rheumatoid arthritis patients is reviewed in G. F. Solomon (1981): "Emotional and Personality Factors in the Onset and Course of Autoimmune Disease, Particularly Rheumatoid Arthritis." In R. Ader (ed.): *Psychoneuroimmunology.* Academic Press, New York.

pp. 209–210 My research collaboration with Dr. George Solomon in the study of patients with AIDS and ARC has been detailed in a number of published papers and talks. Among them are G. F. Solomon, L. Temoshok, A. O'Leary, and J. Zich (1987): "An intensive psychoimmunologic study of long-surviving persons with AIDS." *Annals of the New York Academy of Sciences,* 496, pp. 647–55. G. F. Solomon, M. E. Kemeny, and L. Temoshok (1991): "Psychoneuroimmunologic Aspects of Human Immunodeficiency Virus Infection." In R. Ader (ed): *Psychoneuroimmunology II.* Academic Press, New York. L. Temoshok, D. M. Sweet, S. Jenkins, et al. (1988): "Psychoneuroimmunologic studies of men with AIDS and ARC." Paper presented at the IV International Conference on AIDS; Stockholm, Sweden, June 12–16, 1988. G. F. Solomon and L. Temoshok (1990): "A Psychoneuroimmunologic Perspective on AIDS Research: Questions, Preliminary Findings, and Suggestions." In L. Temoshok and A. Baum (eds.): *Psychosocial Perspectives on AIDS*. Lawrence Erlbaum Associates, Hillsdale, New Jersey. H. Dreher (1988): "The healthy elderly and long-term survivors of AIDS: psychoimmune connections; a conversation with George F. Solomon, M.D." *Advances* 5(1), pp. 6–14.

p. 212 The recent study that showed that distress can affect DNA repair mechanisms, which help protect us from cancer development, was reported in J. K. Kiecolt-Glaser, R. E. Stephens, P. D. Liepetz, et al. (1985): "Distress and DNA repair in human lymphocytes." *Journal of Behavioral Medicine,* 8(4), pp. 311–20.

Chapter 10: Blaming the Victim and Other Traps

pp. 221–224 Treya Wilber's story, and the quotes that appear on these pages, are from a piece she wrote that first appeared in *New Age Journal,* 1988, *When Bad Things Happen to Good People: A Compassionate Response to Illness,* September/October 1988. This piece, along with her diaries of her entire journey, was later published in her husband's excellent 1991 book, *Grace and Grit: Spirituality and Healing in the Life and Death of Treya Killam Wilber.* Shambhala, Boston.

p. 224 G. Radner (1990): *It's Always Something.* Simon and Schuster, New York.

pp. 224–225 The case of "Leah" was reported by Dr. Roger Dafter (1990): "Individuation in illness: moving beyond blame in mind-body healing." *Psychological Perspectives,* 22, pp. 24–37. The quotes from Dr. Dafter are taken from this article.

pp. 226–227 The study discussed in this section is B. R. Cassileth, E. J. Lusk, D. S. Miller, L. L. Brown, and C. Miller (1985): "Psychosocial correlates of survival in advanced malignant disease?" *New England Journal of Medicine,* 312, pp. 1551–555. The controversial editorial appeared in the same issue: M. Angell (1985): "Disease as a reflection of the psyche." *New England Journal of Medicine,* 312, pp. 1570–572.

The letters to the *New England Journal of Medicine* regarding the Cassileth study appeared in: "Letters: Psychosocial variables and the course of cancer," (1985). *New England Journal of Medicine,* 313(21), pp. 354–59.

Here are a few brief excerpts from a few of these letters. A group of five physicians and researchers, including Sandra Levy, Ph.D., and Marc Lippman, M.D., a leading U.S. expert on breast cancer, wrote, "We believe that the conclusion drawn by Cassileth et al.—that psychosocial factors do not predict the outcome of cancer in patients with advanced disease—was unwarranted by the study as it was conducted . . . in our view, it was methodologically limited on two counts: the patient sample and the measures that were used." Peter Vitaliano, Ph.D., and colleagues at the University of Washington School of Medicine, wrote, "In assessing coping and distress, more sophisticated measures with documented reliability and validity must be used, rather than the one-item indexes employed by the authors. In their belief that psychosocial factors can be adequately represented by seven poor measures, the authors ignore the dynamic richness and variety of human experience."

Several letters were aimed directly at Dr. Angell's editorial. Shmuel Livnat, Ph.D., and David L. Felten, Ph.D., of the University of Rochester Medical Center, wrote, "Angell imposes her own definitions on the basic tenets of behavioral medicine, implying that serious researchers and clinicians in this field believe that 'certain mental states bring on certain diseases.' Clearly, such misrepresentation, which is based on anecdote, metaphor, and overstatement garnered from the popular press, does not belong on the editorial pages of the *New England Journal of Medicine*. Angell urges us to throw out the baby with the bathwater. However, a growing body of scientific literature indicates that biobehavioral factors influence a host of physiologic functions that lie at the foundation of homeostasis and resistance to disease."

pp. 229–230 S. Sontag (1977–8): *Illness as Metaphor*. Farrar, Straus and Giroux, New York.

pp. 231–232 Dr. Barrie Cassileth, who was at the time a sociologist at the University of Pennsylvania, delivered a talk regarding the social implications of mind-cancer research at a conference entitled "Current Concepts in Psycho-oncology and AIDS," sponsored by and held at the Memorial Sloan-Kettering Cancer Center, New York, in September 1987. For a review of the conference and Cassileth's presentation, see H. Dreher (1988): "Cancer and the mind: current concepts in psycho-oncology." *Advances,* 4(3), pp. 27–43. The quotes by Cassileth were taken from her written presentation distributed at the conference.

pp. 232–233 LeShan quote from author interview; also cited in H. Dreher (1989): *Your Defense Against Cancer*. Harper & Row, New York.

p. 233 Quotes from K. Horney (1950): *Neurosis and Human Growth*. W. W. Norton, New York.

pp. 236–237 N. Cousins (1979): *Anatomy of an Illness as Perceived by the Patient*. W. W. Norton, New York.

p. 239 Quote from Ken Wilber on visualization and "magical thinking" from Ken Wilber, in "Do We Make Ourselves Sick?" article/interview in *New Age Journal,* September–October 1988.

Chapter 11: Type C Transformation—For Recovery

p. 250 Dr. David Spiegel's important study of psychosocial treatment and survival in breast cancer patients was published in D. Spiegel, J. Bloom, H. C. Kraemer, et al. (1989): "Effect of psychosocial treatment on survival of patients with metastatic breast cancer." *Lancet,* 2, pp. 888–91. See also D. Spiegel (1991): "A psychosocial intervention and survival time of patients with metastatic breast cancer." *Advances* 7(3), pp. 10–19.

For Dr. Spiegel's earlier report on group expression of negative and positive emotions in the same population of advanced breast cancer patients in group treatment, see D. Spiegel and M. C. Glafkides (1983): "Effects of group confrontation with death and dying." *International Journal of Group Psychotherapy,* 33(4), pp. 433–47.

pp. 251–252 The excerpt concerning David Spiegel's therapy groups, which includes quotes from Spiegel, is from an article in *The New York Times,* November 23, 1989: "Therapy Groups Yield Surprising Benefits for Cancer Patients."

p. 253 The preliminary findings of Dr. Levy and colleagues (showing better NK cell activity in patients who received behavior therapy as opposed to a control group) were reported in an article in *The New York Times,* April 20, 1989: "Researchers Find that Optimism Helps the Body's Defense System." Their findings were also reported by Dr. Martin Seligman in his 1991 book, *Learned Optimism,* Alfred A. Knopf, New York.

Dr. Fawzy's findings on the psychologic and immunologic effects of psychiatric therapy for cancer patients is reported in F. I. Fawzy, M. E. Kemeny, N. W. Fawzy, et al. (1990): "A structured psychiatric intervention for cancer patients, II. Changes over time in immunological measures." *Archives of General Psychiatry,* 47, pp. 729–35.

Dr. Steven Greer has reported to the authors on his development and study of a psychological therapy for cancer patients, which he calls Adjuvant Psychological Therapy (APT). Papers on his findings are currently being reviewed for publication.

p. 254 Drs. O. Carl Simonton and Stephanie Simonton-Atchley reported their results in treating cancer patients with imagery and psychotherapy in O. C. Simonton, S. Matthews-Simonton, and J. Creighton (1978): *Getting Well Again.* J. P. Tarcher, Los Angeles. See also J. Achterberg, G. F. Lawlis, O. C. Simonton, and S. Simonton (1977): "Psychological factors and blood chemistries as disease outcome predictors for cancer patients." *Multivariate Experimental Clinical Research,* 3, pp. 107–122. Lawrence LeShan reports results from his psychotherapeutic work with cancer patients in L. LeShan (1977): *You Can Fight For Your Life.* M. Evans, New York, and L. LeShan (1989): *Cancer As a Turning Point.* E. P. Dutton, New York. See also L. LeShan and M. Gassman (1958): "Some observations on psychotherapy with patients with neoplastic disease." *American Journal of Psychotherapy,* 12, pp. 723–34. L. LeShan and E. LeShan (1961): "Psychotherapy and the patient with a limited life span." *Psychiatry,* 24, pp. 318–23.

The study that showed the survival effects of an educational program for medical compliance in a group of patients with hematologic cancers was reported in: J. L. Richardson, D. R. Shelton, M. Krailo, et al. (1990): "The effect of compliance with treatment on survival among patients with hematologic malignancies." *Journal of Clinical Oncology,* 8(2), pp. 356–64.

p. 265 P. Slater (1970): *The Pursuit of Loneliness.* Beacon Press, Boston.

Chapter 12: Small Victories: From Diagnosis to Recovery

p. 275 J. W. Pennebaker (1990): *Opening Up.* William Morrow, New York.

pp. 275–276 S. Levine (1987): *Healing into Life and Death.* Anchor Press/Doubleday, Garden City, New York.

p. 278 N. Cousins (1979): *Anatomy of an Illness as Perceived by the Patient.* W. W. Norton, New York. The lists of questions is from N. Fiore (1984): *The Road Back to Health: Coping with the Emotional Side of Cancer.* Bantam Books, New York.

pp. 279–280 G. F. Solomon and L. Temoshok (1990): "A Psychoneuroimmunologic Perspective on AIDS Research: Questions, Preliminary Findings, and Suggestions." In L. Temoshok and A. Baum (eds.): *Psychosocial Perspectives on AIDS.* Lawrence Erlbaum Associates, Hillsdale, New Jersey. H. Dreher (1988):

"The healthy elderly and long-term survivors of AIDS: psychoimmune connections; a conversation with George F. Solomon, M.D." *Advances,* 5(1), pp. 6–14.

p. 289 A. I. Holleb (ed.) (1986): *The American Cancer Society Cancer Book.* Doubleday, New York. M. Morra and E. Potts (1980): *Choices: Realistic Alternatives in Cancer Treatment.* Avon Books, New York. See also M. Dollinger, E. H. Rosenbaum, and G. Cable (1991): *Everyone's Guide to Cancer Therapy.* Somerville House Books Ltd., Toronto, Canada.

p. 292 A. Storr (1988): *Solitude: A Return to the Self.* The Free Press, New York.

p. 293 Quote from N. Fiore (1984): *The Road Back to Health: Coping with the Emotional Aspects of Cancer.* Bantam Books, New York.

p. 296 Quote from M. Sarton (1980): *Recovering: A Journal.* W. W. Norton, New York.

p. 300 *The Diaries of Franz Kafka—1914–1923* (1949). Schocken Books, New York.

Chapter 13: Stories of Hope, Change, and Survival

pp. 303–305 Dr. Steven Greer has reported to the authors on his development and study of a psychological therapy for cancer patients, which he calls Adjuvant Psychological Therapy (APT). A paper on his findings with 156 patients receiving APT is currently being reviewed for publication.

pp. 310–311 The case report on "Thomas," and the quotation, is from L. LeShan and M. Gassman (1958): "Some observations on psychotherapy with patients with neoplastic disease." *American Journal of Psychotherapy,* 12, pp. 723–34.

pp. 312–314 The expanded discussion of the case of Leah is derived from R. Dafter (1990): "Individuation in illness: moving beyond blame in mind-body healing." *Psychological Perspectives,* 22, pp. 24–37.

pp. 319–322 The case of Irwin is described in an article, G. Levoy (1989): "Inexplicable recoveries from incurable diseases." *Longevity,* October issue, p. 34–42. (The name used there is "Robert M.")

pp. 322–323 Quote from R. C. Cantor (1978): *And a Time to Live.* Harper & Row, New York.

p. 323 Quote from A. Lowen (1980): *Fear of Life.* Macmillan, New York.

Chapter 14: Type C Transformation in Everyday Life

p. 327 This quote from the *Internal Book of Huang Di* comes from I. Veith (1972): *The Yellow Emperor's Classic of Internal Medicine.* University of California Press, Berkeley.

pp. 329–332 Dr. James Pennebaker's important studies are described in J. W. Pennebaker (1990): *Opening Up.* William Morrow, New York. J. W. Pennebaker and S. Beall (1986): "Confronting a traumatic event: toward an understanding of inhibition and disease." *Journal of Abnormal Psychology,* 95, pp. 274–81. The discussion of confiding traumas and immune function, and quote on p. 350, can be found in J. W. Pennebaker, J. K. Kiecolt-Glaser, and R. Glaser (1988): "Disclosure of traumas and immune function: health implications for psychotherapy." *Journal of Consulting and Clinical Psychology,* 56, pp. 239–45.

p. 336 A. Gruen (1986): *The Betrayal of the Self: The Fear of Autonomy in Men and Women.* Grove Press, New York.

p. 339 R. Norwood (1985): *Women Who Love Too Much.* J. P. Tarcher, Los Angeles. M. Beattie (1987): *Codependent No More.* Hazelden Foundation, Harper, San Francisco.

Chapter 15: Expressing Anger: What's Effective?

pp. 343–345 The discussion of Harriet Goldhor Lerner's approach to anger expression, and the quote, are derived from H. G. Lerner (1985): *The Dance of Anger.* Harper & Row, New York.

p. 346 Quote from S. Levine (1987): *Healing into Life and Death.* Anchor Press/Doubleday, Garden City, New York.

p. 356 Quote from G. Roth (1990): *Maps to Ecstasy.* New World Library, San Rafael, California.

Chapter 16: Tending the Mind, Trusting the Body

p. 362 Janice Kiecolt-Glaser and Ronald Glaser have shown the immunological benefits of relaxation techniques in two studies mentioned here. They are J. K. Kiecolt-Glaser, R. Glaser, D. Williger, et al. (1985): "Psychosocial enhancement of immunocompetence in a geriatric population." *Health Psychology,* 4, pp. 25–41. J. K. Kiecolt-Glaser, R. Glaser, E. Strain, et al. (1986): "Modulation of cellular immunity in medical students." *Journal of Behavioral Medicine,* 9, pp. 5–21.

p. 363 The meditation books I recommend include: S. Levine (1979): *A Gradual Awakening.* Anchor Press/Doubleday, Garden City, New York. H. Benson and M. Z. Klipper (1976): *The Relaxation Response.* Avon Books, New York. J. Borysenko (1987): *Minding the Body, Mending the Mind.* Bantam Books, New York. L. LeShan (1974): *How to Meditate.* Little Brown, New York.

Quote from J. Campbell (1988): *The Power of Myth.* Doubleday, New York.

p. 366 William Fry's research on crying is described in W. H. Fry II, D. DeSota-Johnson, C. Hoffman, and J. T. McCall (1981): "Effect of stimulus on the chemical composition of human tears." *American Journal of Ophthalmology,* 92(4), pp. 559–67. Quote by Dr. Fry is from E. Padus et al. (1986): *Emotions and Your Health.* Rodale Press, Emmaus, Pennsylvania.

pp. 366–367 Quote from A. Lowen (1980): *Fear of Life.* Macmillan, New York.

p. 367 Research on the health benefits of laughter described in K. M. Dillon, B. Minchoff, and K. H. Baker (1985–6): "Positive emotional states and enhancement of the immune system." *International Journal of Psychiatry in Medicine,* 15, pp. 13–17. L. S. Berk, S. A. Tan, S. L. Nehlsen-Cannarella, et al. (1988): "Humor associated laughter decreases cortisol and increases spontaneous lymphocyte blastogenesis." *Clinical Research,* 36, p. 435A. L. S. Berk, S. A. Tan, S. L. Nehlsen-Cannarella, et al. (1988): "Mirth modulates adrenocorticomedullary activity: suppression of cortisol and epinephrine." *Clinical Research,* 36, p. 121. Quote by Jane Brody from *The New York Times,* April 7, 1988, "Increasingly, Laughter as Potential Therapy for Patients Is Being Taken Seriously."

p. 368 P. Reynolds and G. A. Kaplan (1986): "Social connections and cancer:

a prospective study of Alameda County residents." Paper presented at the Society of Behavioral Medicine meeting, San Francisco, March 1986.

For a review of the relationship between social connections and the development of cancer, see J. G. Joseph and S. L. Syme (1982): "Social connection and the etiology of cancer: an epidemiological review and discussion." In J. Cohen et al. (eds.): *Psychosocial Aspects of Cancer.* Raven Press, New York.

To quote from the above review: "Many different studies, with a variety of designs and addressing particular forms of social connections, suggest in provocative fashion that an association exists between these two factors. It is now time to improve research methods so that sharpened and more informed inferences can be drawn."

pp. 371–373 For a complete discussion of the "backstage" concept, see E. Goffman (1959): *The Presentation of Self in Everyday Life.* Doubleday, New York.

p. 372 Quote from A. Lowen (1980): *Fear of Life.* Macmillan, New York.

p. 373 Lawrence LeShan discusses his idea of a "third road" in L. LeShan (1977): *You Can Fight for Your Life.* M. Evans, New York.

p. 376 Verse quotation from S. Mitchell (1988): *Tao-te-ching* (Lao-tzu). Harper & Row, New York.

p. 377 Quote from L. Dossey (1984): *Beyond Illness.* New Science Library, Boston.

Chapter 17: The Future of the Type C Connection

p. 383 Quote by Dr. Candace Pert from S. S. Hall (1989): "A molecular code links emotions, mind and health." *Smithsonian,* June issue.

p. 385 J. K. Kiecolt-Glaser, R. E. Stephens, P. D. Liepetz, et al. (1985): "Distress and DNA repair in human lymphocytes." *Journal of Behavioral Medicine,* 8(4), pp. 311–20.

Ernest Lawrence Rossi speculated about a possible mind-gene connection in his article, E. L. Rossi (1988): "A mind-gene connection?" *Psychological Perspectives,* 19(2), pp. 212–21.

p. 387 N. Cousins (1979): *Anatomy of an Illness as Perceived by the Patient.* W. W. Norton, New York.

INDEX

abandonment, fears of, 333
abuse:
  flexibility factor and, 47
  nice-guy syndrome and, 26, 29, 208
Achterberg, Jeanne, 313–14
acting out vs. acting in, 25
active faith, 79–81
Ader, Robert, 185–87
adjustment problems, 98
Adjuvant Psychological Therapy (APT),
  303–9
adolescents, cancer in, 72
adrenaline, 208, 366
Adult Children of Alcoholics (ACOA), 384
aggression, 22–23, 57, 73
  passive, 352–54
aging, 71–72
AIDS, 9, 314, 385
  psychological factors in, 209–10
Alcoholics Anonymous (AA), 384
alcoholism, 58–59, 165–66
Allen, Woody, 24
American Journal of Psychotherapy,
  310–11
amygdala, 192
Anatomy of an Illness (Cousins), 236–37,
  278, 367
And a Time to Live (Cantor), 144, 322–23
Angell, Marcia, 227
anger, 154, 238
  aggression and, 22–23
  in Appelbaum study, 20

awareness of, 262–63, 347–48, 358
biological basis of, 22–24
family interaction patterns and, 58–60
flexibility factor and, 46–47
memories of, 50–51, 89, 91–92, 108–9,
  173, 307–8
naturalness of, 22–24
repression of, 17–25, 31, 38–39, 56–57,
  59–60, 78, 89, 107, 116, 220, 261–63,
  307–8
sadness as defense against, 36
suppression vs. repression of, 49–53
toward parents, 153, 174, 297
anger, expression of, 47, 58, 59, 60, 91,
  307–8
assertiveness and, 349–58
blaming vs., 350–52
decisive action and, 356–57
double-decker anger and, 354–56
effective, 343–59
passive aggression and, 352–54
saying no and, 357–58
skills of, 346–49
Type A behavior and, 344–45
animal experiments:
helplessness in, 137, 205
immune system in, 186–87
with NK cells, 201
antibodies, 189, 195–96
IgA, 367
antigens, cancer-specific
  (tumor-associated), 195–96

426 • INDEX

natural killer (NK) cells *(cont.)*
  metastases and, 200
  mind-body therapy and, 253
  psychological factors and, 202–5
near-death incident, 34
needs:
  expression of, 34, 298–99
  of other people, 19, 27, 38, 39, 48, 168,
    219–20, 361
  staying in contact with, 34, 35, 38, 93,
    175, 317–18
negative emotions:
  expression of, 134–36
  expressors and, 92–93
  hope and, 237–38
  inability to express, 26–31, 36–37, 39,
    43, 81–82, 134–35, 168; *see also*
    specific emotions
  reframing and, 265–66
  Type A and, 38
  use of term, 37
nervous system, 37, 68, 111, 190–91
neuropeptides, 52–53, 68, 184–85, 190–93,
    206
  as informational substances, 193
  as language of brain and body, 192–93
  opiates, 191–92, 205–7
Neurosis and Human Growth (Horney),
    156
neurotransmitters, 68
New Age Journal, 223–24
New Age view of health, 135–36, 221–24,
    228, 239
New England Journal of Medicine, 226–27
New York Psychosomatic Study Group,
    142
New York Times, 199, 200, 250, 251–52,
    367
niceness, excessive, 4–5, 25–30, 208, 220,
    243–46, 299, 332–33, 344
Nietzsche, Friedrich, 272, 302
NK cells, *see* natural killer cells
"no," learning to say, 357–58
nonexpression (nonexpressors), 87–92, 158,
    166–67
  cancer defense and, 95–97
  coping continuum and, 54, 55
  in Greer's study, 107
  negative emotions and, 26–31, 36–37,
    39, 43, 81–82, 134–35, 168
  repressive coping and, 108–12
  as toxic core of Type C, 87–88
  use of term, 50
  see also repression; suppression
nonverbal Type C behavior, 70, 72–79
numbness, 52, 154, 282
nurses, communication with, 284–85

Ohio State University, 204
Old, Lloyd J., 197–98
Opening Up (Pennebaker), 275
opiates, 191–92, 205–7
  helplessness and, 205–6
optimism, 85, 87, 145, 203, 253, 270
O'Regan, Brendan, 141–42
organ transplants, immune suppression
    and, 198–99
other-directed people, 361
  cancer and, 5–6, 17, 27, 28, 30–34
  use of term, 5
others:
  needs of, 19, 27, 38, 39, 48, 168,
    219–220, 361
  pleasing of, *see* niceness, excessive
Our Inner Conflicts (Horney), 28
outrage, 46

parents:
  anger toward, 153, 174, 297
  blaming of, 152–53
  death of, 26–27, 121–22, 140–41, 158,
    165, 297
  see also fathers; mothers
passive aggression, avoiding of, 352–54
passive faith, 71
  active faith vs., 79–81
passivity, 75
Pasternak, Boris, 26
Pathfinders (Sheehy), 80
Penfield, Wilder, 192
Penn, Irving, 198–99
Pennebaker, James W., 275, 329–32
personality:
  arthritis and, 209
  defined, 43
  Type C contrasted with, 43
Pert, Candace, 182, 184–85, 190–93, 383
Pettingale, Keith W., 124–25
phagocytes, 188
physical sensations, 109
  anger expression and, 350, 353
  in emotional expression study, 88, 89,
    91–92
  losing touch with, 27–28, 154
  reframing and, 266
Picasso, Pablo, 360
Pierrakos, John, 42
Pittsburgh Cancer Institute, 202, 203–4
plans, recovery, 279–82
positive attitude trap, 236–40
powerlessness, 79–80, 127, 138
Power of Myth, The (Campbell), 178,
    363
prayer, 79
pregnancy, 89–90

ABOUT THE AUTHORS

LYDIA TEMOSHOK, Ph.D., is a clinical psychologist recognized worldwide as a scientist at the forefront of research in the fields of behavioral medicine, psychosocial oncology, and HIV/AIDS. Educated at Yale College and the University of Michigan, and previously on the faculty at the University of California at San Francisco School of Medicine, she currently heads the U.S. military's research program on the influence of behavior on the prevention and consequences of HIV/AIDS.

HENRY DREHER is a science writer specializing in health and mind-body interactions. He is a frequent contributor to *East West/Natural Health* and *Advances: The Journal of Mind-Body Health.* He is the author of *Your Defense Against Cancer: The Complete Guide to Cancer Prevention.* Mr. Dreher received his master's degree in fine arts from Columbia University. He lives in New York City.